# MRI *of*
# Head & Neck
# Anatomy

# MRI of Head & Neck Anatomy

**William T.C. Yuh**, M.D., M.S.E.E.
Associate Professor, Department of Radiology
University of Iowa College of Medicine, Iowa City, Iowa

**E. Turgut Talı**, M.D.
Visiting Neuroradiology Fellow, Department of Radiology
University of Iowa College of Medicine, Iowa City, Iowa
Assistant Professor, Department of Radiology
Gazi University Faculty of Medicine, Ankara, Turkey

**Adel K. Afifi**, M.D.
Professor, Departments of Pediatrics, Anatomy, and Neurology
University of Iowa College of Medicine, Iowa City, Iowa

**Kayıhan Şahinoğlu**, M.D.
Associate Professor, Department of Anatomy
University of Istanbul Faculty of Medicine, Istanbul, Turkey

**Feng Gao**, M.D.
Assistant Professor, Department of Radiology
Shandong Medical Imaging Research Institute, Shandong, China

**Ronald A. Bergman**, Ph.D.
Professor, Department of Anatomy
University of Iowa College of Medicine, Iowa City, Iowa

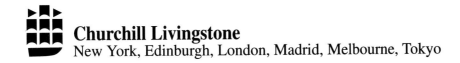
**Churchill Livingstone**
New York, Edinburgh, London, Madrid, Melbourne, Tokyo

**Library of Congress Cataloging-in-Publication Data**

MRI of head and neck anatomy / William T.C. Yuh ... [et al.].
      p.   cm.
    Includes index.
    ISBN 0-443-08892-6
    1.  Head—Magnetic resonance imaging—Atlases.  2. Neck—Magnetic
resonance imaging—Atlases.     I. Yuh, William T. C.
    [DNLM: 1. Head—anatomy & histology—atlases.  2. Neck—anatomy &
histology—atlases.  3. Magnetic Resonance Imaging—atlases.
4. Angiography—atlases.  WE 17 M9394 1994]
QM535.M75  1994
611′91′0222—dc20
DNLM/DLC
for Library of Congress                   93-28308
                                              CIP

© **Churchill Livingstone Inc. 1994**

Distributed in the United Kingdom by Churchill Livingstone, Robert Stevenson House, 1–3 Baxter's Place, Leith Walk, Edinburgh EH1 3AF, and by associated companies, branches, and representatives throughout the world.

The Publishers have made every effort to trace the copyright holders for borrowed material. If they have inadvertently overlooked any, they will be pleased to make the necessary arrangements at the first opportunity.

Acquisitions Editor: *Nancy Mullins*
Copy Editor: *David Terry*
Production Supervisor: *Sharon Tuder*
Cover Design: *Jeannette Jacobs*

Printed in the United States of America

First published in 1994   7 6 5 4 3 2 1

*For P.S.B.*
*for minding the p's and q's,*
*for dotting the i's,*
*and for crossing the t's.*

*What would we have ever done without you?*

# PREFACE

Significant advances in imaging technology have allowed us to examine the head and neck in such detail that the results approach cadaver sections in quality. Many normal anatomic details that may not be visualized by other imaging techniques can now be shown readily by magnetic resonance imaging (MRI). It is important, therefore, to develop an understanding of normal anatomy in order to identify abnormal structures. Because of the increased application of MRI in clinical problem solving, an atlas identifying each division and component of the brain and cerebellum, the cranial nerves, and many of their end organs, as well as their blood supply, is clinically useful.

For those interested in head and neck MRI techniques, including radiologic technicians and medical students as well as physicians and medical specialists, an understanding of the structural components of the head and neck and their topographic relationships is essential. It is important to develop an understanding of head and neck anatomy in three dimensions and to be able to recognize structures viewed in different planes and with various signal characteristics. With different imaging parameters, multisectional anatomy has become increasingly important for the interpretation of computed images that have a growing clinical usefulness. Pathologic structures and their localization and relation to surrounding normal structures may be understood with a resource such as we hope to provide with this book.

In particular, the study of the head and neck is founded on a mastery of anatomy. It is on that foundation that an understanding of physiology and pathology can be built. We are convinced that learning the normal anatomy by frequent reference to an MRI atlas is the most fundamental and rewarding means of understanding and interpreting neuroradiologic images.

The present work is a high-quality atlas of sequential sectional anatomy in three dimensions. Each image is labeled and described. The terminology used is a compromise between usual radiologic and anatomic usage and Nomina Anatomica. We have chosen to use what we think is the most commonly employed terminology in our labeling of figures, but have included other commonly used synonyms in the index. We have done this to facilitate the rapid location of structures of interest; those who may be familiar with or are biased in favor of terms not appearing among the labels on the figures will find such terms listed as cross references in the index. Our goal has been to produce a head and neck atlas with brief annotations sufficiently detailed to facilitate difficult imaging interpretations in this rapidly evolving technology.

We are grateful for the interest of Churchill Livingstone and specifically Ms. Toni Tracy, President. The fastidious work of David Terry and Kamely Dahir is greatly appreciated.

The completion of this work depended on the contributions of many people. In particular, the invaluable contribution of Dr. David J. Fisher, who solved difficult computer problems and devised the high-resolution imaging protocols used in our atlas, is acknowledged with gratitude. Others making significant contributions include Phyllis S. Bergman, Heide Muller Berns, Dr. Steven Cornell, Dr. Hanna Damasio, Dr. Brad Jansen, Beth McCabe, Rena Olsen, and Paul Reimann.

*W.T.C.Y.*
*E.T.T.*
*A.K.A.*
*K.S.*
*F.G.*
*R.A.B.*

Iowa City, Iowa, 1993

# INTRODUCTION

The pulse sequence used in the imaging of the head included three-dimensional (3-D) spoiled gradient-recalled-echo (SPGR) volume, conventional spin-echo, and fast spin-echo sequences. T1-weighted images of the head were obtained using 3-D SPGR volume imaging technique (TR/TE/NEX = 25/5/4) with a 1.6-mm slice thickness and 26-cm FOV. This technique provides thin-sliced, high-resolution images that can be displayed in 3-D projection. SPGR images also provide excellent tissue contrast between the gray and white matter of brain parenchyma. However, the susceptibility artifacts present in the extracranial head and neck regions limit the application of SPGR in these regions. For this reason, extracranial head and neck regions were imaged using conventional spin-echo pulse sequences.

T2-weighted images (TR/TE/NEX = 3,200/105/4) of the head were obtained using fast spin-echo imaging with a 5-mm slice thickness and 26-cm FOV. With the application of an increased matrix (512 x 384), multiple signal averages (NEX), and a spin-echo pulse sequence, images of the head were obtained with high resolution and high contrast that demonstrated fine anatomic detail.

The pulse sequence used in the imaging of the neck consisted of both conventional spin-echo T1-weighted and fast spin-echo T2-weighted sequences. Both sequences have less susceptibility artifact than SPGR sequences. On T1-weighted images (TR/TE/NEX = 500/14/4), the slice thickness was 4 mm for coronal and sagittal planes and 5 mm for the axial plane. These T1-weighted images were obtained with a 512 x 384 matrix and 24-cm FOV. Fine anatomic detail was demonstrated because of the distinctive tissue contrast between muscle (dark) and fat (bright) anatomy.

T2-weighted images (TR/TE/NEX = 4,000/95/4) of the neck were obtained using fast spin-echo pulse sequences with a 24-cm FOV, 5-mm slice thickness, and 512 x 384 matrix. With the application of these parameters, increased anatomic detail could be resolved. As compared with conventional T2-weighted images, the cerebrospinal fluid pulsation artifact decreased significantly with fast spin-echo sequences, and the spinal cord was better visualized. The signal of fat on fast spin-echo sequences is generally higher than that in conventional T2-weighted images but does not interfere with the quality of the images.

In general, cranial nerves can be difficult to demonstrate because of their size, orientation, and anatomic location. Orthogonal and reformatted images were used to obtain optimal visualization.

Postcontrast T1-weighted images (TR/TE/NEX = 350/20/2) of the normal head and neck, which are used routinely in practice, are also provided in this atlas in order to demonstrate the expected normal changes after contrast material administration. The contrast studies were performed immediately after the intravenous injection of 0.1 mmol/kg of Gd-DTPA (Magnevist, Berlex Laboratories).

Although magnetic resonance angiography (MRA) does not match the resolution of conventional angiography, intracranial vascular structures can be demonstrated by MRA, which uses the signal characteristics of flowing blood without injection of a contrast agent. MRA images of the head, including arterial and venous structures, were obtained using 3-D time-of-flight technique sequences. MRA images of the neck, including both arterial and venous structures, were obtained using the two-dimensional time-of-flight technique. The images presented are primarily in the coronal and oblique planes. The MRA images are courtesy of Drs. Evan Fram and Paul Keller, Barrow Neurologic Institute.

Those images of cranial nerves appearing in Chapter 3 as Figures 3-3, 3-4, 3-6, 3-8, 3-9, and 3-15 to 3-21 are presented by courtesy of Philips Medical Systems, Shelton, Connecticut.

# CONTENTS

# 1

# HEAD

# AXIAL VIEWS

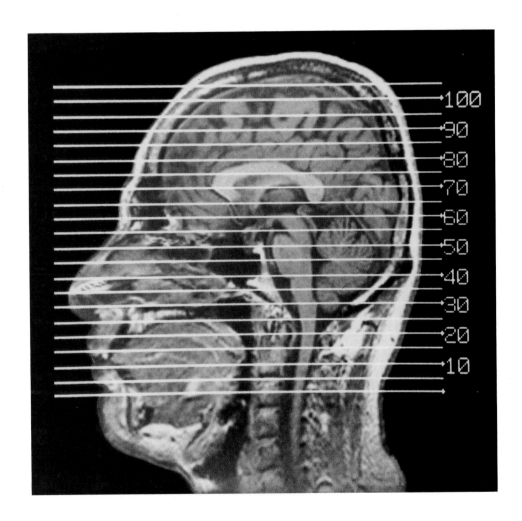

Key to the axial planes of inspection for T1-weighted images.

## Figure 1-1

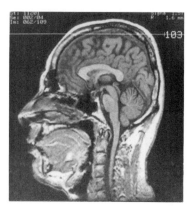

Axial T1-weighted image of the brain showing the superficial frontal cerebral cortex. Surrounding the cerebral cortex is the dura mater. The bright signal intensities of the subcutaneous fatty tissue of the skin and diploë are seen surrounding the lamina externa of the parietal bone. The lamina interna of the parietal bone is seen medial to the diploë. The falx cerebri, the interhemispheric fold of the dura mater, is seen between the two hemispheres. On both ends of the falx cerebri is the superior sagittal sinus.

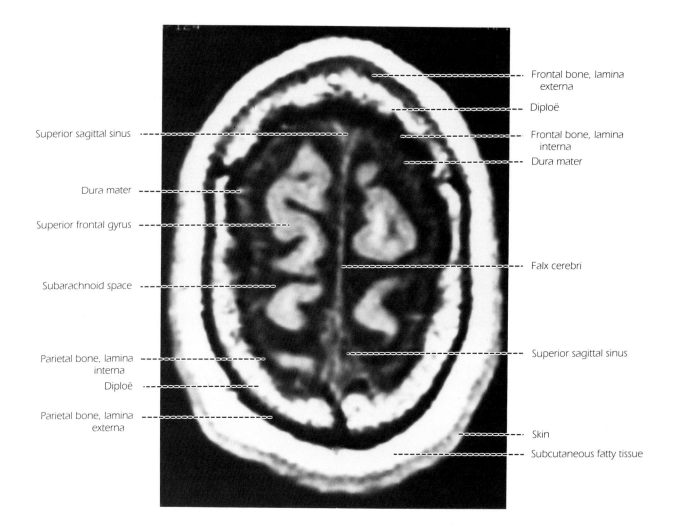

Superficial axial T1-weighted image of the cerebral hemispheres. The two hemispheres are separated by the falx cerebri, a dural fold of meninges between the two hemispheres. On both ends of the falx cerebri is the superior sagittal sinus. The subarachnoid space is seen between cerebral gyri. The cerebral cortex is surrounded by the dura mater. The bright signal intensities of the subcutaneous fatty tissue of the skin and the diploë are found on both ends of the lamina externa of bone.

## Figure 1-2

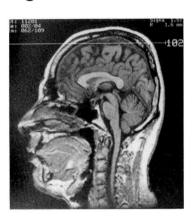

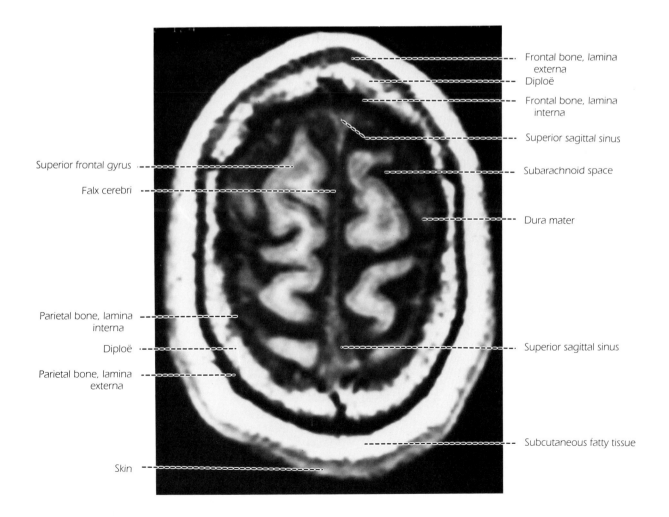

- Frontal bone, lamina externa
- Diploë
- Frontal bone, lamina interna
- Superior sagittal sinus
- Subarachnoid space
- Dura mater
- Superior sagittal sinus
- Subcutaneous fatty tissue

- Superior frontal gyrus
- Falx cerebri
- Parietal bone, lamina interna
- Diploë
- Parietal bone, lamina externa
- Skin

# Figure 1-3

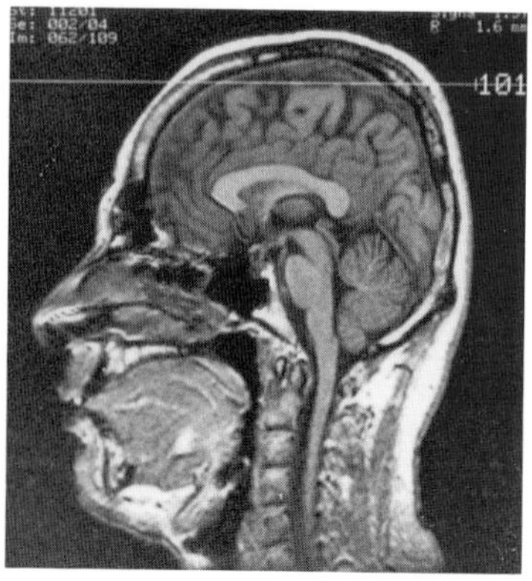
101

Superficial axial T1-weighted image through the frontal and parietal cortices. The falx cerebri, a dural fold, separates the two hemispheres. The central (rolandic) sulcus separates the frontal and parietal lobes. Posterior to the central sulcus is the postcentral gyrus. The postcentral sulcus delineates the posterior boundary of the postcentral gyrus and separates it from the superior parietal lobule. In the frontal lobe, the superior frontal sulcus separates the superior and middle frontal gyri. The superior sagittal sinus is seen on both ends of the falx cerebri.

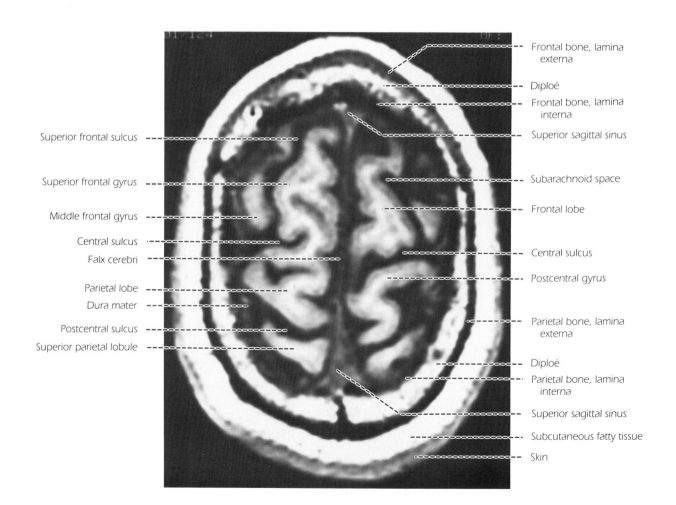

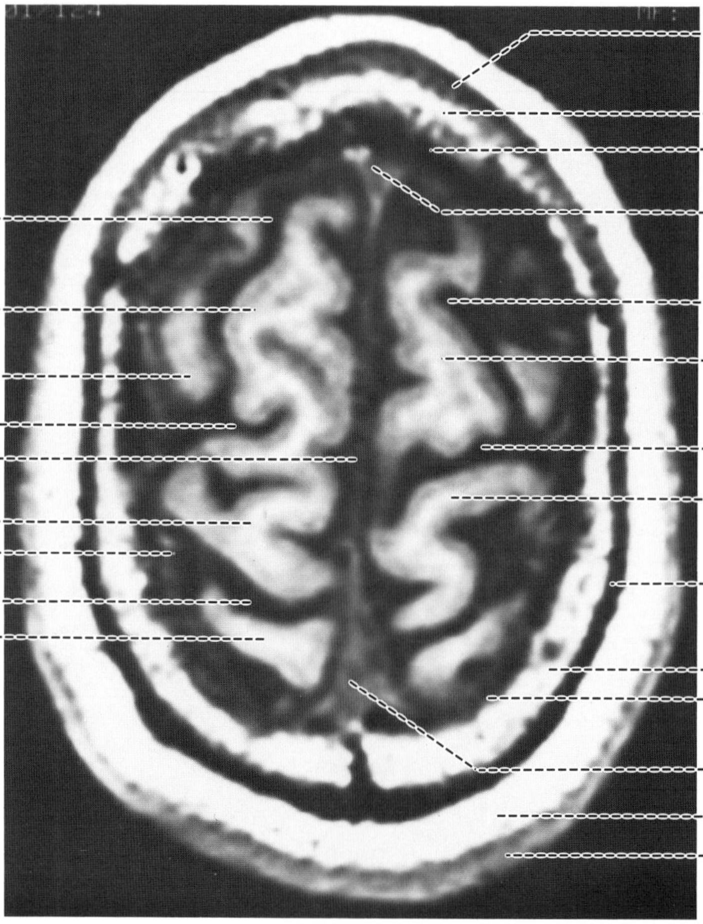
Superior frontal sulcus
Superior frontal gyrus
Middle frontal gyrus
Central sulcus
Falx cerebri
Parietal lobe
Dura mater
Postcentral sulcus
Superior parietal lobule
Frontal bone, lamina externa
Diploë
Frontal bone, lamina interna
Superior sagittal sinus
Subarachnoid space
Frontal lobe
Central sulcus
Postcentral gyrus
Parietal bone, lamina externa
Diploë
Parietal bone, lamina interna
Superior sagittal sinus
Subcutaneous fatty tissue
Skin

Superficial axial T1-weighted image through the frontal and parietal lobes. The dura mater surrounds the cerebral hemisphere medial to the lamina interna of the parietal and frontal bones. A dural fold, the falx cerebri, separates the two hemispheres. On each end of the falx cerebri is the superior sagittal sinus. The superior frontal sulcus separates the superior and middle frontal gyri in the frontal lobe. The central (rolandic) sulcus separates the frontal and parietal lobes. Posterior to the central sulcus is the postcentral gyrus. The postcentral sulcus separates the postcentral gyrus from the superior parietal lobule. The subarachnoid space surrounds the cerebral hemisphere and is seen between gyri.

## Figure 1-4

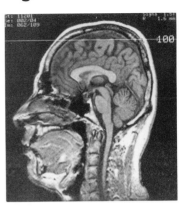

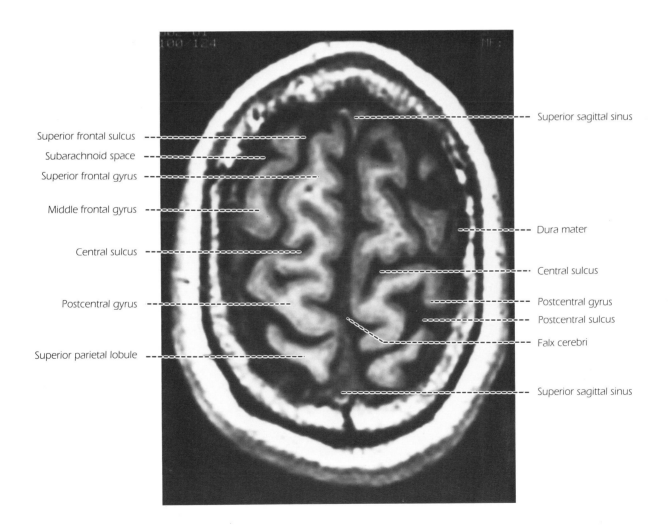

## Figure 1-5

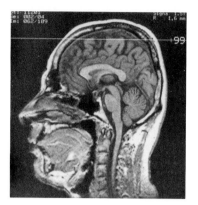

Superficial axial T1-weighted image through the frontal and parietal lobes. The two hemispheres are separated by the falx cerebri, a dural fold in the interhemispheric fissure. The superior sagittal sinus is found on each end of the falx cerebri. The central sulcus separates the frontal and parietal lobes. In the frontal lobe, the superior and middle frontal gyri are separated by the superior frontal sulcus. The paracentral lobule is located on the medial surface within the frontal and parietal lobes. In the posterior part of the parietal lobe is the superior parietal lobule.

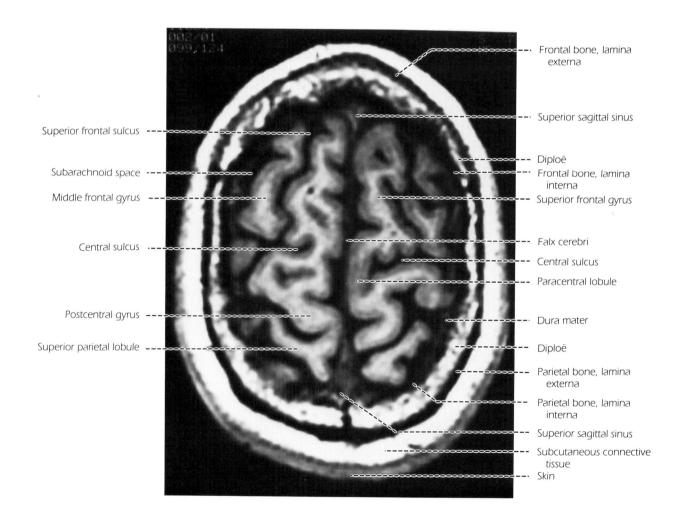

Superficial axial T1-weighted image through the frontal and parietal lobes. The cerebral hemispheres are surrounded by the dura mater. The central (rolandic) sulcus separates the frontal and parietal lobes. Rostral to the central sulcus is the precentral gyrus and caudal to it is the postcentral gyrus. The postcentral sulcus delineates the posterior boundary of the postcentral gyrus. Deep and medial to the central sulcus is the paracentral lobule, occupying adjacent parts of the frontal and parietal lobes. The marginal sulcus delineates the posterior boundary of the paracentral lobule. The superior parietal lobule is located in the caudal part of the parietal cortex. The superior frontal sulcus separates the superior and middle frontal gyri.

## Figure 1-6

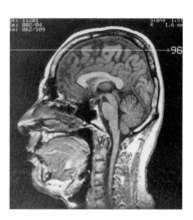

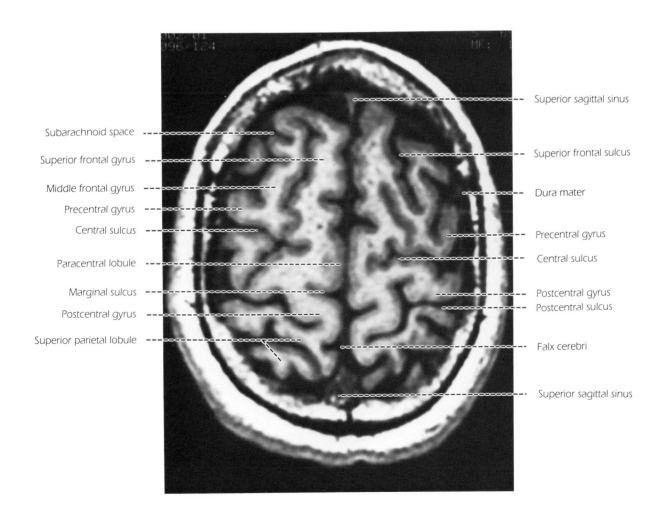

## Figure 1-7

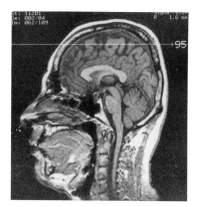

Axial T1-weighted image through the superficial parts of the frontal and parietal lobes. The falx cerebri separates the two hemispheres. The superior sagittal sinus is cut on both ends of the falx cerebri. The central (rolandic) sulcus separates the precentral and postcentral gyri. Medial to the central sulcus is the paracentral lobule, between the paracentral sulcus anteriorly and the marginal sulcus posteriorly. Caudal to the postcentral gyrus is the postcentral sulcus, separating the gyrus from the superior parietal lobule. The superior frontal sulcus separates the superior and middle frontal gyri.

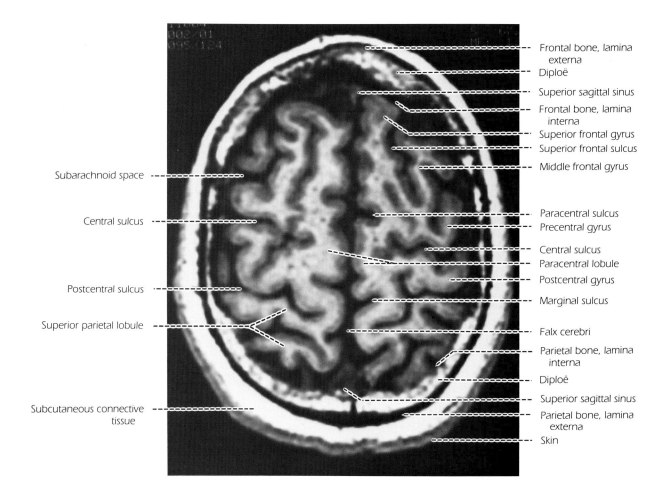

Axial T1-weighted image through the frontal and parietal lobes. The central sulcus separates the pre- and postcentral gyri. Rostral to the precentral gyrus is the precentral sulcus. Caudal to the postcentral gyrus is the postcentral sulcus, separating the gyrus from the superior parietal lobule. The paracentral lobule is located between the paracentral sulcus rostrally and the marginal sulcus caudally. It occupies adjacent portions of the frontal and parietal lobes. The superior frontal sulcus separates the superior and middle frontal gyri.

## Figure 1-8

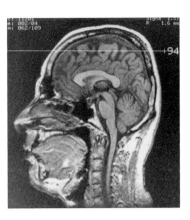

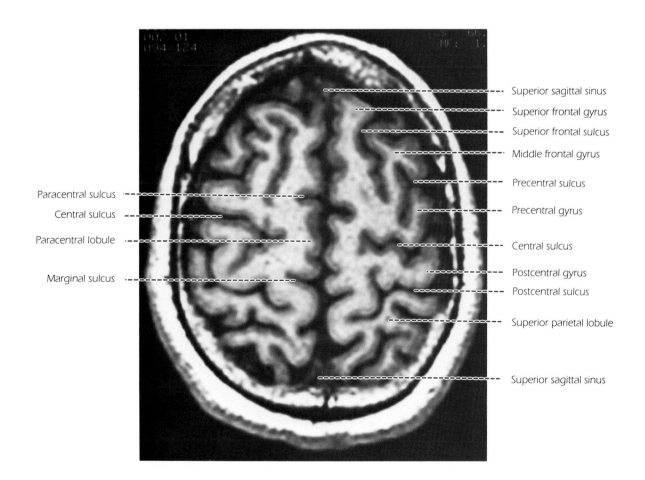

# Figure 1-9

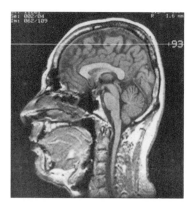

Axial T1-weighted image through the frontal and parietal lobes. The central sulcus separates the pre- and postcentral gyri. The postcentral sulcus separates the postcentral gyrus from the superior parietal lobule. The subarachnoid space surrounds the cerebral hemispheres and insinuates between gyri. Branches of the superficial temporal artery are seen within the subcutaneous tissue of the skin. The brain is protected by the following layers of tissue from medial to lateral: the dura mater, lamina interna of bone, diploë, lamina externa of bone, subcutaneous connective tissue, and skin.

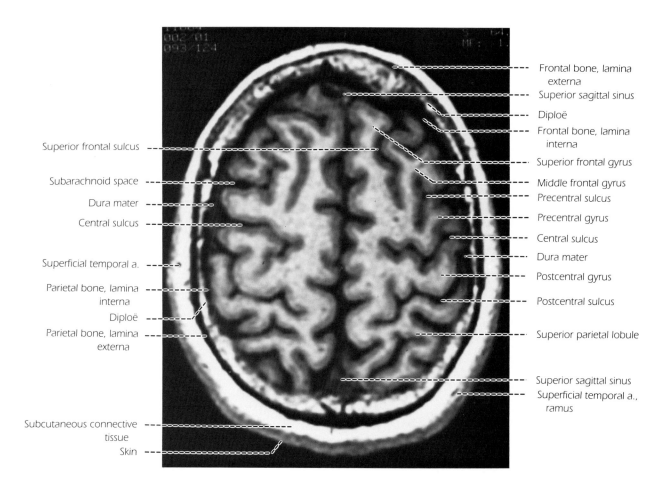

Axial T1-weighted image through the centrum semiovale. The central sulcus separates the pre- and postcentral gyri. Caudal to the postcentral gyrus is the postcentral sulcus. In the parietal lobe, the inferior parietal lobule and the precuneus are seen. In the frontal lobe, the superior frontal sulcus separates the superior and middle frontal gyri. The occipitofrontalis muscle is seen rostrally. The superior sagittal sinus is cut caudally. The superficial temporal artery is located external to the lamina externa of bone within the subcutaneous tissue.

## Figure 1-10

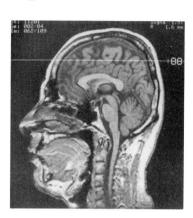

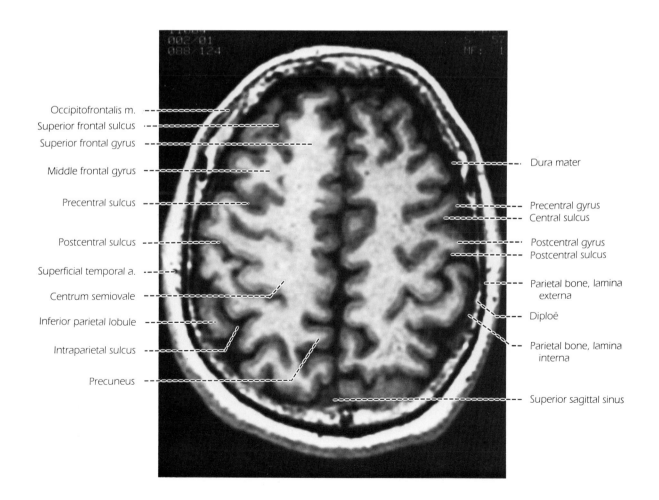

## Figure 1-11

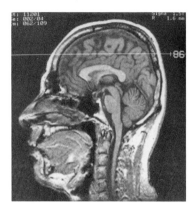

Axial T1-weighted image through the centrum semiovale of the frontal and parietal lobes. The dura mater surrounds the cerebral hemispheres. The fold of the dura, the falx cerebri, fills the space between the two hemispheres. The superior sagittal sinus is seen caudal to the falx cerebri. The temporalis muscle is located lateral to the lamina externa of bone. The central sulcus is anterior to the postcentral gyrus. The superior frontal sulcus separates the superior and middle frontal gyri. The precuneus is seen rostral to the parieto-occipital sulcus.

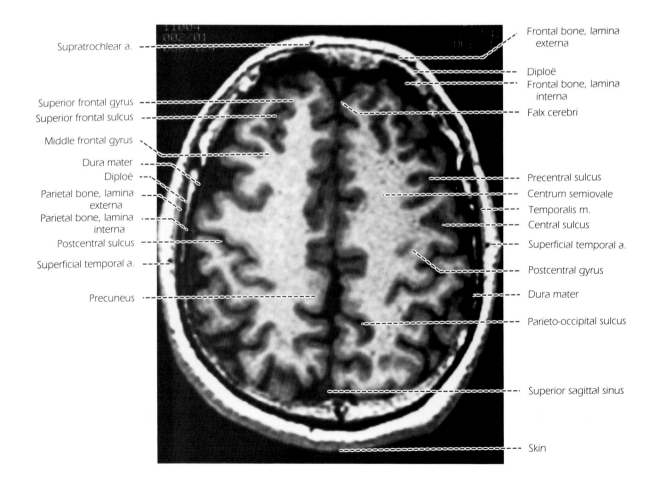

Axial T1-weighted image at the level of the centrum semiovale. The centrum semiovale occupies the deep white matter core of the frontal and parietal lobes. On each side of the midline is the cingulate gyrus. The cingulum is the deep white matter core of the cingulate gyrus. The central sulcus is rostral to the postcentral gyrus. Caudal to the postcentral gyrus is the postcentral sulcus. The inferior parietal lobule is located within the parietal lobe. The parieto-occipital sulcus is caudal to the cingulate gyrus. In the frontal lobe, the superior frontal sulcus separates the superior and middle frontal gyri.

## Figure 1-12

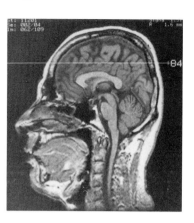

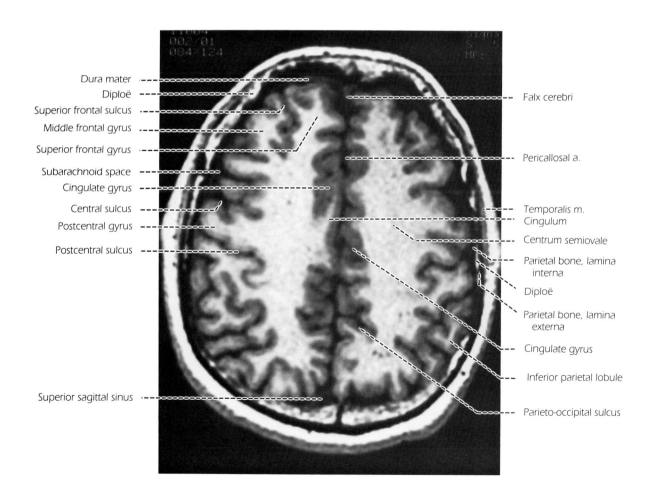

## Figure 1-13

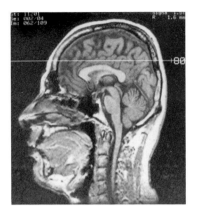

Axial T1-weighted image of the cerebral hemispheres at the level of the centrum semiovale. The centrum semiovale occupies the deep white matter core of the cerebral hemispheres. The postcentral gyrus is located between the central and postcentral sulci. The cingulum, the deep white matter core of the cingulate gyrus, is found on each side of the midline, medial to the centrum semiovale. The parieto-occipital sulcus delineates the posterior boundary of the precuneus. Caudally, the cuneus, part of the occipital lobe, is seen. The superior sagittal sinus is located both rostrally and caudally. The temporalis muscle is outside the lamina externa of bone. The subarachnoid space surrounds the cerebral hemispheres and is located between gyri. In the frontal lobe, the superior frontal sulcus separates the superior and middle frontal gyri.

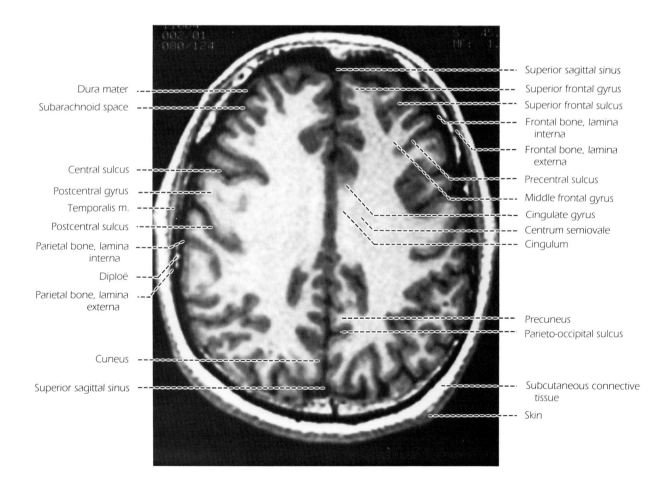

Axial T1-weighted image through the most superficial part of the lateral ventricle. The lateral ventricles are seen on both sides of the midline. Medial to the lateral ventricle is the cingulum, the deep white matter core of the cingulate gyrus. The central sulcus is between the pre- and postcentral gyri. Rostral to the precentral gyrus is the precentral sulcus. Caudal to the postcentral gyrus is the postcentral sulcus. The superior frontal sulcus separates the superior and middle frontal gyri. The lateral fissure separates the supramarginal and angular gyri, both gyri of the parietal lobe. Rostral to the parieto-occipital sulcus is the precuneus. Caudal to the parieto-occipital sulcus is the cuneus. The temporalis muscle is lateral to the lamina externa of bone and medial to the subcutaneous connective tissue. The supratrochlear artery is seen within the subcutaneous connective tissue rostrally.

## Figure 1-14

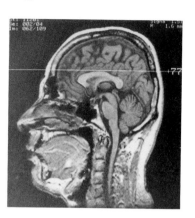

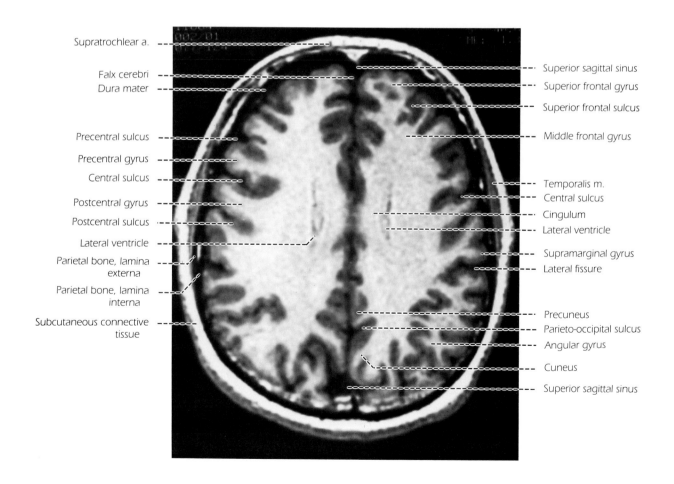

Supratrochlear a.

Falx cerebri
Dura mater

Precentral sulcus
Precentral gyrus
Central sulcus
Postcentral gyrus
Postcentral sulcus
Lateral ventricle
Parietal bone, lamina externa
Parietal bone, lamina interna
Subcutaneous connective tissue

Superior sagittal sinus
Superior frontal gyrus
Superior frontal sulcus
Middle frontal gyrus
Temporalis m.
Central sulcus
Cingulum
Lateral ventricle
Supramarginal gyrus
Lateral fissure
Precuneus
Parieto-occipital sulcus
Angular gyrus
Cuneus
Superior sagittal sinus

# Figure 1-15

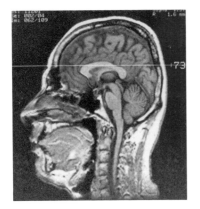

Axial T1-weighted image through the head of the caudate nucleus and corpus callosum. The head of the caudate nucleus is seen bulging into the lateral ventricle. The corpus callosum extends into the frontal pole (forceps minor) and occipital pole (forceps major). Branches of the pericallosal artery are located rostral to the corpus callosum, in the interhemispheric fissure. In the frontal lobe, the superior frontal sulcus separates the superior and middle frontal gyri. The postcentral gyrus is located between the central and postcentral sulci. The parieto-occipital sulcus separates the precuneus and cuneus. Branches of the supratrochlear artery are seen in the subcutaneous connective tissue rostrally. The temporalis muscle is located lateral to the lamina externa of bone and medial to the subcutaneous connective tissue.

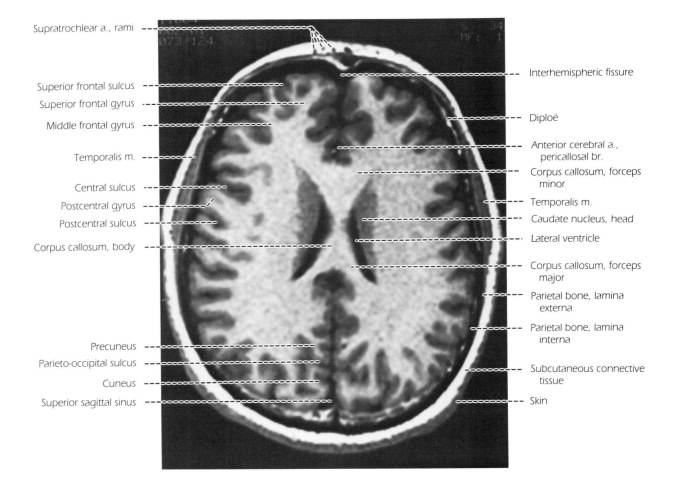

Supratrochlear a., rami

Superior frontal sulcus
Superior frontal gyrus
Middle frontal gyrus

Temporalis m.

Central sulcus
Postcentral gyrus
Postcentral sulcus

Corpus callosum, body

Precuneus
Parieto-occipital sulcus
Cuneus
Superior sagittal sinus

Interhemispheric fissure

Diploë

Anterior cerebral a., pericallosal br.
Corpus callosum, forceps minor
Temporalis m.
Caudate nucleus, head
Lateral ventricle
Corpus callosum, forceps major
Parietal bone, lamina externa
Parietal bone, lamina interna

Subcutaneous connective tissue
Skin

Axial T1-weighted image through the genu and splenium of the corpus callosum. The head of the caudate nucleus is in the lateral wall of the cavity of the lateral ventricle. The septum pellucidum separates the two cavities of the lateral ventricle. The choroid plexus is seen caudally in the lateral ventricle. Lateral to the caudate nucleus is the internal capsule. The genu delineates the lateral ventricles rostrally, and the splenium of the corpus callosum delineates them caudally. The forceps major of the splenium extends toward the occipital pole posteriorly. Rostral and dorsal to the genu of the corpus callosum is the cingulate gyrus. The cingulate sulcus separates the cingulate gyrus from the rest of the frontal lobe. Within the frontal lobe, the superior frontal sulcus separates the superior and middle frontal gyri. The central sulcus separates the pre- and postcentral gyri. The lateral fissure is seen rostral to the supramarginal gyrus. Caudally, the parieto-occipital sulcus separates the precuneus from the cuneus. Branches of the supratrochlear arteries are seen in the subcutaneous connective tissue rostrally. The temporalis muscle is located lateral to the lamina externa of bone and medial to the subcutaneous connective tissue.

## Figure 1-16

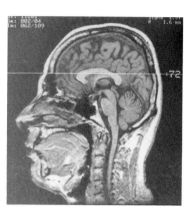

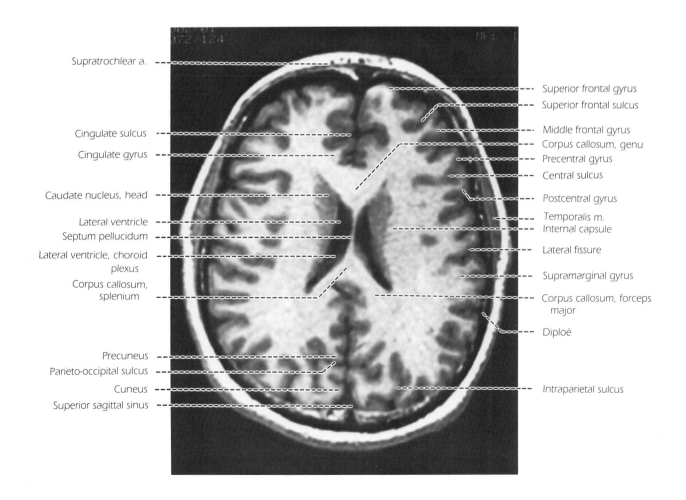

# Figure 1-17

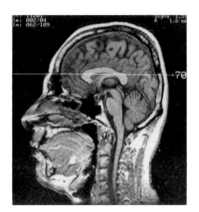

Axial T1-weighted image through the anterior horn and trigone of the lateral ventricle. The genu and splenium of the corpus callosum are seen. The septum pellucidum separates the two cavities of the lateral ventricle. Ventral to the septum pellucidum is the fornix. The caudate nucleus is in the lateral wall of the anterior horn of the lateral ventricle. Rostral and dorsal to the genu of the corpus callosum is the cingulate gyrus. Also dorsal to the genu are the pericallosal branches of the anterior cerebral artery. The thalamus is seen ventral to the caudate nucleus. Dorsal to the trigone of the lateral ventricle is the tail of the caudate nucleus. The parieto-occipital sulcus separates the precuneus and cuneus. In the depth of the lateral fissure is the insular cortex (island of Reil). Branches of the supratrochlear artery are found within the subcutaneous connective tissue anteriorly.

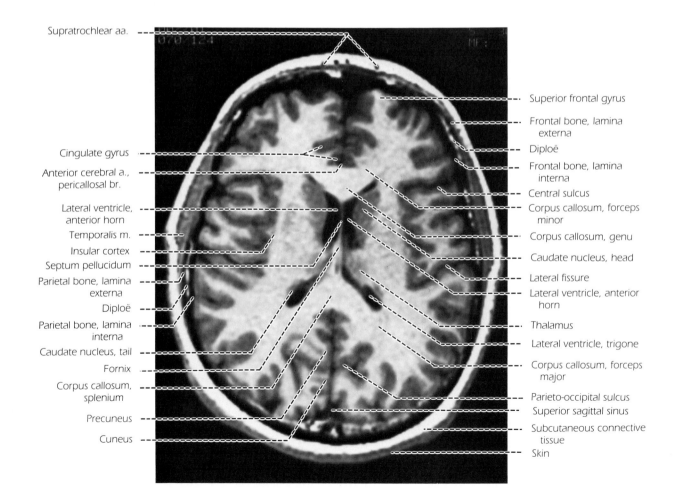

Axial T1-weighted image through the basal ganglia and thalamus. The corpus callosum is sectioned rostrally through the genu and caudally through the splenium. The septum pellucidum separates the two cavities of the anterior horn of the lateral ventricle. The head of the caudate nucleus bulges into the anterior horn of the lateral ventricle. The anterior limb of the internal capsule separates the caudate nucleus from the putamen. Lateral to the putamen is the external capsule. The thalamus is medial to the putamen. Dorsal to the trigone of the lateral ventricle is the tail of the caudate nucleus. The insular cortex (island of Reil) is located deep within the lateral fissure. Caudal to the lateral fissure is the superior temporal gyrus. The parieto-occipital sulcus separates the precuneus and cuneus. Branches of the pericallosal artery are dorsal and rostral to the genu of the corpus callosum.

## Figure 1-18

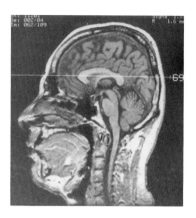

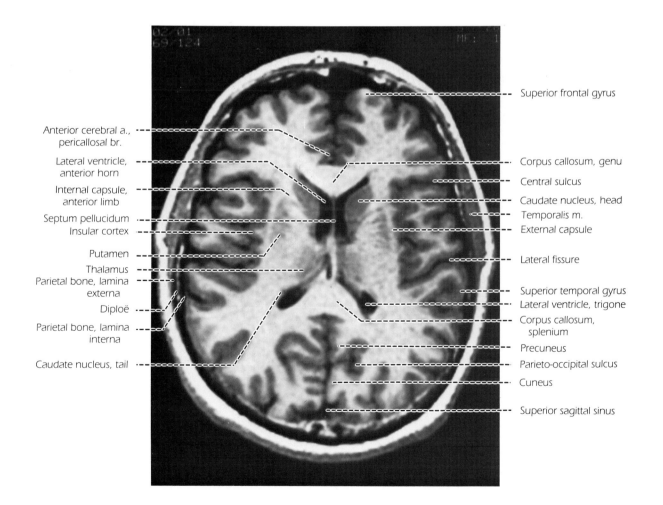

Superior frontal gyrus

Anterior cerebral a., pericallosal br.

Lateral ventricle, anterior horn

Internal capsule, anterior limb

Septum pellucidum
Insular cortex

Putamen
Thalamus
Parietal bone, lamina externa

Diploë

Parietal bone, lamina interna

Caudate nucleus, tail

Corpus callosum, genu
Central sulcus
Caudate nucleus, head
Temporalis m.
External capsule

Lateral fissure

Superior temporal gyrus
Lateral ventricle, trigone
Corpus callosum, splenium
Precuneus
Parieto-occipital sulcus
Cuneus
Superior sagittal sinus

## Figure 1-19

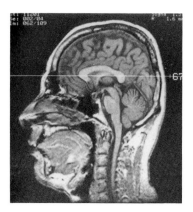

Axial T1-weighted image through the basal ganglia and thalamus. The third ventricle is in the midline between the two thalami. Within the thalamus, the anterior thalamic nucleus is located rostrally, the dorsomedial nucleus medially, and the lateral nucleus laterally. The posterior limb of the internal capsule separates the thalamus from the putamen. The anterior limb of the internal capsule separates the caudate nucleus from the putamen. The genu of the internal capsule is between the anterior and posterior limbs. The head of the caudate nucleus bulges into the anterior horn of the lateral ventricle. The tail of the caudate nucleus is dorsal to the trigone of the lateral ventricle. The septum pellucidum separates the two cavities of the anterior horn of the lateral ventricle. Ventral to the septum pellucidum is the body of the fornix. More caudally, within the trigone of the lateral ventricle, is the crus of the fornix. The corpus callosum is sectioned anteriorly (the genu) and posteriorly (the splenium). The insular cortex (island of Reil) is located deep within the lateral fissure. The cingulate gyrus is rostral to the genu of the corpus callosum. The parieto-occipital sulcus delineates the anterior boundary of the cuneus gyrus. The interventricular foramen (foramen of Monro) joins the lateral ventricle with the third ventricle. The choroid plexus is found within the trigone of the lateral ventricle.

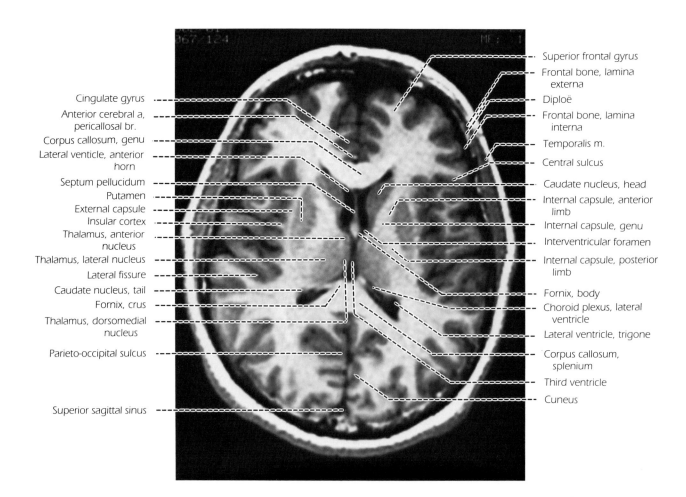

Axial T1-weighted image through the basal ganglia and thalamus. The thalamus is seen on each side of the midline separated from the putamen by the posterior limb of the internal capsule. The anterior limb of the internal capsule separates the caudate from the putamen. Between the anterior and posterior limbs of the internal capsule is the genu of the internal capsule. The head of the caudate nucleus bulges into the anterior horn of the lateral ventricle. The septum pellucidum separates the two cavities of the anterior horn of the lateral ventricle. Ventral to the septum pellucidum is the fornix. The trigone of the lateral ventricle is found caudally. The crus of the fornix is seen in the trigone. The corpus callosum is sectioned both rostrally at the genu and caudally at the splenium. The cingulate gyrus is rostral to the genu of the corpus callosum. The pericallosal branches of the anterior cerebral artery are rostral to the genu of the corpus callosum within the longitudinal cerebral fissure. Lateral to the putamen is the external capsule. The claustrum is lateral to the external capsule. The optic radiation is located lateral and posterior to the trigone. The interventricular foramen (foramen of Monro) joins the lateral ventricle with the third ventricle.

## Figure 1-20

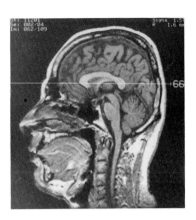

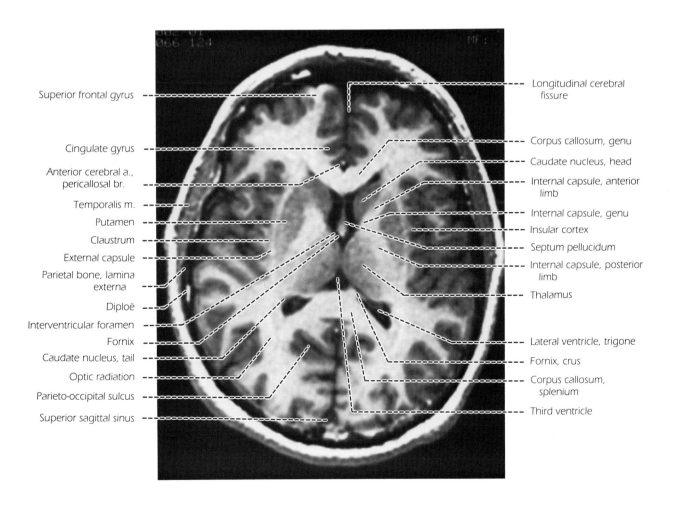

Superior frontal gyrus

Cingulate gyrus

Anterior cerebral a., pericallosal br.

Temporalis m.

Putamen

Claustrum

External capsule

Parietal bone, lamina externa

Diploë

Interventricular foramen

Fornix

Caudate nucleus, tail

Optic radiation

Parieto-occipital sulcus

Superior sagittal sinus

Longitudinal cerebral fissure

Corpus callosum, genu

Caudate nucleus, head

Internal capsule, anterior limb

Internal capsule, genu

Insular cortex

Septum pellucidum

Internal capsule, posterior limb

Thalamus

Lateral ventricle, trigone

Fornix, crus

Corpus callosum, splenium

Third ventricle

## Figure 1-21

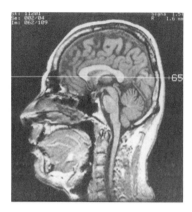

Axial T1-weighted image through the basal ganglia and thalamus. The two thalami are connected across the midline by the massa intermedia. The posterior limb of the internal capsule separates the thalamus from the putamen nucleus. The anterior limb of the internal capsule separates the putamen and caudate nuclei. The genu of the internal capsule is found between the anterior and posterior limbs of the internal capsule. External to the putamen is the external capsule. The claustrum is located between the external and extreme capsules. Lateral to the extreme capsule and deep within the lateral fissure is the insular cortex (island of Reil). The corpus callosum is sectioned both rostrally at the level of the genu and caudally at the level of the splenium. Rostral to the genu of the corpus callosum, within the interhemispheric fissure, are the pericallosal branches of the anterior cerebral artery. The septum pellucidum separates the two cavities of the anterior horn of the lateral ventricle. The caudate nucleus bulges into the cavity of the anterior horn of the lateral ventricle. Inferior to the septum pellucidum is the fornix. The interventricular foramen (foramen of Monro) connects the lateral ventricle with the third ventricle. The crus of the fornix is located within the trigone of the lateral ventricle. The choroid plexus is also seen within the trigone. The optic radiation is found lateral and caudal to the trigone of the lateral ventricle. The parieto-occipital sulcus delineates the posterior boundary of the precuneus. The frontal sinus is seen anteriorly.

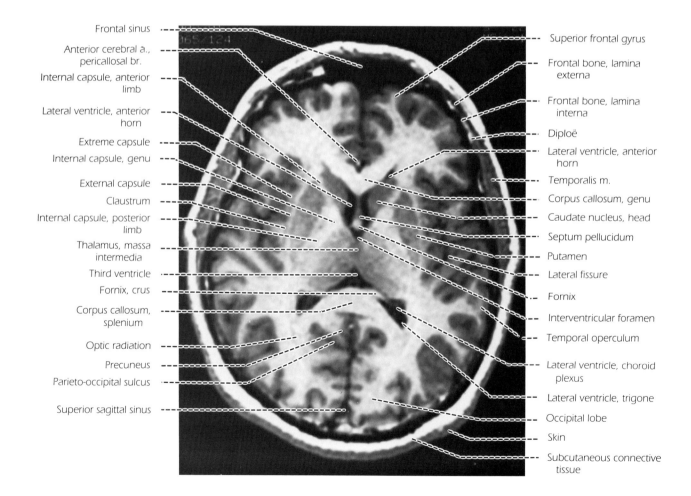

Frontal sinus

Anterior cerebral a., pericallosal br.

Internal capsule, anterior limb

Lateral ventricle, anterior horn

Extreme capsule

Internal capsule, genu

External capsule

Claustrum

Internal capsule, posterior limb

Thalamus, massa intermedia

Third ventricle

Fornix, crus

Corpus callosum, splenium

Optic radiation

Precuneus

Parieto-occipital sulcus

Superior sagittal sinus

Superior frontal gyrus

Frontal bone, lamina externa

Frontal bone, lamina interna

Diploë

Lateral ventricle, anterior horn

Temporalis m.

Corpus callosum, genu

Caudate nucleus, head

Septum pellucidum

Putamen

Lateral fissure

Fornix

Interventricular foramen

Temporal operculum

Lateral ventricle, choroid plexus

Lateral ventricle, trigone

Occipital lobe

Skin

Subcutaneous connective tissue

Axial T1-weighted image through the basal ganglia and thalamus. The thalamus is seen on each side of the third ventricle. Within the thalamus, the mamillothalamic tract is seen in cross section. The caudate nucleus bulges into the anterior horn of the lateral ventricle. The septum pellucidum separates the two cavities of the lateral ventricle. Ventral to the septum pellucidum are the columns of the fornix. Between the caudate nucleus and thalamus are the thalamostriate vein and stria terminalis. The anterior limb of the internal capsule separates the caudate from the putamen. Medial to the putamen is the globus pallidus. The posterior limb of the internal capsule separates the globus pallidus from the thalamus. The genu of the internal capsule is found between the anterior and posterior limbs. Lateral to the putamen is the external capsule. The claustrum is sandwiched between the external and extreme capsules. The corpus callosum is sectioned rostrally at the level of the genu and caudally at the level of the splenium. The pericallosal branches of the anterior cerebral artery are rostral to the genu of the corpus callosum within the interhemispheric fissure. The fimbria is seen within the trigone of the lateral ventricle. The tail of the caudate nucleus is dorsal to the trigone. The parieto-occipital sulcus delineates the posterior boundary of the precuneus. The occipital lobe is seen caudally. The temporal operculum overlies the lateral fissure. The choroid plexus is seen within the trigone of the lateral ventricle. The optic radiation is located lateral and caudal to the trigone of the lateral ventricle in the direction of the occipital lobe.

## Figure 1-22

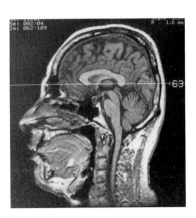

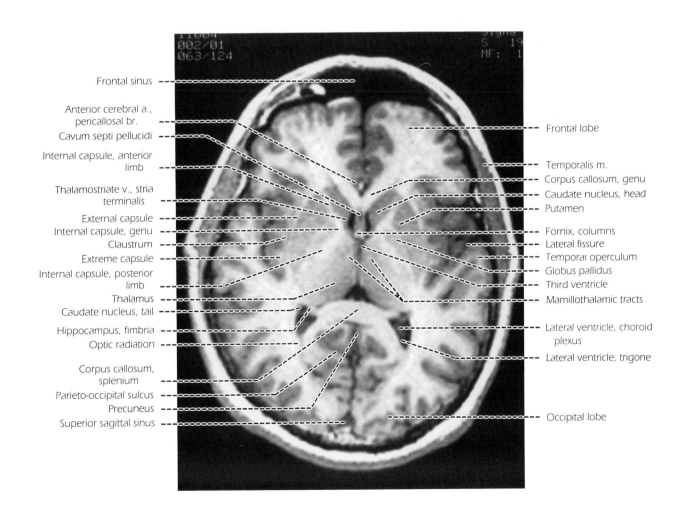

# Figure 1-23

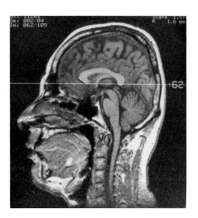

Axial T1-weighted image through the basal ganglia and thalamus. The thalamus is found on each side of the third ventricle. Within the thalamus, the dorsomedial nucleus is seen medially. The stria medullaris thalami lines the medial and dorsal boundary of the thalamus. The head of the caudate nucleus bulges into the lateral ventricle. The two cavities of the lateral ventricle are separated by the septum pellucidum. The cavum septum pellucidum is seen within the septum. Ventral to the septum pellucidum is the fornix. The caudate nucleus is separated from the putamen by the anterior limb of the internal capsule. Medial to the putamen is the globus pallidus. The posterior limb of the internal capsule separates the globus pallidus from the thalamus. The genu of the internal capsule is between the anterior and posterior limbs. Lateral to the putamen is the external capsule. The claustrum is sandwiched between the external and extreme capsules. The insular cortex is seen deep within the lateral fissure. Overlying the lateral fissure on one side is the transverse gyrus of Heschl. Within the trigone of the lateral ventricle is the fimbria of the fornix. The pericallosal branches of the anterior cerebral artery are in the interhemispheric fissure rostral to the corpus callosum.

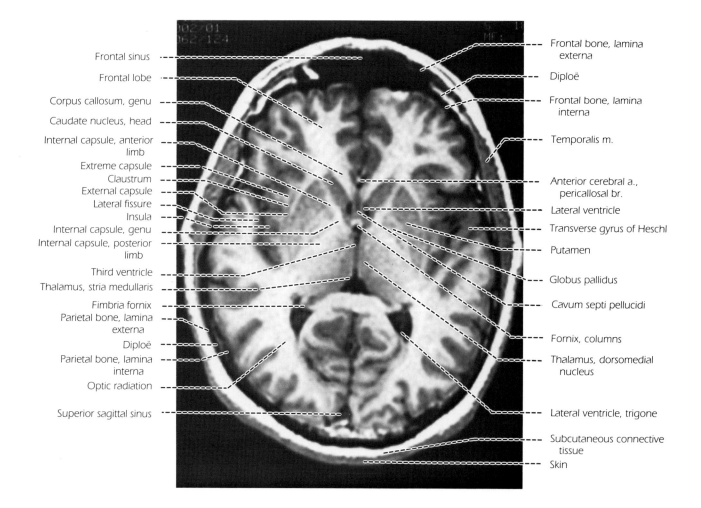

Frontal sinus

Frontal lobe

Corpus callosum, genu

Caudate nucleus, head

Internal capsule, anterior limb

Extreme capsule

Claustrum

External capsule

Lateral fissure

Insula

Internal capsule, genu

Internal capsule, posterior limb

Third ventricle

Thalamus, stria medullaris

Fimbria fornix

Parietal bone, lamina externa

Diploë

Parietal bone, lamina interna

Optic radiation

Superior sagittal sinus

Frontal bone, lamina externa

Diploë

Frontal bone, lamina interna

Temporalis m.

Anterior cerebral a., pericallosal br.

Lateral ventricle

Transverse gyrus of Heschl

Putamen

Globus pallidus

Cavum septi pellucidi

Fornix, columns

Thalamus, dorsomedial nucleus

Lateral ventricle, trigone

Subcutaneous connective tissue

Skin

Axial T1-weighted image through the basal ganglia and thalamus. The thalamus is found on each side of the third ventricle. The stria medullaris thalami is seen as a bright signal intensity on the medial and caudal border of the thalamus. The posterior limb of the internal capsule separates the thalamus from the globus pallidus. The anterior limb of the internal capsule separates the caudate and putamen nuclei. The genu of the internal capsule is seen between the anterior and posterior limbs. The columns of the fornix are located ventral and caudal to the caudate nucleus overlying the cavity of the third ventricle. Deep within the lateral fissure is the insular cortex. The tail of the caudate nucleus is dorsal to the trigone of the lateral ventricle. Medial and dorsal to the trigone is the hippocampus. The pericallosal branches of the anterior cerebral artery are seen in the interhemispheric fissure.

## Figure 1-24

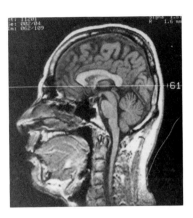

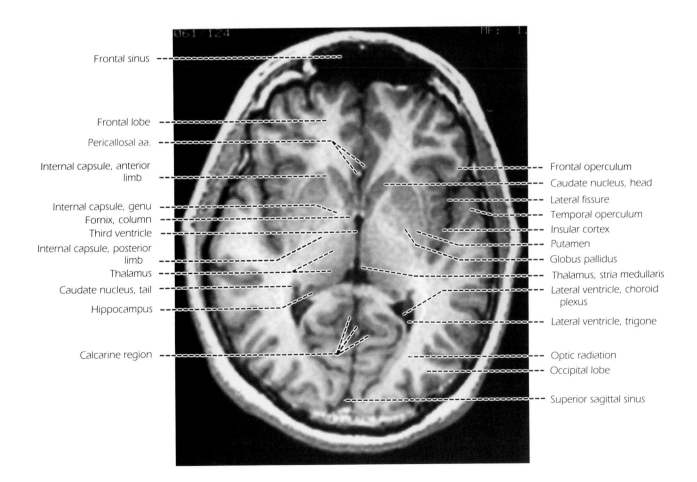

Frontal sinus

Frontal lobe

Pericallosal aa.

Internal capsule, anterior limb

Internal capsule, genu
Fornix, column
Third ventricle
Internal capsule, posterior limb
Thalamus
Caudate nucleus, tail
Hippocampus

Calcarine region

Frontal operculum
Caudate nucleus, head
Lateral fissure
Temporal operculum
Insular cortex
Putamen
Globus pallidus
Thalamus, stria medullaris
Lateral ventricle, choroid plexus

Lateral ventricle, trigone

Optic radiation
Occipital lobe

Superior sagittal sinus

# Figure 1-25

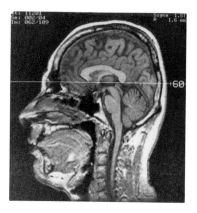

Axial T1-weighted image through the basal ganglia and thalamus. The thalamus is seen on each side of the third ventricle. The stria medullaris thalami is seen as a bright signal intensity at the caudal border of the thalamus. The anterior commissure is visualized rostrally beneath the caudate nucleus. Ventral to the anterior commissure are the columns of the fornix. The caudate nucleus is separated from the putamen by the anterior limb of the internal capsule. Medial to the putamen is the globus pallidus. The posterior limb of the internal capsule separates the globus pallidus from the thalamus. Lateral to the putamen is the external capsule. The claustrum is found between the external and extreme capsules. The insular cortex is located deep within the lateral fissure. The hippocampus with its alveus is rostral and medial to the trigone of the lateral ventricle. The optic radiation is located lateral and caudal to the trigone. The pericallosal branches of the anterior cerebral artery are seen within the interhemispheric fissure. The frontal and temporal opercula overlie the lateral fissure.

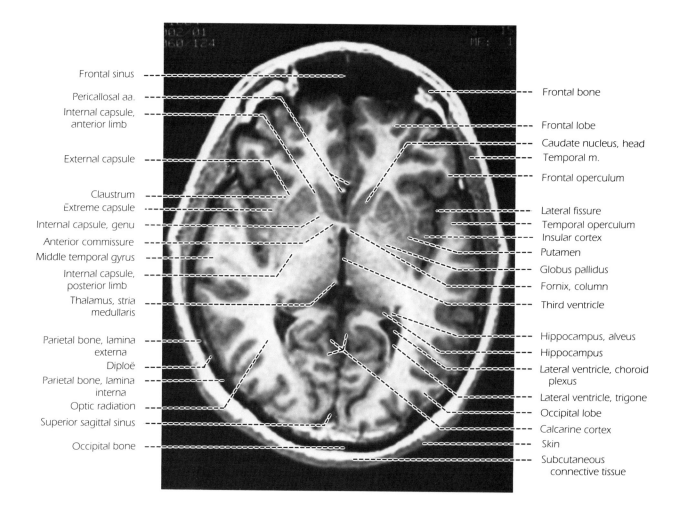

Axial T1-weighted image through the basal ganglia and thalamus. The third ventricle is in the midline. On each side of the third ventricle is the thalamus. The pineal gland is seen caudally. Ventral to the pineal gland is the habenular commissure. Adjacent to the pineal gland is the pineal cistern. The caudate nucleus is separated from the putamen by the anterior limb of the internal capsule. Medial to the putamen is the globus pallidus. The hippocampus is medial to the trigone of the lateral ventricle. The insular cortex is located deep within the lateral fissure. The transverse gyrus of Heschl extends from the superior temporal lobe into the lateral fissure. The frontal operculum overlies the lateral fissure. The pericallosal branches of the anterior cerebral artery are seen in the inter-hemispheric fissure. The gyrus rectus is located in the frontal lobe. The superior oblique and levator palpebrae superioris muscles are seen within the orbit.

# Figure 1-26

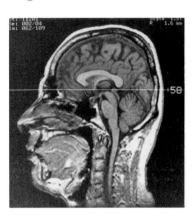

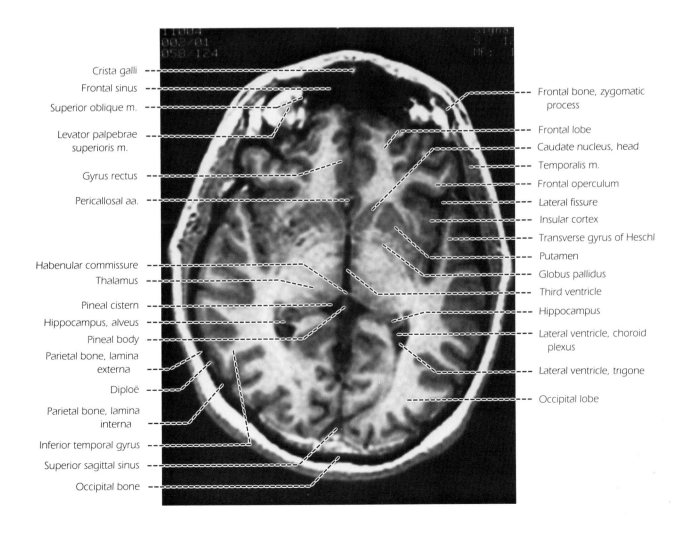

Crista galli
Frontal sinus
Superior oblique m.
Levator palpebrae superioris m.
Gyrus rectus
Pericallosal aa.
Habenular commissure
Thalamus
Pineal cistern
Hippocampus, alveus
Pineal body
Parietal bone, lamina externa
Diploë
Parietal bone, lamina interna
Inferior temporal gyrus
Superior sagittal sinus
Occipital bone

Frontal bone, zygomatic process
Frontal lobe
Caudate nucleus, head
Temporalis m.
Frontal operculum
Lateral fissure
Insular cortex
Transverse gyrus of Heschl
Putamen
Globus pallidus
Third ventricle
Hippocampus
Lateral ventricle, choroid plexus
Lateral ventricle, trigone
Occipital lobe

# Figure 1-27

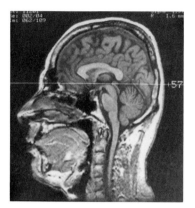

Axial T1-weighted image through the basal ganglia and thalamus. The third ventricle is in the midline. On each side of the third ventricle is the thalamus. In the caudal part of the thalamus are the habenular nuclei. Ventral to the habenular nuclei is the habenular commissure. The head of the caudate nucleus and the putamen are seen rostrally. The frontal and temporal opercula overlie the lateral fissure. The insular cortex is located deep within the lateral fissure. The pericallosal branches of the anterior cerebral artery are seen in the interhemispheric fissure. The hippocampus is seen within the lateral ventricle posteriorly. In the bony orbit, the lacrimal gland and the superior rectus and levator palpebrae superioris muscles are found.

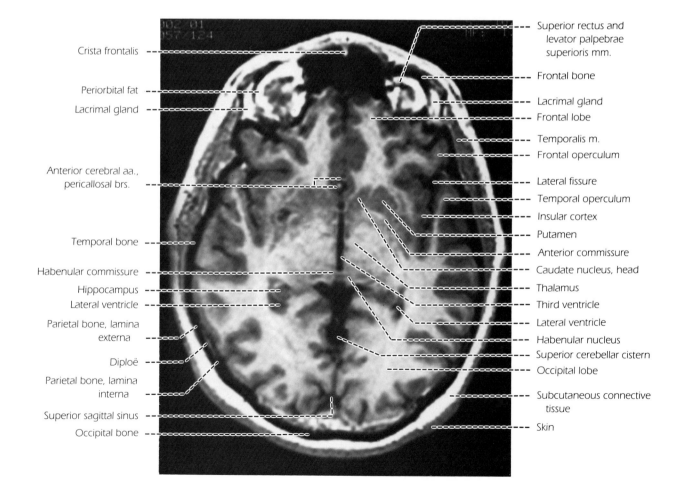

Axial T1-weighted image through the midbrain. Within the frontal lobe are the orbital and rectus gyri. Anterior cerebral artery branches are found in the interhemispheric fissure. The frontal and temporal opercula overlie the lateral fissure. Deep within the lateral fissure is the insular cortex. The putamen nucleus is still seen. Within the midbrain, the cerebral aqueduct (aqueduct of Sylvius) is seen surrounded by the periaqueductal gray. Dorsal to the midbrain is the quadrigeminal cistern overlying the superior colliculus. The superior vermis of the cerebellum is seen between the two occipital lobes.

## Figure 1-28

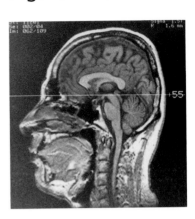

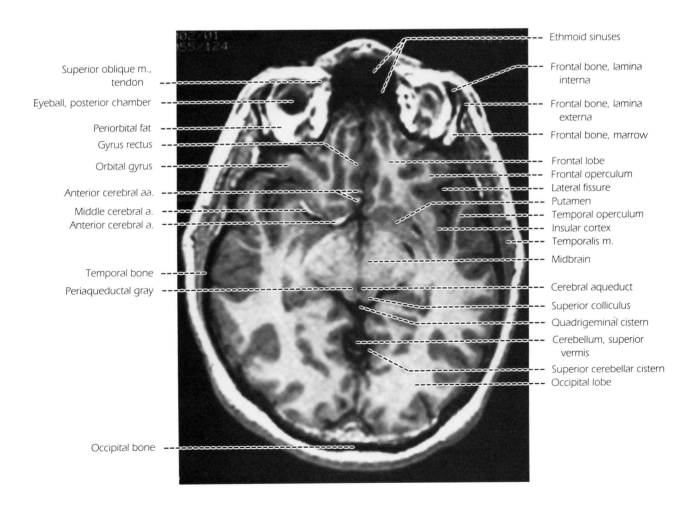

Superior oblique m., tendon

Eyeball, posterior chamber

Periorbital fat

Gyrus rectus

Orbital gyrus

Anterior cerebral aa.

Middle cerebral a.

Anterior cerebral a.

Temporal bone

Periaqueductal gray

Occipital bone

Ethmoid sinuses

Frontal bone, lamina interna

Frontal bone, lamina externa

Frontal bone, marrow

Frontal lobe

Frontal operculum

Lateral fissure

Putamen

Temporal operculum

Insular cortex

Temporalis m.

Midbrain

Cerebral aqueduct

Superior colliculus

Quadrigeminal cistern

Cerebellum, superior vermis

Superior cerebellar cistern

Occipital lobe

# Figure 1-29

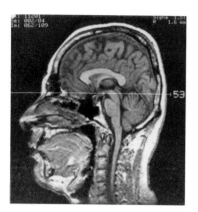

Axial T1-weighted image through the midbrain. In the frontal lobe, the gyrus rectus and the medial orbital gyrus are seen. Between the two frontal lobes rostrally is the bony crista galli. The optic nerve is caudal to the orbit within the periorbital fat. The superior oblique muscle and its tendon are medial to the globe. The lacrimal artery and nerve as well as the ophthalmic artery are seen within the periorbital fat. The middle cerebral artery is located in the lateral fissure. The anterior cerebral artery is found between the two frontal lobes. The optic tract appears as a bright signal intensity beneath the midbrain. The infundibular recess of the third ventricle is located between the two optic tracts. Within the midbrain, the crus cerebri (cerebral peduncle), substantia nigra, red nucleus, tegmentum, cerebral aqueduct (aqueduct of Sylvius), and superior colliculus are seen. Between the cerebral peduncle and the temporal lobe is the crural cistern. Within the temporal lobe, the superior and inferior temporal gyri are found. The hippocampus is in the medial part of the inferior (temporal) horn of the lateral ventricle. The quadrigeminal cistern overlies the superior colliculus. The superior cerebellar vermis is seen in the midline posteriorly. The uncus of the temporal lobe is in close proximity to the midbrain.

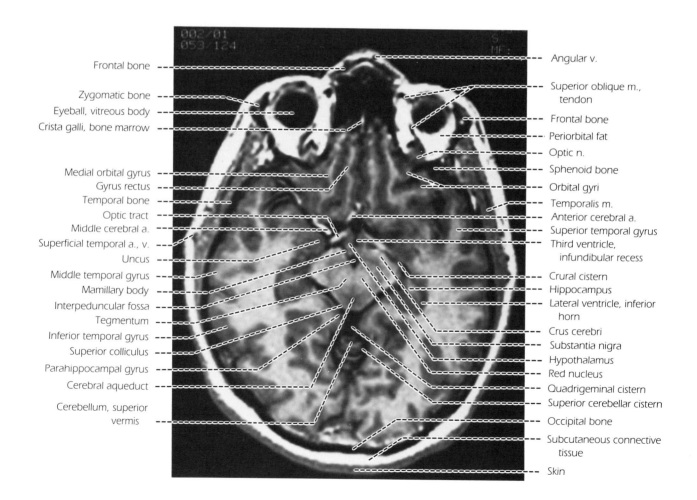

Axial T1-weighted image through the midbrain. In the frontal lobe, the orbital gyrus is lateral to the gyrus rectus. In between the two frontal lobes anteriorly is the bony crista galli, the anterior attachment of the falx cerebri. In the temporal lobe, the amygdaloid nucleus is found within the uncus. The hippocampus is located within the inferior or temporal horn of the lateral ventricle. The parahippocampal gyrus is adjacent to the hippocampus. The bright signal intensities of the anterior and middle cerebral arteries are seen. The anterior cerebral artery is found in the space between the frontal lobes, whereas the middle cerebral artery is seen in the lateral fissure. Within the midbrain, the crus cerebri, substantia nigra, red nucleus, superior colliculus, and the cerebral aqueduct (aqueduct of Sylvius) are also seen. Dorsal to the superior colliculus is the quadrigeminal cistern. Dorsal to the quadrigeminal cistern is the superior vermis of the cerebellum. Close to the mamillary body is the infundibulum. On each side of the infundibulum are the optic tracts. The superior rectus muscle is seen within periorbital fat. The vitreous body of the eyeball is identified.

# Figure 1-30

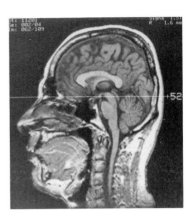

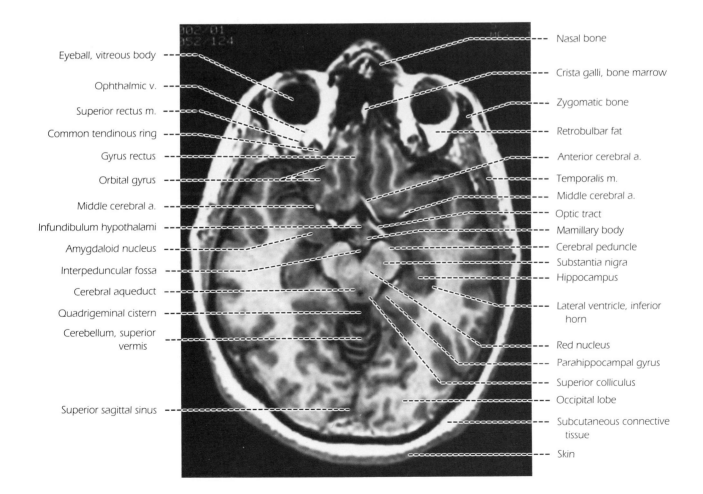

# Figure 1-31

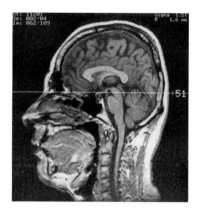

Axial T1-weighted image through the midbrain. In the frontal lobe, the gyrus rectus is medial to the medial orbital gyrus. Anterior to the frontal lobe is the crista galli. The eyelid is seen within the orbit. The vitreous body of the eyeball is also seen. The medial rectus muscle is visualized within the periorbital fat. Caudal to the orbit is the common tendinous ring (Zinn's ring). Caudal to the frontal lobes is the optic chiasma. Extending from the optic chiasma caudally is the optic tract. Several arterial channels are seen as bright signal intensities including the internal carotid, middle cerebral, and posterior cerebral arteries. The posterior cerebral artery is seen near the midbrain. Close to the optic chiasma is the infundibulum of the hypothalamus. Within the temporal lobe, the amygdaloid nucleus is seen medially. The inferior horn of the lateral ventricle is caudal to the amygdaloid nucleus. Within the midbrain, the crus cerebri, substantia nigra, cerebral aqueduct (aqueduct of Sylvius), and inferior colliculus are seen. Dorsal to the inferior colliculus is the quadrigeminal cistern. Close to the quadrigeminal cistern in the midline is the superior vermis of the cerebellum.

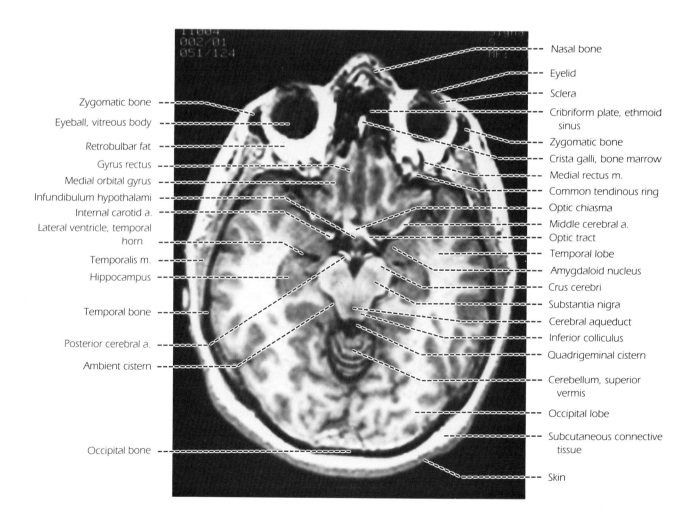

Axial T1-weighted image through the midbrain. Within the midbrain, the crus cerebri, substantia nigra, cerebral aqueduct, and inferior colliculus are seen. Dorsal to the inferior colliculus is the quadrigeminal cistern. In the midline of the midbrain is the decussation of the superior cerebellar peduncle (brachium conjunctivum). Ventral to the midbrain, in the interpeduncular cistern, is the basilar artery. Beneath the crus cerebri is the posterior cerebral artery. The internal carotid artery is found more rostrally. The optic nerve and optic chiasma are seen as bright signal intensities. The uncus of the temporal lobe is located in the medial aspect of the temporal lobe close to the midbrain. The vermis of the cerebellum is dorsal to the midbrain. Close to the optic chiasma and dorsal to it is the infundibulum. Within the orbit, the lateral and medial rectus muscles are seen. The optic nerve is located in the optic canal. The cribriform plate of the ethmoid and the crista galli are seen in the midline anteriorly.

## Figure 1-32

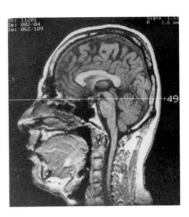

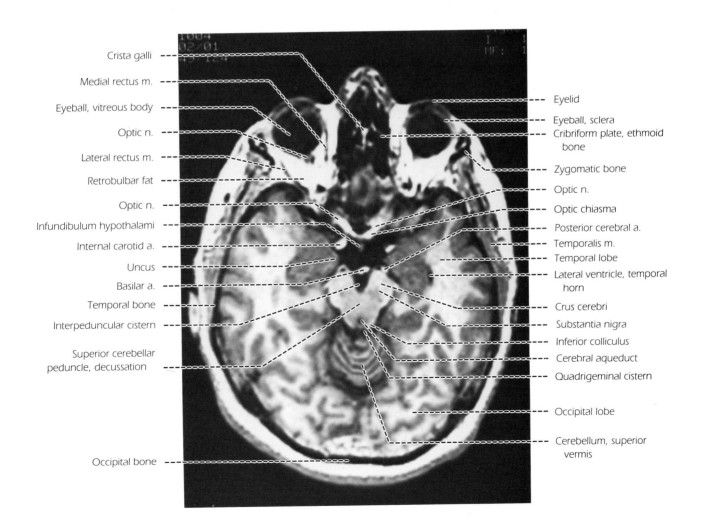

# Figure 1-33

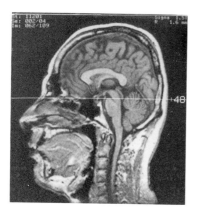

Axial T1-weighted image through the midbrain. Within the midbrain, the crus cerebri, substantia nigra, cerebral aqueduct, and the decussation of the superior cerebellar peduncle are seen. Dorsal to the cerebral aqueduct is the superior medullary velum. Superior to the midbrain is the cerebellum. Ventral to the midbrain is the basilar artery, and close to the crus cerebri is the posterior cerebral artery. The internal carotid artery is seen rostrally. The uncus of the temporal lobe is in the medial part of the temporal lobe, close to the midbrain. The oculomotor nerve is seen exiting from the ventral aspect of the midbrain. Within the eyeball are seen the anterior chamber, lens, and vitreous body. The medial and lateral rectus muscles are found within periorbital fat. Extending from the globe caudally is the optic nerve. The ethmoid sinuses are seen on each side of the midline anteriorly.

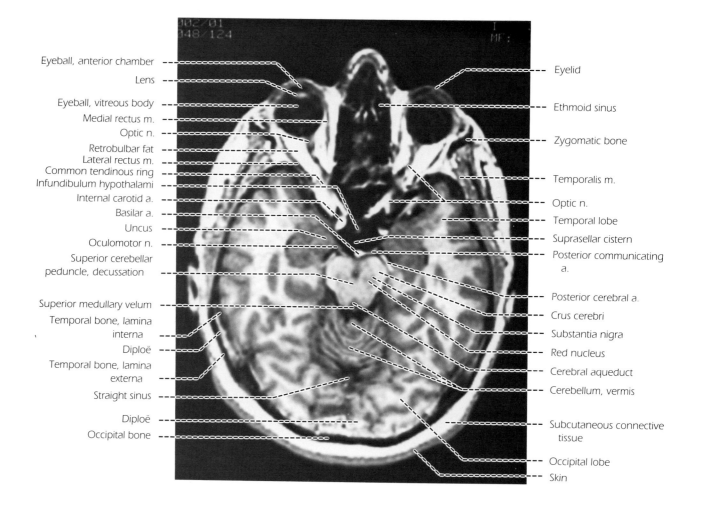

Axial T1-weighted image through the pons. The basilar artery is ventral to the pons. The uncus of the temporal lobe is located medially within the temporal lobe. Lateral to the uncus is the temporal horn of the lateral ventricle. Dorsal to the pons is the cerebellum. Within the cerebellum, the vermis is in the midline, and the cerebellar hemisphere is more laterally placed. The anterior chamber, lens, and vitreous body are seen within the eyeball. The lateral and medial rectus muscles are located within the periorbital fat. The optic nerve extends from the eyeball posteriorly. The internal carotid artery is a bright signal intensity close to the uncus.

## Figure 1-34

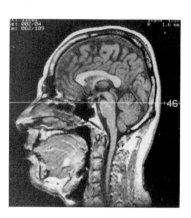

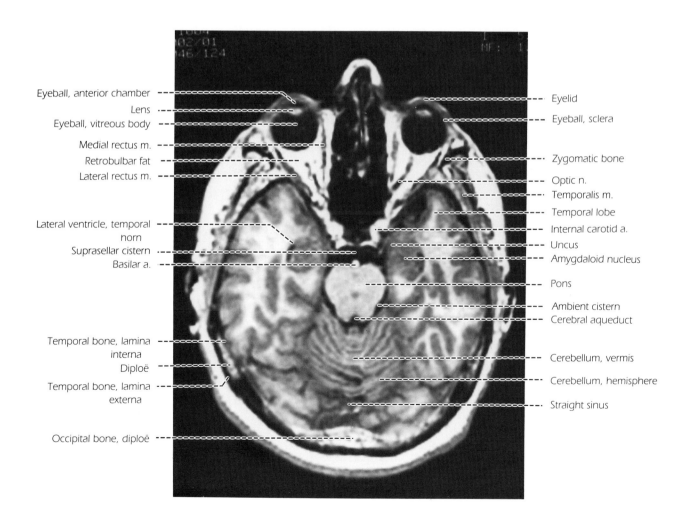

Eyeball, anterior chamber
Lens
Eyeball, vitreous body
Medial rectus m.
Retrobulbar fat
Lateral rectus m.
Lateral ventricle, temporal horn
Suprasellar cistern
Basilar a.
Temporal bone, lamina interna
Diploë
Temporal bone, lamina externa
Occipital bone, diploë

Eyelid
Eyeball, sclera
Zygomatic bone
Optic n.
Temporalis m.
Temporal lobe
Internal carotid a.
Uncus
Amygdaloid nucleus
Pons
Ambient cistern
Cerebral aqueduct
Cerebellum, vermis
Cerebellum, hemisphere
Straight sinus

# Figure 1-35

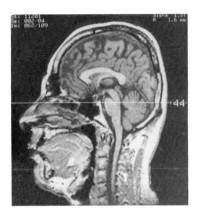

Axial T1-weighted axial image through the temporal lobes, cerebellum, and pons. Ventral to the pons is the basilar artery. Surrounding the pons are the prepontine and lateral pontine cisterns. The superior medullary velum is seen in the dorsal aspect of the pons overlying the fourth ventricle. The bright signal intensity of the superior cerebellar peduncle is seen in the dorsal part of the pons. Ventrolateral to the fourth ventricle is the locus ceruleus. Dorsal to the pons is the cerebellum. The vermis of the cerebellum is in the midline, whereas the cerebellar hemispheres are located laterally. The parahippocampal gyrus is medially located within the temporal lobe. The hypophysis is dorsal to the basiocciput. Close to the hypophysis is the bright signal intensity of the internal carotid artery. Within the eyeball, the lens and the vitreous body are seen. The medial and lateral rectus muscles are within retrobulbar fat. The ethmoid sinuses are medial to the orbit.

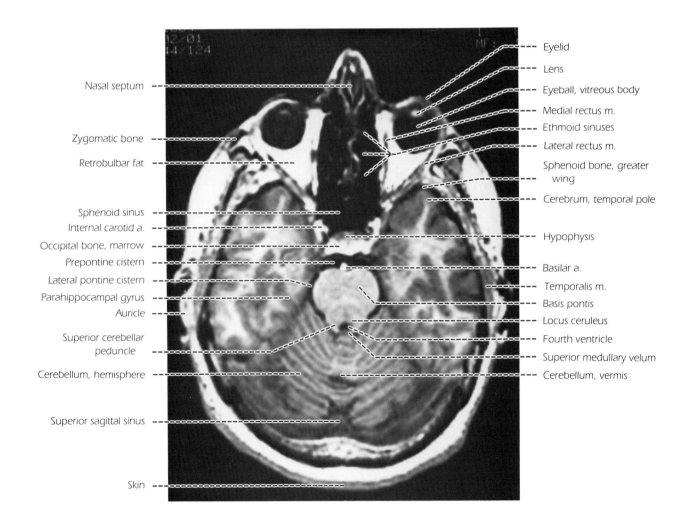

Axial T1-weighted image through the temporal poles, cerebellum, and pons. Ventral to the pons is the basilar artery. Surrounding the pons are the prepontine and lateral pontine cisterns. Within the pons, the superior cerebellar peduncle is seen. The fourth ventricle is superior to the pons. Dorsal to the pons is the cerebellum showing the vermis, which is in the midline, and the cerebellar hemispheres, which are more laterally placed. Within the eyeball the posterior chamber is seen. Two muscles of extraocular movement are seen, the inferior oblique and rectus muscles. The ethmoid sinuses and the perpendicular plate of the ethmoid bone are more rostrally placed.

## Figure 1-36

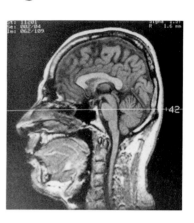

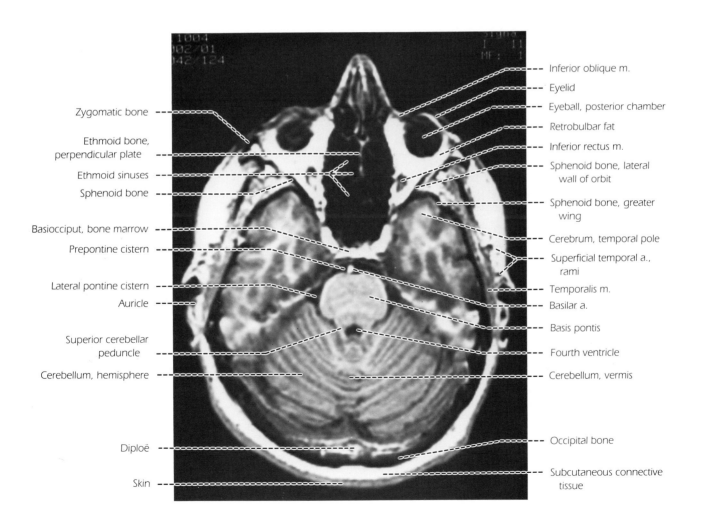

Inferior oblique m.

Eyelid

Eyeball, posterior chamber

Retrobulbar fat

Inferior rectus m.

Sphenoid bone, lateral wall of orbit

Sphenoid bone, greater wing

Cerebrum, temporal pole

Superficial temporal a., rami

Temporalis m.

Basilar a.

Basis pontis

Fourth ventricle

Cerebellum, vermis

Occipital bone

Subcutaneous connective tissue

Zygomatic bone

Ethmoid bone, perpendicular plate

Ethmoid sinuses

Sphenoid bone

Basiocciput, bone marrow

Prepontine cistern

Lateral pontine cistern

Auricle

Superior cerebellar peduncle

Cerebellum, hemisphere

Diploë

Skin

# Figure 1-37

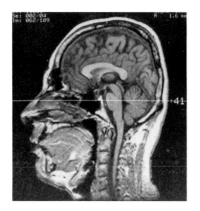

Axial T1-weighted image through the temporal poles, cerebellum, and pons. Ventral to the pons is the bright signal intensity of the basilar artery. Surrounding the pons are the prepontine and lateral pontine cisterns. The basis pontis is found in the ventral aspect of the pons. Located laterally and dorsally in the pons are the middle and superior cerebellar peduncles. The fourth ventricle is dorsal to the pons. Overlying the pons and fourth ventricle is the cerebellum. The posterior chamber of the eyeball is seen within the orbit. The inferior oblique and rectus muscles are seen surrounding the eyeball. Several venous sinuses are visualized including the transverse sinus, straight sinus, and confluence of sinuses (torcular herophili).

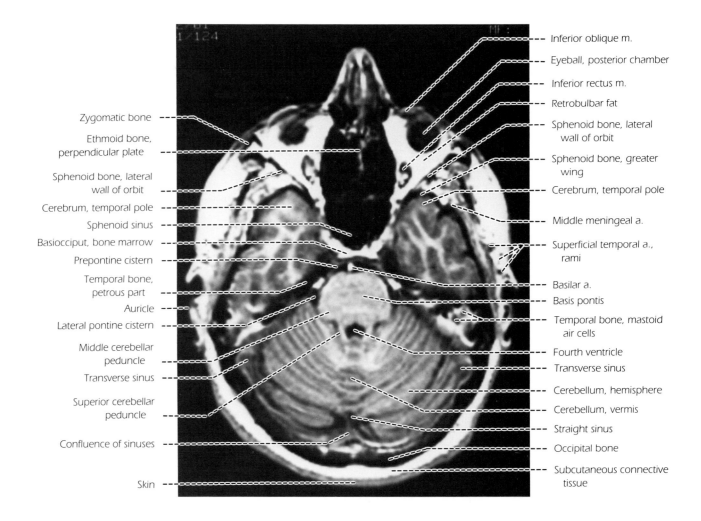

Axial T1-weighted image through the temporal pole, pons, and cerebellum. Ventral to the pons is the basilar artery. The middle and superior cerebellar peduncles are seen dorsolaterally in the pons. The fourth ventricle overlies the pons. Dorsal to the pons and the fourth ventricle is the cerebellum. The straight and transverse venous sinuses are identified. The sphenoid air sinus is in close proximity to the basiocciput.

## Figure 1-38

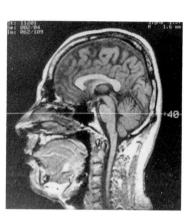

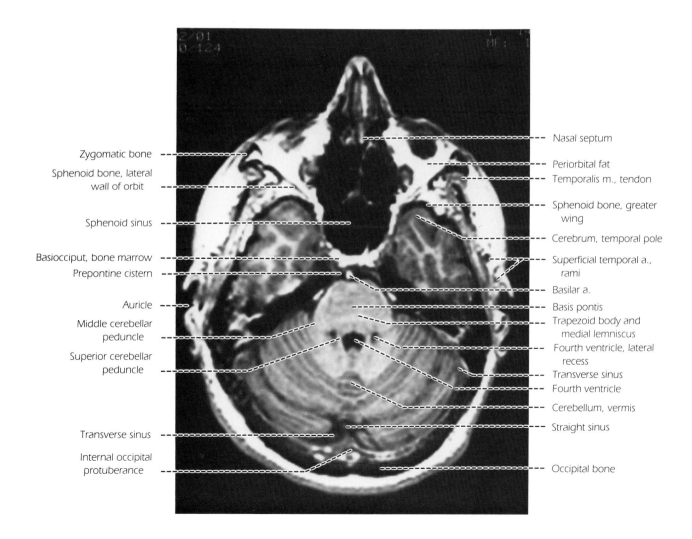

Zygomatic bone

Sphenoid bone, lateral wall of orbit

Sphenoid sinus

Basiocciput, bone marrow

Prepontine cistern

Auricle

Middle cerebellar peduncle

Superior cerebellar peduncle

Transverse sinus

Internal occipital protuberance

Nasal septum

Periorbital fat

Temporalis m., tendon

Sphenoid bone, greater wing

Cerebrum, temporal pole

Superficial temporal a., rami

Basilar a.

Basis pontis

Trapezoid body and medial lemniscus

Fourth ventricle, lateral recess

Transverse sinus

Fourth ventricle

Cerebellum, vermis

Straight sinus

Occipital bone

# Figure 1-39

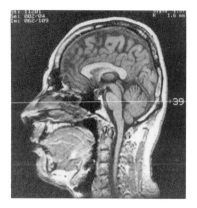

Axial T1-weighted image through the temporal pole, pons, and cerebellum. The basilar artery is ventral to the pons. The basis pontis occupies the ventral part of the pons. The middle cerebellar peduncle joins the basis pontis and cerebellum. The fourth ventricle is located dorsal to the pons. Dorsal to the fourth ventricle is the cerebellum. Farther rostrally, the nasal septum is seen in the midline, and the ethmoid sinuses are located on each side of the nasal septum. More caudally, the mastoid air cells are seen. Exiting from the midpons is the trigeminal nerve.

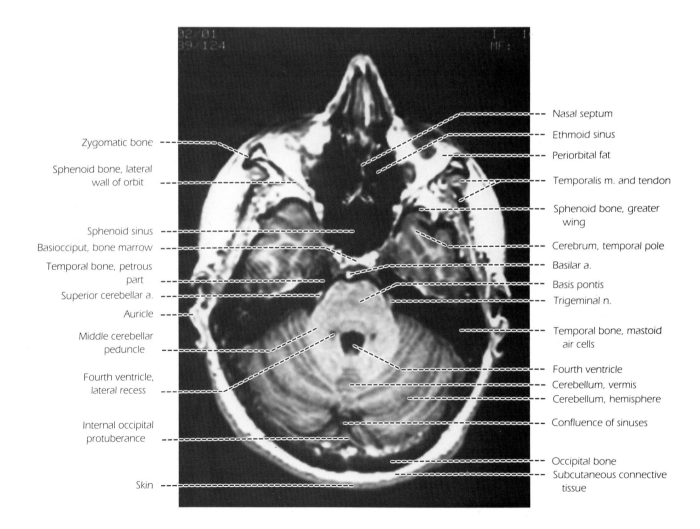

Axial T1-weighted image through the temporal pole, pons, and cerebellum. The basilar artery occupies a cavity ventral to the pons. The basis pontis is the ventral part of the pons. Connecting the basis pontis and cerebellum is the middle cerebellar peduncle. The fourth ventricle and cerebellum are dorsal to the pons. The nasal cavity, nasal septum, and ethmoid labyrinth are seen more rostrally. The mastoid air sinuses are located caudally in the temporal bone. The sphenoid sinus is seen close to the temporal pole in the midline.

## Figure 1-40

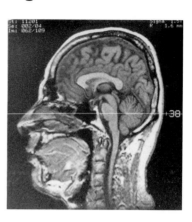

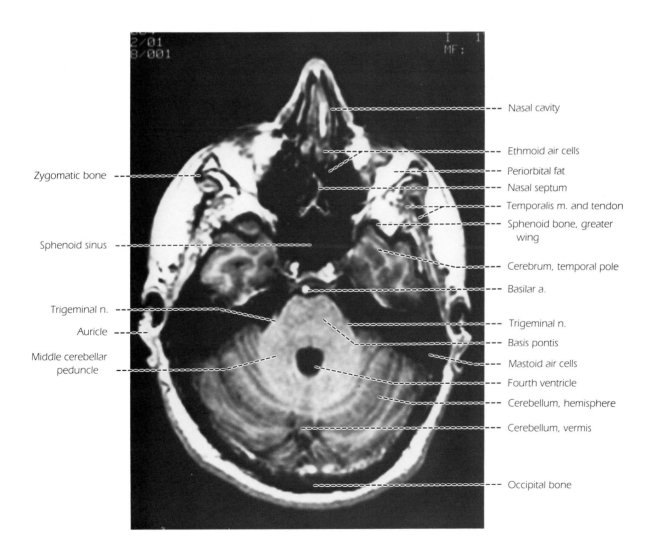

## Figure 1-41

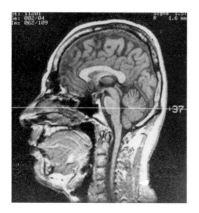

Axial T1-weighted image through the temporal pole, pons, and cerebellum. The basilar artery is ventral to the pons. The basis pontis occupies the ventral part of the pons. The middle cerebellar peduncle joins the basis pontis and cerebellum. Dorsal to the pons are the fourth ventricle and cerebellum. The internal carotid artery is medial to the temporal pole. The sphenoid sinus is also found medial to the temporal pole in the midline. The nasal septum, ethmoid sinus, and nasolacrimal duct are seen rostrally. Bony landmarks include the greater wing of the sphenoid bone, occipital bone, petrous part of the temporal bone, and zygomatic bone.

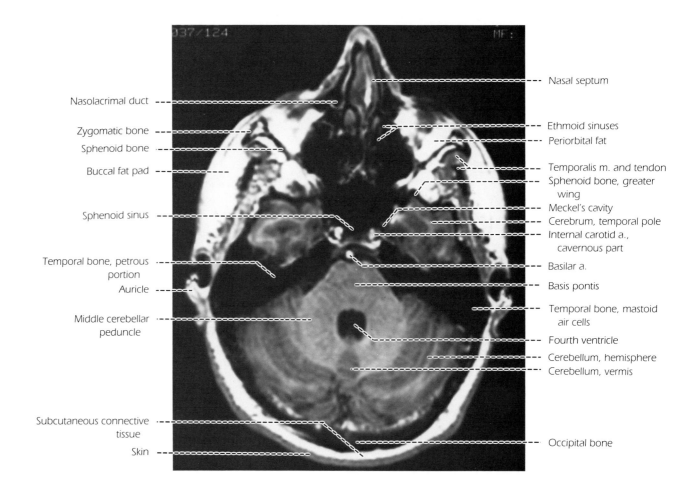

Axial T1-weighted image through the temporal pole, pons, and cerebellum. The basilar artery is a bright signal intensity ventral to the basis pontis. The middle cerebellar peduncle joins the basis pontis and cerebellum. The nodule of the vermis overlies the fourth ventricle. The internal carotid arteries are seen as bright signal intensities medial to the temporal pole. Also close to the temporal pole is Meckel's cavity, the location of the trigeminal ganglion. The nasal septum and ethmoid sinus are in the midline rostrally.

## Figure 1-42

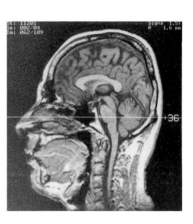

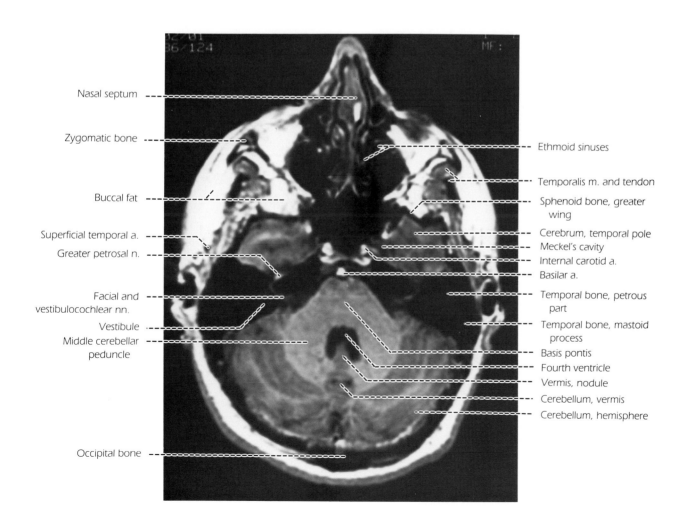

Nasal septum

Zygomatic bone

Buccal fat

Superficial temporal a.

Greater petrosal n.

Facial and vestibulocochlear nn.

Vestibule

Middle cerebellar peduncle

Occipital bone

Ethmoid sinuses

Temporalis m. and tendon

Sphenoid bone, greater wing

Cerebrum, temporal pole

Meckel's cavity

Internal carotid a.

Basilar a.

Temporal bone, petrous part

Temporal bone, mastoid process

Basis pontis

Fourth ventricle

Vermis, nodule

Cerebellum, vermis

Cerebellum, hemisphere

# Figure 1-43

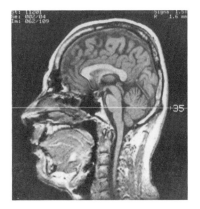

Axial T1-weighted image through the temporal pole, pons, and cerebellum. The basilar artery is ventral to the basis pontis. The middle cerebellar peduncle joins the basis pontis and cerebellum. The nodule of the vermis overlies the fourth ventricle. Meckel's cavity, site of the trigeminal ganglion, is located medial to the temporal pole. The nasal septum and nasal cavity are seen farther rostrally, in the midline. The maxillary, sphenoid, and mastoid sinuses are seen. The cochlea, vestibule, and vestibulocochlear nerve (cranial nerve VIII) are located in close proximity to each other.

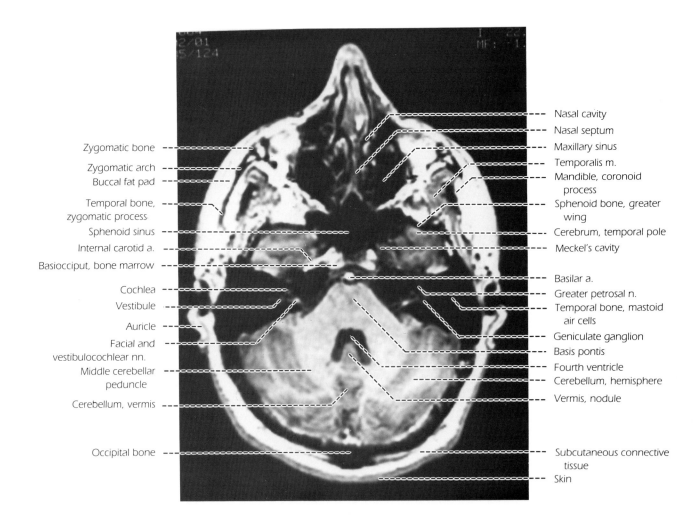

Axial T1-weighted image through the pons and cerebellum. The basilar artery is ventral to the basis pontis. The middle cerebellar peduncle joins the basis pontis and cerebellum. The nodule of the vermis overlies the fourth ventricle. The deep white matter of the cerebellum (corpus medullare) is seen. The facial and vestibulocochlear nerves (cranial nerves VII and VIII) are found exiting from the pons laterally. The nasal septum and nasal cavity are seen rostrally in the midline.

## Figure 1-44

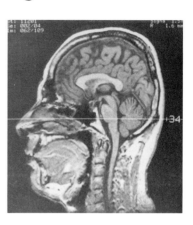

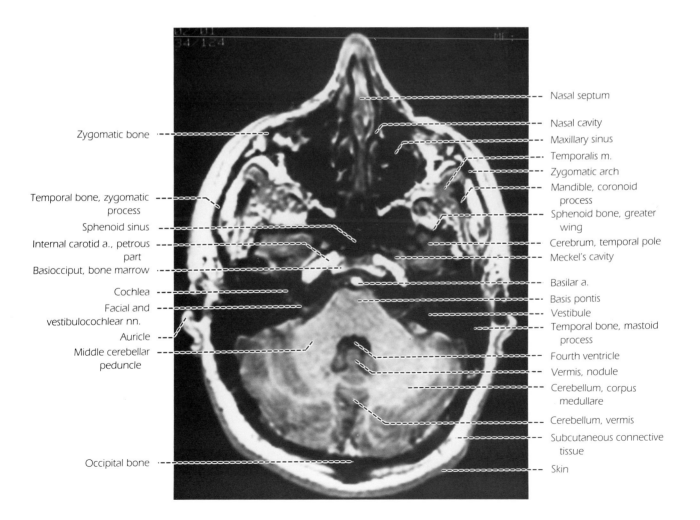

# Figure 1-45

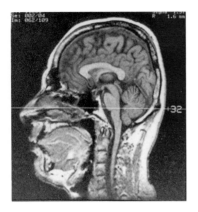

Axial T1-weighted image through the pons and cerebellum. The basis pontis occupies the ventral portion of the pons. The cerebellar tonsils, inferior cerebellar vermis, and cerebellar hemispheres are seen dorsal to the pons. The vertebral artery is ventral and lateral to the pons. The internal carotid artery is a bright signal intensity on each side of the basiocciput. The nasal septum and adjacent nasal cavity are seen rostrally.

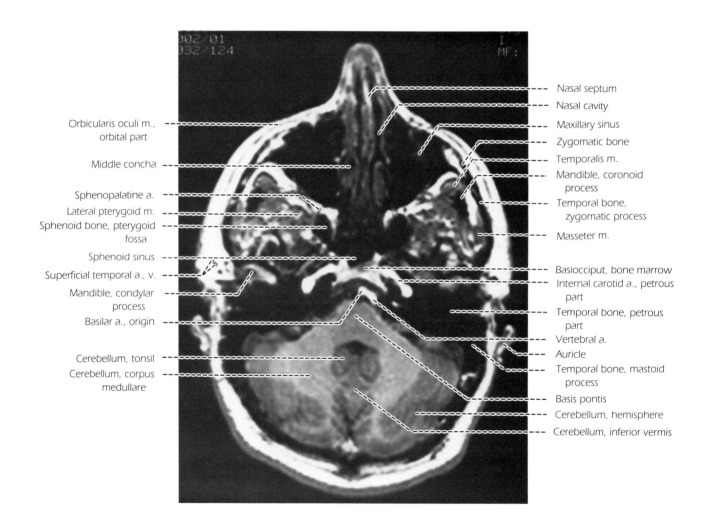

Orbicularis oculi m., orbital part

Middle concha

Sphenopalatine a.

Lateral pterygoid m.

Sphenoid bone, pterygoid fossa

Sphenoid sinus

Superficial temporal a., v.

Mandible, condylar process

Basilar a., origin

Cerebellum, tonsil

Cerebellum, corpus medullare

Nasal septum

Nasal cavity

Maxillary sinus

Zygomatic bone

Temporalis m.

Mandible, coronoid process

Temporal bone, zygomatic process

Masseter m.

Basiocciput, bone marrow

Internal carotid a., petrous part

Temporal bone, petrous part

Vertebral a.

Auricle

Temporal bone, mastoid process

Basis pontis

Cerebellum, hemisphere

Cerebellum, inferior vermis

Axial T1-weighted image through the medulla oblongata and cerebellum. Bright signal intensities of the vertebral arteries are seen ventral and lateral to the medulla oblongata. The medullary pyramids occupy a ventral position within the medulla oblongata. Exiting from the medulla dorsolaterally are the glossopharyngeal, vagus, and accessory nerves (cranial nerves IX, X, and XI). Bulging into the fourth ventricle are the cerebellar tonsils. Dorsal to the fourth ventricle is the cerebellar vermis. The cerebellar hemispheres are located laterally within the cerebellum. The deep white matter core of the cerebellum (corpus medullare) is found on each side of the fourth ventricle. Several muscles are seen in this section including the temporalis, masseter, and lateral pterygoid. Bony landmarks include the condylar head of the mandible, occipital bone, basiocciput, and coronoid process of the mandible.

## Figure 1-46

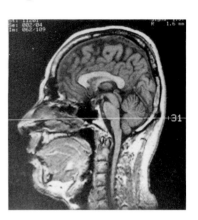

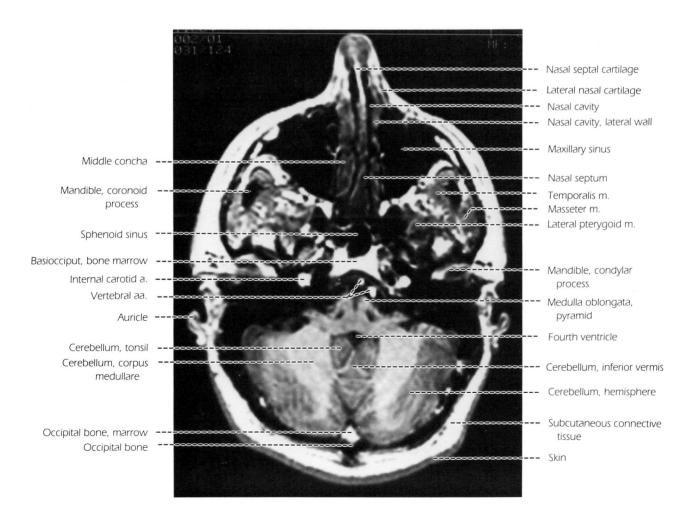

## Figure 1-47

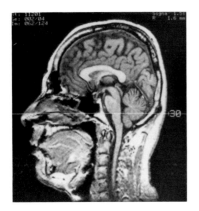

Axial T1-weighted image through the medulla oblongata and cerebellum. Ventral and lateral to the medulla oblongata are the vertebral arteries. Ventral within the medulla are the medullary pyramids. Dorsolateral in the medulla is the restiform body (inferior cerebellar peduncle). Exiting from the dorsolateral part of the medulla are the glosso-pharyngeal, vagus, and accessory nerves (cranial nerves IX, X, and XI). The fourth ventricle is located dorsal to the medulla oblongata. The cerebellar tonsils are located medially within the cerebellum. The inferior cerebellar vermis and corpus medullare of the cerebellum are also seen. The temporalis, masseter, and lateral pterygoid muscles are identified. Several bony landmarks are present including the zygomatic bone, condylar head of the mandible, coronoid process of the mandible, petrous part of the temporal bone, and basiocciput.

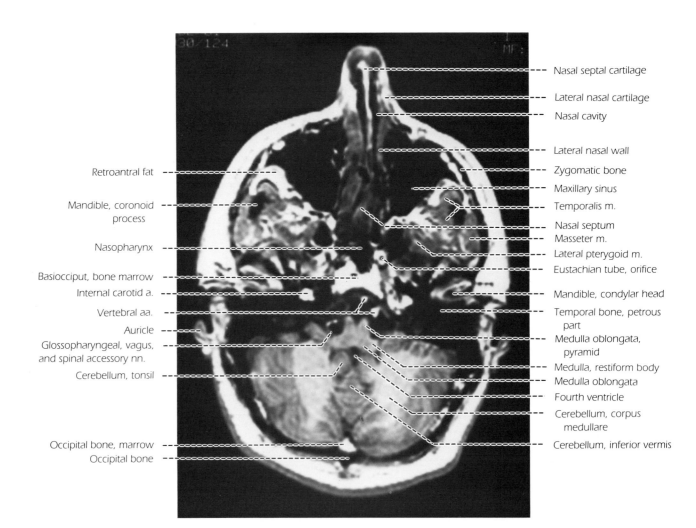

Axial T1-weighted image through the base of the skull showing the basiocciput, medulla oblongata, and cerebellum. The vertebral arteries are seen ventral and lateral to the medulla oblongata. Dorsolateral within the medulla oblongata are the restiform bodies. The medullary pyramids occupy a ventral position in the medulla oblongata. The fourth ventricle is located dorsal to the medulla oblongata. The cerebellar tonsils are found in the medial aspect of the cerebellum. The inferior vermis and corpus medullare are also seen within the cerebellum. The internal carotid artery is seen as a bright signal intensity lateral to the basiocciput. Bony landmarks include the zygomatic bone, condylar and coronoid processes of the mandible, occipital bone, and basiocciput. Skeletal muscles include the temporalis, masseter, and lateral pterygoid. The nasal septum, septal nasal cartilage, and lateral nasal cartilage are seen more rostrally.

## Figure 1-48

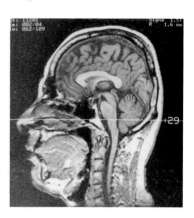

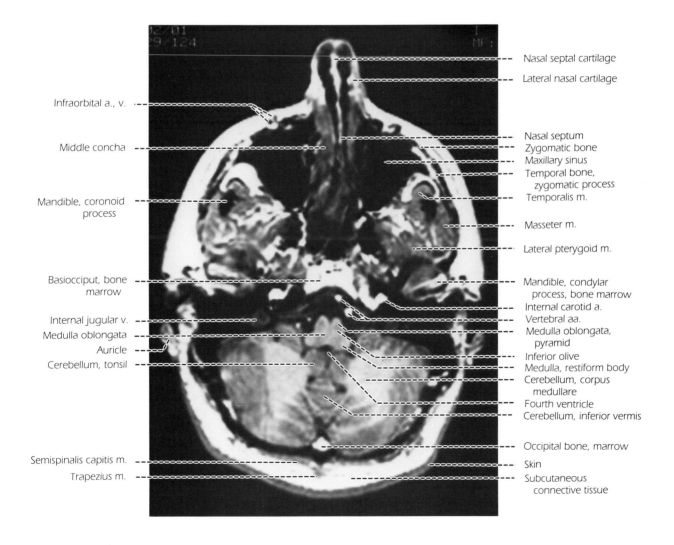

Nasal septal cartilage

Lateral nasal cartilage

Infraorbital a., v.

Middle concha

Mandible, coronoid process

Basiocciput, bone marrow

Internal jugular v.
Medulla oblongata
Auricle
Cerebellum, tonsil

Semispinalis capitis m.
Trapezius m.

Nasal septum
Zygomatic bone
Maxillary sinus
Temporal bone, zygomatic process
Temporalis m.

Masseter m.

Lateral pterygoid m.

Mandible, condylar process, bone marrow
Internal carotid a.
Vertebral aa.
Medulla oblongata, pyramid
Inferior olive
Medulla, restiform body
Cerebellum, corpus medullare
Fourth ventricle
Cerebellum, inferior vermis

Occipital bone, marrow

Skin

Subcutaneous connective tissue

# Figure 1-49

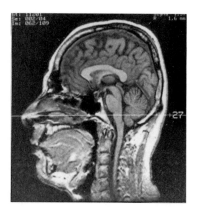

Axial T1-weighted image through the base of the skull at the level of the medulla oblongata and cerebellum. The medullary pyramids occupy a ventral position within the medulla oblongata. The fourth ventricle is located between the medulla oblongata and cerebellum. The cerebellar tonsils are medially located within the cerebellum. The inferior cerebellar vermis is in the midline, and the cerebellar hemispheres are laterally located. Vertebral arteries are seen ventrolateral to the medulla oblongata. The internal carotid arteries are identified lateral to the basiocciput, the facial artery is found anteriorly within the subcutaneous connective tissue, and the occipital arteries are located in the occipital subcutaneous connective tissue. The septal nasal cartilage and lateral nasal cartilage are seen rostrally. The temporalis, masseter, and lateral pterygoid muscles are identified. Bony landmarks include the condylar and coronoid processes of the mandible, mastoid process, occipital bone, and basiocciput.

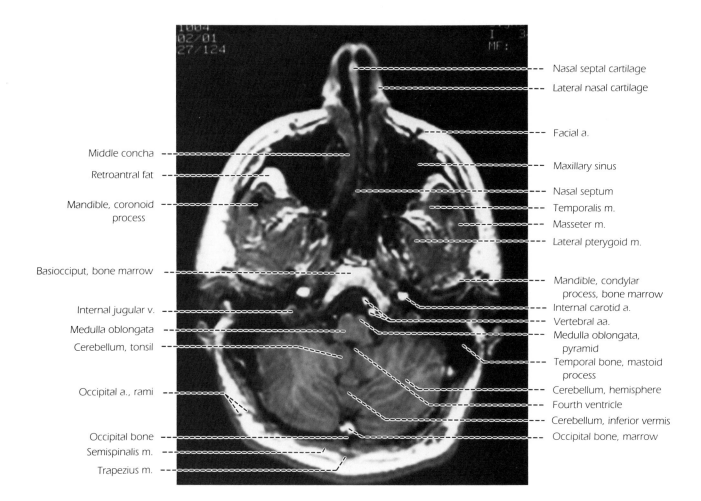

Axial T1-weighted image through the base of the skull showing the medulla oblongata and cerebellum. The vertebral arteries are ventral and lateral to the medulla oblongata. The internal carotid artery is located lateral to the basiocciput. The septal cartilage, lateral nasal cartilage, and nasal septum are seen in the midline and lateral part of the nose anteriorly. The facial artery is found in the subcutaneous connective tissue rostrally. The posterior inferior cerebellar artery is ventrolateral to the medulla oblongata. The nasopharynx is close to the vomer and choana. The posterior inferior cerebellar artery is seen arising from the vertebral artery. Muscles in this section include the medial and lateral pterygoid.

## Figure 1-50

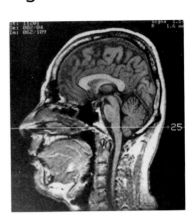

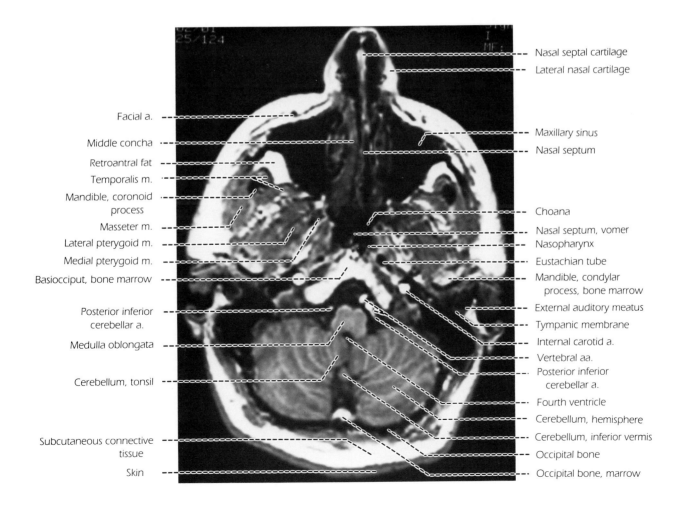

## Figure 1-51

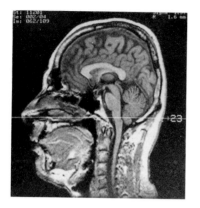

Axial T1-weighted image through the base of the skull. The vertebral arteries are ventral and lateral to the medulla oblongata. Dorsal to the medulla oblongata are the fourth ventricle and cerebellum. The mastoid process is lateral to the cerebellum. The internal carotid arteries are lateral to the basiocciput. The internal jugular vein is close to the internal carotid artery. The facial artery is seen in the subcutaneous connective tissue anteriorly. The inferior and middle conchae are located within the nasal cavity. The maxillary air sinus is lateral to the nasal cavity. Muscles identified in this section include the masseter, lateral and medial pterygoids, tensor veli palatini, semispinalis capitis, trapezius, and temporalis.

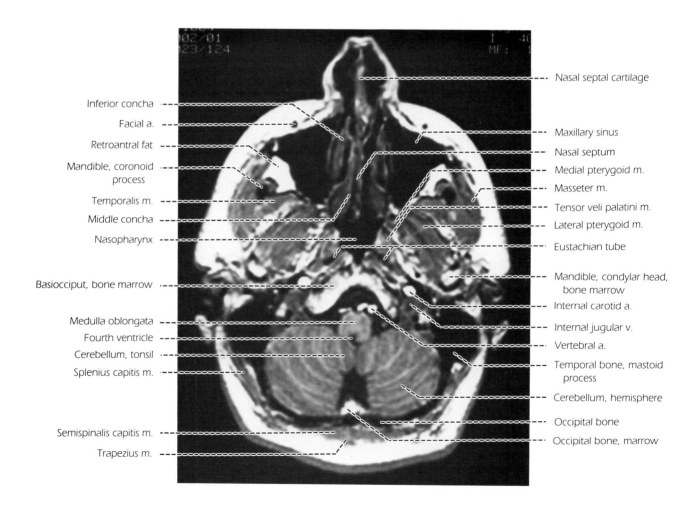

Axial T1-weighted image through the base of the skull showing the medulla oblongata and cerebellum. The vertebral arteries are ventral and lateral to the medulla oblongata. The fourth ventricle and cerebellum are dorsal to the medulla oblongata. The internal carotid artery and internal jugular vein are in close proximity lateral to the basiocciput. The nasopharynx and lateral pharyngeal recess (Rosenmüller's fossa) are seen. Muscles found in this section include the masseter, temporalis, medial and lateral pterygoids, longus capitis, trapezius, semispinalis capitis, and splenius capitis.

## Figure 1-52

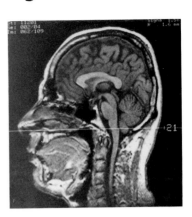

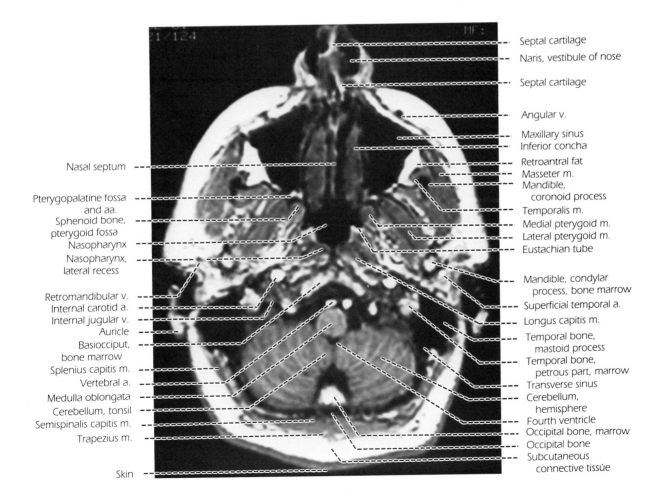

## Figure 1-53

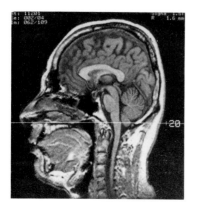

Axial T1-weighted image through the base of the skull. Nasal structures seen in this section include the septal nasal cartilage, lateral nasal cartilage, nares, inferior conchae, and nasal septum. The maxillary sinuses are on each side of the nasal cavity. The nasopharynx and lateral recess (Rosenmüller's fossa) are seen caudal to the nasal cavity. The vertebral arteries are ventral to the medulla oblongata. The cerebellum is dorsal and lateral to the medulla oblongata. Muscles seen in this section include the temporalis, masseter, medial and lateral pterygoids, trapezius, semispinalis capitis, and longus capitis. Bony landmarks in this section include the condylar and coronoid processes of the mandible, mastoid process, occipital bone, and sphenoid bone.

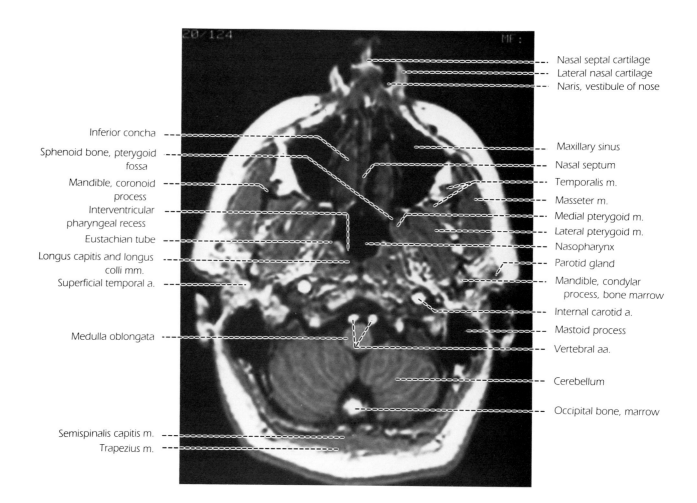

Axial T1-weighted image through the base of the skull. Neural structures seen in this section include the medulla oblongata and cerebellum. Ventral to the medulla oblongata are the two vertebral arteries. The internal carotid artery is seen as a bright signal intensity. Muscles identified in this section include the temporalis, masseter, medial and lateral pterygoids, semispinalis capitis, splenius capitis, and longus capitis. The nasopharynx occupies the midline caudal to the nasal septum. The maxillary sinuses are lateral to nasal structures. Bony landmarks include the mandible, condylar process of the mandible, occipital bone, and mastoid process.

## Figure 1-54

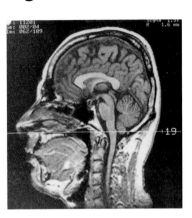

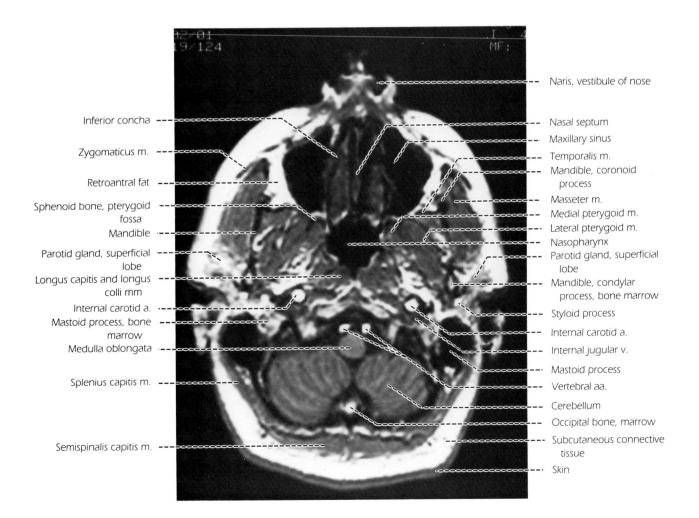

Inferior concha

Zygomaticus m.

Retroantral fat

Sphenoid bone, pterygoid fossa

Mandible

Parotid gland, superficial lobe

Longus capitis and longus colli mm

Internal carotid a.

Mastoid process, bone marrow

Medulla oblongata

Splenius capitis m.

Semispinalis capitis m.

Naris, vestibule of nose

Nasal septum

Maxillary sinus

Temporalis m.

Mandible, coronoid process

Masseter m.

Medial pterygoid m.

Lateral pterygoid m.

Nasopharynx

Parotid gland, superficial lobe

Mandible, condylar process, bone marrow

Styloid process

Internal carotid a.

Internal jugular v.

Mastoid process

Vertebral aa.

Cerebellum

Occipital bone, marrow

Subcutaneous connective tissue

Skin

## Figure 1-55

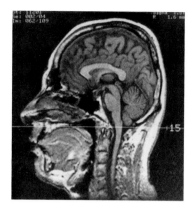

Axial T1-weighted image through the base of the skull. Neural structures seen are the medulla oblongata and inferior surface of the cerebellum. The vertebral arteries are ventral to the medulla oblongata. The internal carotid arteries are seen as bright signal intensities close to the internal jugular vein. Bony landmarks in this section include the mandible, condylar process of the mandible, styloid process of the temporal bone, mastoid process, occipital condyle, and hard palate. Muscles identified in this section include the masseter and lateral and medial pterygoids. The nasopharynx is found in the midline.

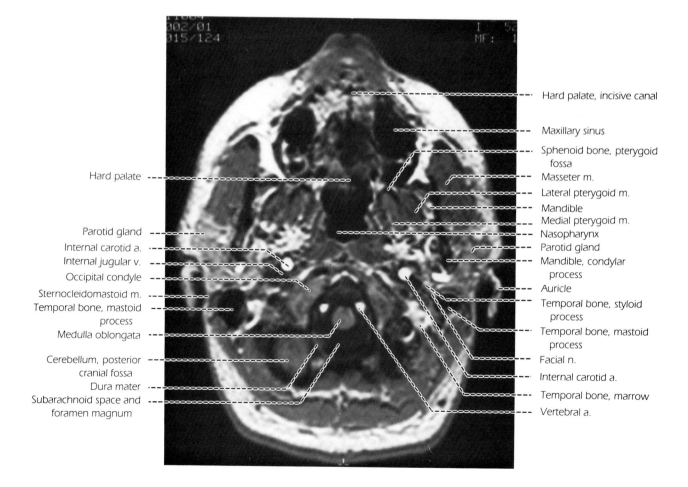

Hard palate

Parotid gland
Internal carotid a.
Internal jugular v.
Occipital condyle
Sternocleidomastoid m.
Temporal bone, mastoid process
Medulla oblongata

Cerebellum, posterior cranial fossa
Dura mater
Subarachnoid space and foramen magnum

Hard palate, incisive canal

Maxillary sinus

Sphenoid bone, pterygoid fossa

Masseter m.
Lateral pterygoid m.
Mandible
Medial pterygoid m.
Nasopharynx
Parotid gland
Mandible, condylar process
Auricle
Temporal bone, styloid process
Temporal bone, mastoid process
Facial n.
Internal carotid a.
Temporal bone, marrow
Vertebral a.

Axial T1-weighted image through the base of the skull. Neural structures seen in this section include the medulla oblongata and cerebellum. The vertebral arteries are located ventrolateral to the medulla oblongata. The internal carotid arteries are seen as bright signal intensities medial to the external carotid arteries. The nasopharynx is in the midline caudal to the hard palate. The internal jugular vein is adjacent to the internal carotid artery. Muscles identified in this section include the masseter and lateral and medial pterygoids. The parotid gland is also seen.

## Figure 1-56

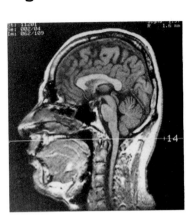

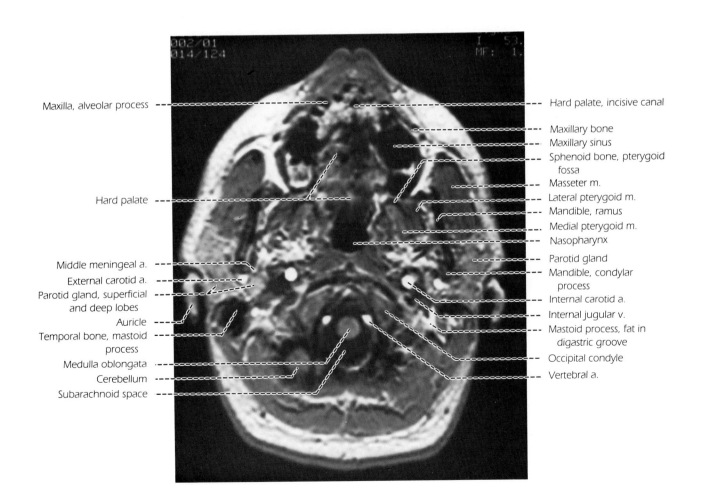

Maxilla, alveolar process

Hard palate

Middle meningeal a.
External carotid a.
Parotid gland, superficial and deep lobes
Auricle
Temporal bone, mastoid process
Medulla oblongata
Cerebellum
Subarachnoid space

Hard palate, incisive canal
Maxillary bone
Maxillary sinus
Sphenoid bone, pterygoid fossa
Masseter m.
Lateral pterygoid m.
Mandible, ramus
Medial pterygoid m.
Nasopharynx
Parotid gland
Mandible, condylar process
Internal carotid a.
Internal jugular v.
Mastoid process, fat in digastric groove
Occipital condyle
Vertebral a.

# Figure 1-57

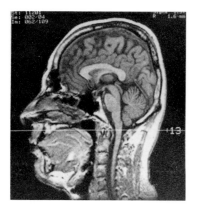

Axial T1-weighted image through the base of the skull. This section is at the junction of the spinal cord and medulla oblongata. Vertebral arteries are located on either side of these neural structures. Other structures identified in this section include the maxillary sinus, masseter muscle, medial and lateral pterygoid muscles, pterygoid process of the sphenoid bone, mandible, parotid gland, internal and external carotid arteries, internal jugular vein, occipital condyle, oropharynx, pharyngeal raphe, and hard palate.

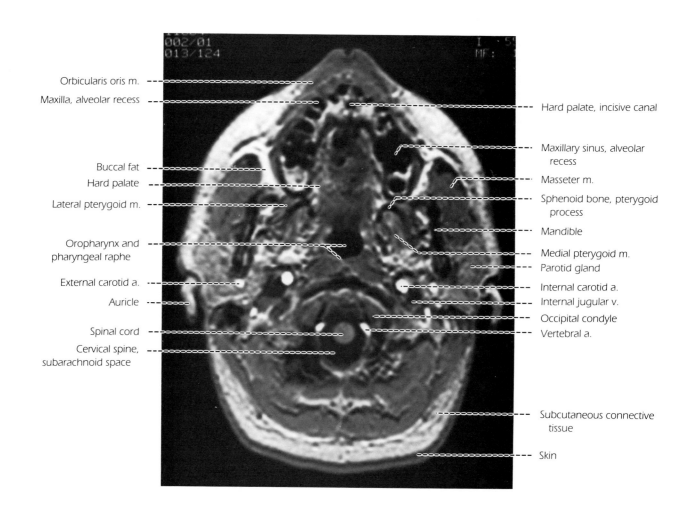

Orbicularis oris m.

Maxilla, alveolar recess

Hard palate, incisive canal

Maxillary sinus, alveolar recess

Buccal fat

Masseter m.

Hard palate

Sphenoid bone, pterygoid process

Lateral pterygoid m.

Mandible

Oropharynx and pharyngeal raphe

Medial pterygoid m.

Parotid gland

External carotid a.

Internal carotid a.

Auricle

Internal jugular v.

Occipital condyle

Spinal cord

Vertebral a.

Cervical spine, subarachnoid space

Subcutaneous connective tissue

Skin

Axial T2-weighted image showing the superior sagittal sinus cut both anteriorly and posteriorly. The falx cerebri separates the two hemispheres. The central (rolandic) sulcus separates the pre- and postcentral gyri. Caudal to the postcentral gyrus is the postcentral sulcus. The precentral sulcus is anterior to the precentral gyrus. The superior frontal sulcus is shown separating the superior and middle frontal gyri.

Figure 1-58

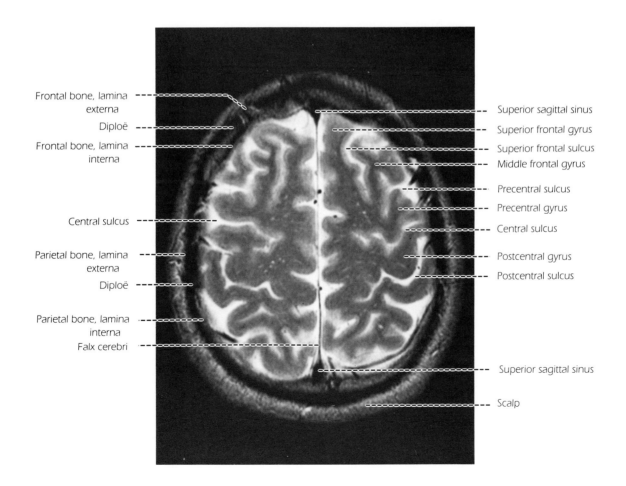

# Figure 1-59

Axial T2-weighted image through the upper part of the brain showing the falx cerebri separating the two hemispheres. The superior sagittal sinus is cut both rostrally and caudally. The centrum semiovale, the deep white matter core of the hemispheres, is shown. The central sulcus is seen separating the pre- and postcentral gyri. Rostral to the precentral gyrus is the precentral sulcus. Caudal to the postcentral gyrus is the postcentral sulcus. On the medial surface of the hemisphere is the parieto-occipital sulcus. The superior frontal sulcus separates the superior and middle frontal gyri. The dura mater and frontal bone are seen. Virchow-Robin spaces are identified.

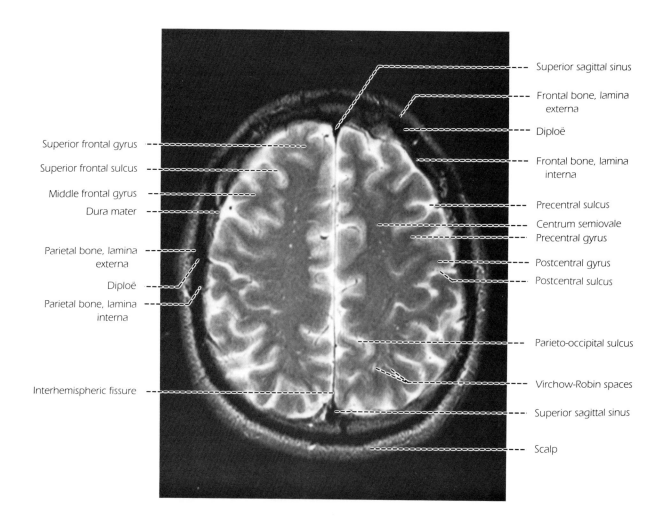

Axial T2-weighted image showing the superior sagittal sinus both rostrally and caudally. The centrum semiovale, the deep white matter core of the hemispheres, is shown. The cingulate gyrus is seen on each side of the midline. Caudal to the cingulate gyrus is the precuneus. The parieto-occipital sulcus is caudal to the precuneus. The falx cerebri separates the two hemispheres. The central sulcus separates the pre- and postcentral gyri. Rostral to the precentral gyrus is the precentral sulcus. Caudal to the postcentral gyrus is the postcentral sulcus. The superior frontal sulcus separates the superior and middle frontal gyri. Virchow-Robin spaces are shown.

# Figure 1-60

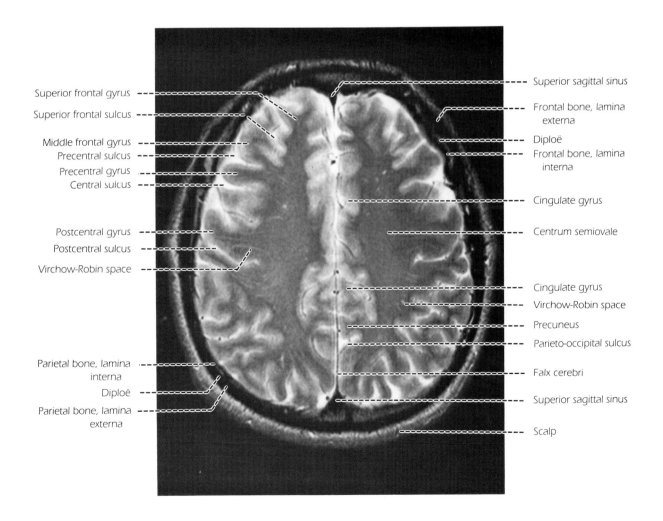

# Figure 1-61

Axial T2-weighted image through the hemisphere just above the lateral ventricles. The superior sagittal sinus is seen both rostrally and caudally. The superior surface of the lateral ventricles is seen on each side of the midline. The pericallosal branch of the anterior cerebral artery is in the interhemispheric fissure. On each side of the midline rostrally is the cingulate gyrus. Caudally, the parieto-occipital sulcus separates the precuneus and cuneus. The central sulcus separates the pre- and postcentral gyri. The precentral sulcus is rostral to the precentral gyrus, whereas the postcentral sulcus is posterior to the postcentral gyrus. The superior frontal sulcus separates the superior and middle frontal gyri. The middle meningeal artery is seen coursing in the dura lateral to the brain.

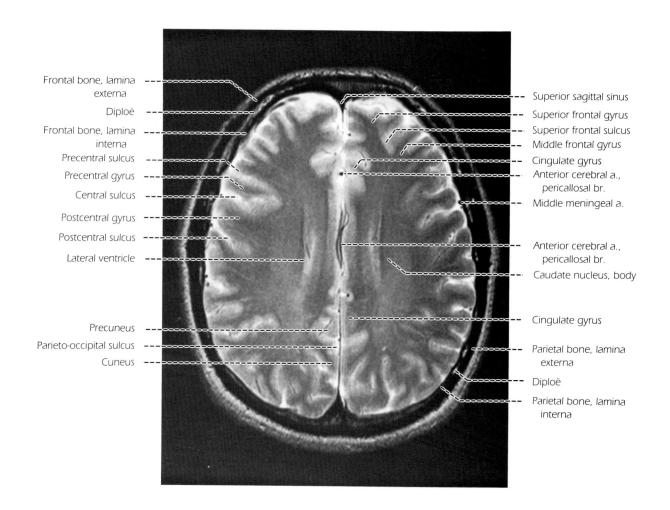

Axial T2-weighted image through the lateral ventricles. The septum pellucidum separates the two lateral ventricles. Within the lateral ventricle is the choroid plexus. The head of the caudate nucleus is in the lateral wall of the anterior horn of the lateral ventricle. The corpus callosum is seen rostral to the lateral ventricle. The forceps minor and major of the corpus callosum extend to the frontal and occipital poles, respectively. Dorsal to the corpus callosum and within the interhemispheric fissure is the pericallosal branch of the anterior cerebral artery. Also dorsal to the corpus callosum is the cingulate gyrus. The superior sagittal sinus is seen both rostrally and caudally. The parieto-occipital sulcus separates the precuneus and cuneus.

Figure 1-62

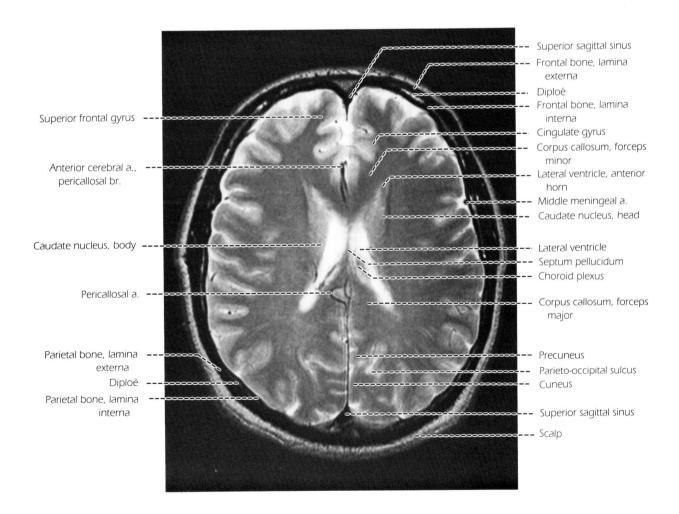

# Figure 1-63

Axial T2-weighted image at the level of the genu and splenium of the corpus callosum. Extending from the genu toward the frontal pole is the forceps minor of the corpus callosum. Extending from the splenium of the corpus callosum toward the occipital pole is the forceps major of the corpus callosum. Superior to the corpus callosum are the pericallosal and callosomarginal branches of the anterior cerebral artery. The caudate nucleus is in the lateral wall of the anterior horn of the lateral ventricle. The two anterior horns are separated by the septum pellucidum. The putamen and caudate nuclei are separated by the anterior limb of the internal capsule. The genu of the internal capsule connects the anterior and posterior limbs. The posterior limb separates the putamen and thalamus. The parieto-occipital sulcus separates the precuneus and cuneus. The external capsule is seen lateral to the putamen. Lateral to the external capsule is the insular cortex. The optic radiation is lateral to the trigone of the lateral ventricle.

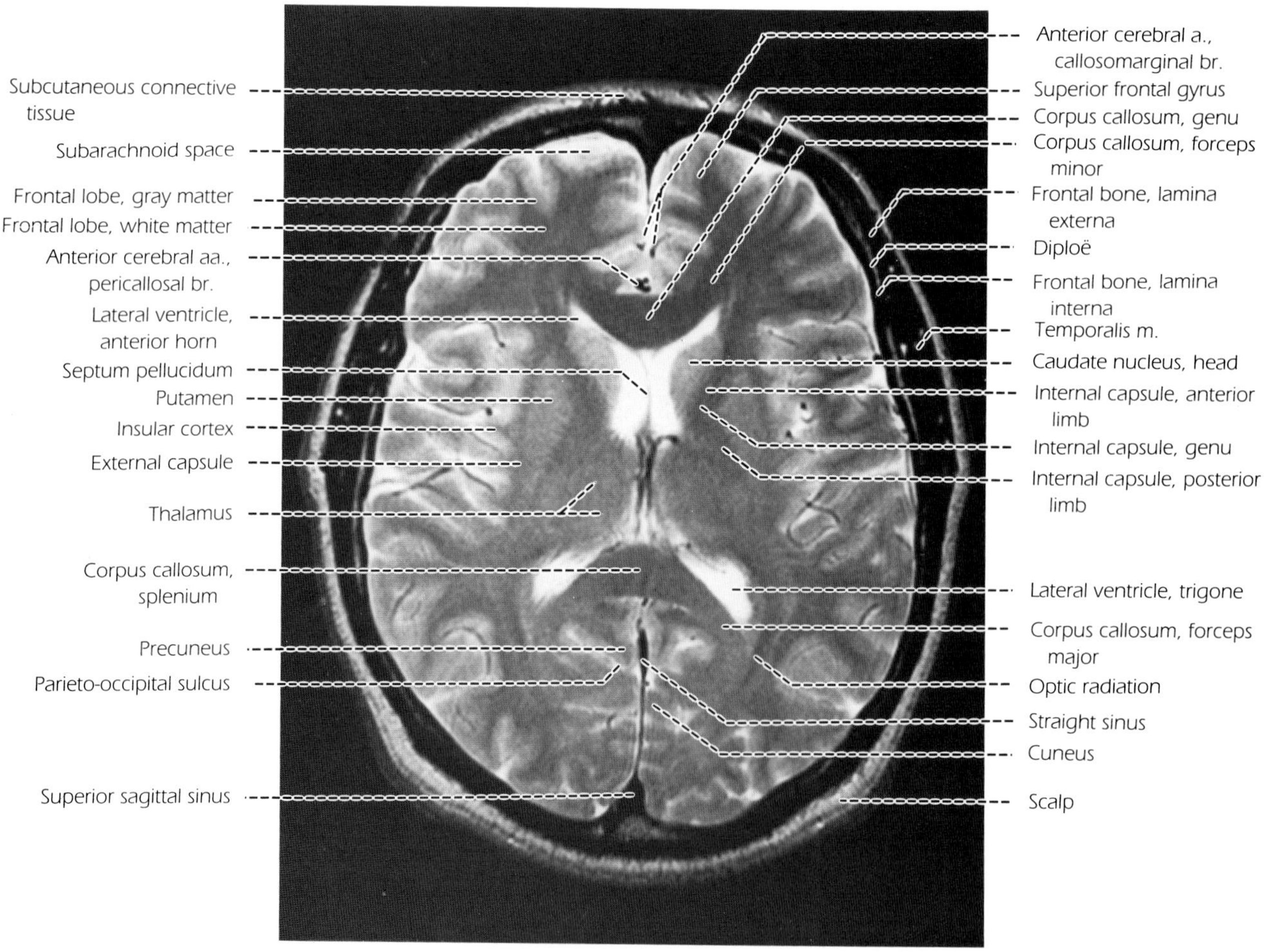
Subcutaneous connective tissue
Subarachnoid space
Frontal lobe, gray matter
Frontal lobe, white matter
Anterior cerebral aa., pericallosal br.
Lateral ventricle, anterior horn
Septum pellucidum
Putamen
Insular cortex
External capsule
Thalamus
Corpus callosum, splenium
Precuneus
Parieto-occipital sulcus
Superior sagittal sinus
Anterior cerebral a., callosomarginal br.
Superior frontal gyrus
Corpus callosum, genu
Corpus callosum, forceps minor
Frontal bone, lamina externa
Diploë
Frontal bone, lamina interna
Temporalis m.
Caudate nucleus, head
Internal capsule, anterior limb
Internal capsule, genu
Internal capsule, posterior limb
Lateral ventricle, trigone
Corpus callosum, forceps major
Optic radiation
Straight sinus
Cuneus
Scalp

Axial T2-weighted image through the thalamus. The third ventricle is in the midline separating the two thalami. Within the thalamus, the mamillothalamic tract is seen in cross section. Also seen in this section is the caudate nucleus in the lateral wall of the lateral ventricle. The anterior limb of the internal capsule separates the caudate nucleus and putamen. The posterior limb of the internal capsule separates the putamen and thalamus. The genu of the internal capsule is between the anterior and posterior limbs. The pulvinar nucleus of the thalamus is caudally located in the thalamus. The optic radiation is lateral to the trigone of the lateral ventricle. The columns of the fornix are seen just above the third ventricle. Lateral to the putamen is the external capsule. The claustrum is located between the external and extreme capsules. In the interhemispheric fissure rostrally are the pericallosal branches of the anterior cerebral artery.

Figure 1-64

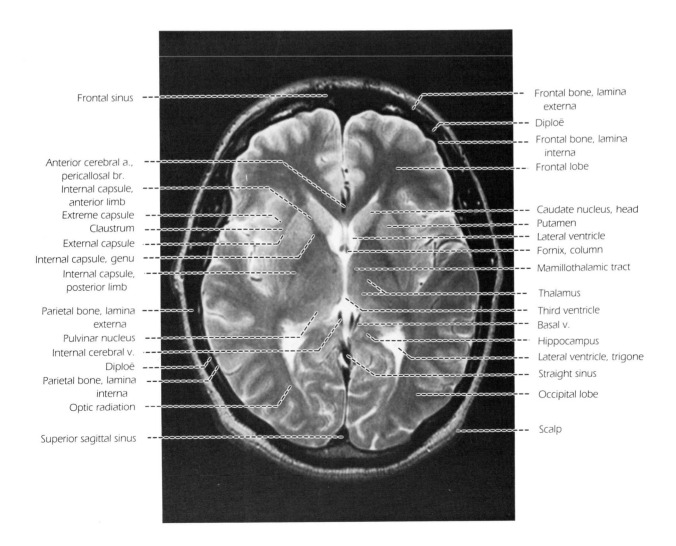

## Figure 1-65

Axial T2-weighted image through the thalamus and anterior commissure. The anterior commissure is seen coursing from the midline laterally. Inferior to the anterior commissure are the columns of the fornix cut in cross section. Beneath the fornix is the mamillothalamic tract. The third ventricle is in the midline between the two thalami. Caudal to the thalamus is the pineal cistern. Caudal to the pineal cistern is the superior cerebellar cistern. The trigone of the lateral ventricle is still seen. The superior sagittal sinus and straight sinus are seen caudally. The putamen and caudate are separated by the anterior limb of the internal capsule. In the interhemispheric fissure are pericallosal branches of the anterior cerebral artery. The hippocampus is medial to the trigone of the lateral ventricle. The frontal and temporal opercula overlie the lateral fissure.

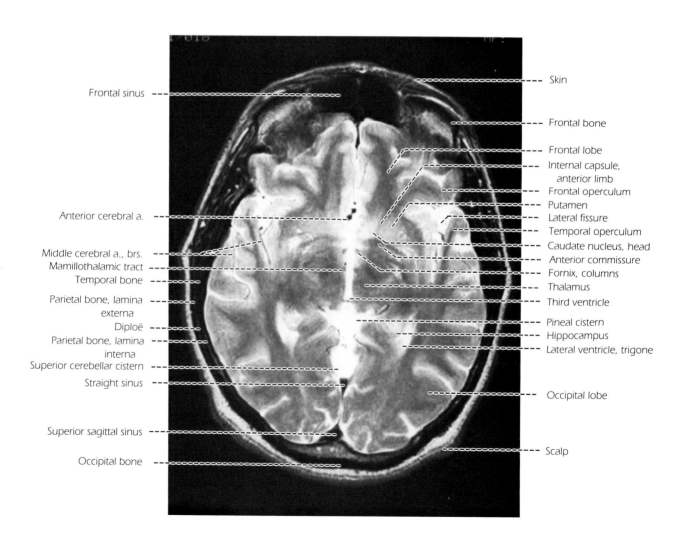

Frontal sinus

Anterior cerebral a.

Middle cerebral a., brs.
Mamillothalamic tract
Temporal bone

Parietal bone, lamina externa
Diploë
Parietal bone, lamina interna
Superior cerebellar cistern
Straight sinus

Superior sagittal sinus

Occipital bone

Skin

Frontal bone

Frontal lobe
Internal capsule, anterior limb
Frontal operculum
Putamen
Lateral fissure
Temporal operculum
Caudate nucleus, head
Anterior commissure
Fornix, columns
Thalamus
Third ventricle

Pineal cistern
Hippocampus
Lateral ventricle, trigone

Occipital lobe

Scalp

Axial T2-weighted image through the brain stem. The eyeball is seen anteriorly. The superior oblique muscle, one of the muscles of extraocular movement, is seen within the orbit. In the midline, the crista galli of the ethmoid bone is seen. The medial orbital gyrus and gyrus rectus of the frontal lobe are seen rostrally. Several vascular channels are identified including the anterior cerebral, middle cerebral, internal carotid, and posterior cerebral arteries. Two venous sinuses are seen: the superior sagittal sinus and straight sinus. In the midbrain, the crus cerebri, substantia nigra, and red nucleus are identified. The cerebral aqueduct (aqueduct of Sylvius) is within the tectum of the midbrain. Around the cerebral aqueduct is the periaqueductal gray. The superior vermis of the cerebellum is seen. Superior to the midbrain is the quadrigeminal cistern containing cerebrospinal fluid. Between the two cerebral peduncles, or crus cerebri, is the interpeduncular fossa with its cistern also containing cerebrospinal fluid.

# Figure 1-66

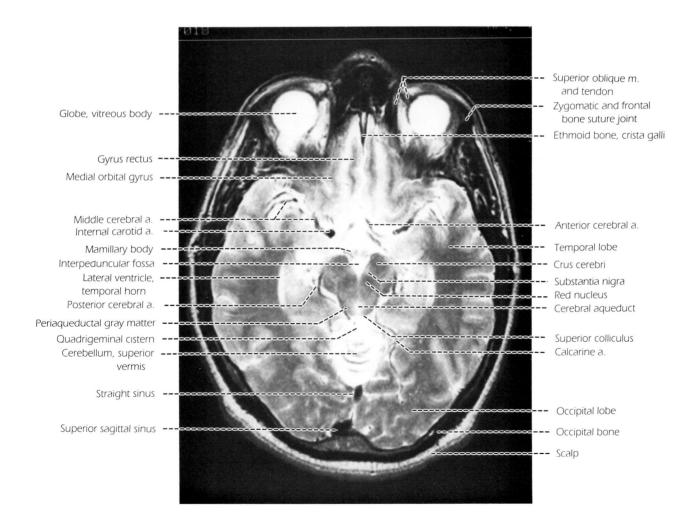

Superior oblique m. and tendon

Zygomatic and frontal bone suture joint

Ethmoid bone, crista galli

Globe, vitreous body

Gyrus rectus

Medial orbital gyrus

Middle cerebral a.
Internal carotid a.

Mamillary body
Interpeduncular fossa
Lateral ventricle, temporal horn
Posterior cerebral a.

Periaqueductal gray matter
Quadrigeminal cistern
Cerebellum, superior vermis

Straight sinus

Superior sagittal sinus

Anterior cerebral a.

Temporal lobe

Crus cerebri

Substantia nigra
Red nucleus
Cerebral aqueduct

Superior colliculus
Calcarine a.

Occipital lobe

Occipital bone

Scalp

# Figure 1-67

Axial T2-weighted image at the level of the brain stem. Rostrally, the ethmoid sinuses are found on each side of the midline. Several structures are seen within the orbit. Within the globe, the vitreous body is identified. The optic nerve is found coursing in the optic canal. Of the muscles of extraocular movement, the medial rectus muscles is identified. The suprasellar cistern is seen to good advantage. Lateral to the suprasellar cistern is the internal carotid artery. The basilar artery is ventral to the brain stem, and the posterior cerebral artery courses around the brain stem. The ambient cistern is in continuity with the quadrigeminal cistern. The cerebellar vermis and hemispheres are identified.

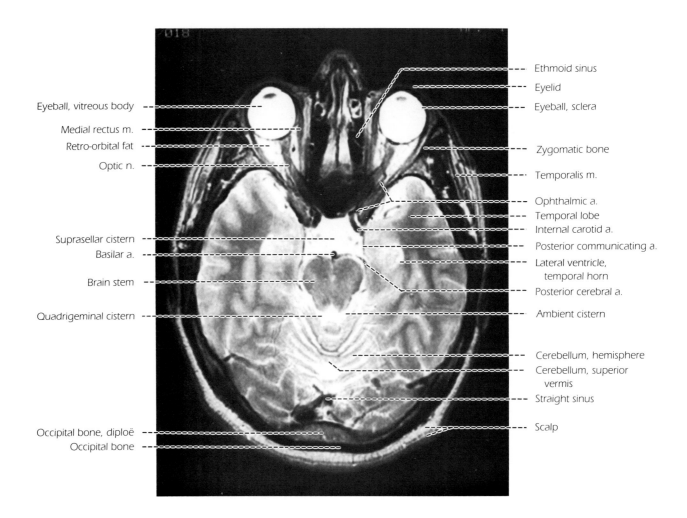

Eyeball, vitreous body

Medial rectus m.

Retro-orbital fat

Optic n.

Suprasellar cistern

Basilar a.

Brain stem

Quadrigeminal cistern

Occipital bone, diploë

Occipital bone

Ethmoid sinus

Eyelid

Eyeball, sclera

Zygomatic bone

Temporalis m.

Ophthalmic a.

Temporal lobe

Internal carotid a.

Posterior communicating a.

Lateral ventricle, temporal horn

Posterior cerebral a.

Ambient cistern

Cerebellum, hemisphere

Cerebellum, superior vermis

Straight sinus

Scalp

Axial T2-weighted image at the level of the pons. The basis pontis is in the ventral part of the pons. The basilar artery is underneath the basis pontis. The prepontine and lateral pontine cisterns are identified. The cerebellar vermis and cerebellar hemispheres are shown. Between the cerebellum and the pons is the fourth ventricle. The straight and transverse venous sinuses are seen. In the temporal lobe, the parahippocampal gyrus is identified. Within the eyeball, the anterior chamber and lens are visualized. The periorbital fat is seen to good advantage. The vitreous body is located within the eyeball. Other structures in this section include the lateral wall of the orbital cavity, greater wing of the sphenoid bone, temporalis muscle, internal carotid artery, bone marrow of the basiocciput, auricle, scalp, and occipital bone.

Figure 1-68

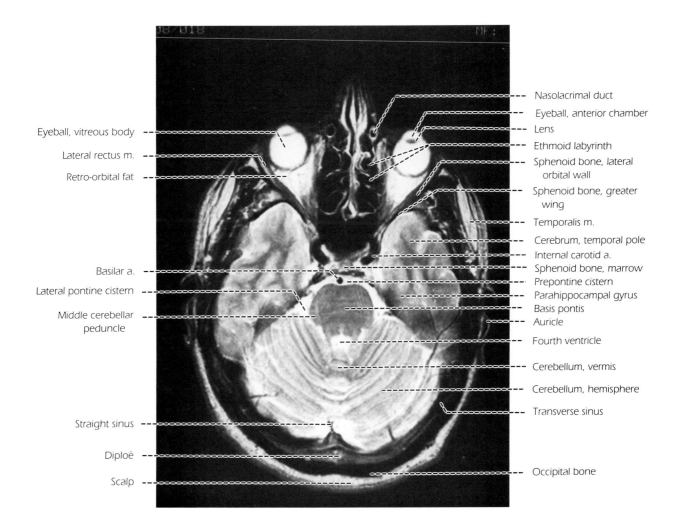

## Figure 1-69

Axial T2-weighted image through the temporal pole, brain stem, and cerebellum. The portion of the brain stem shown here is the pons. The basis pontis is identified. Ventral to the basis pontis is the basilar artery. The middle cerebellar peduncle connects the pons with the cerebellum. The fourth ventricle is between the cerebellum and pons. The nodule of the vermis is dorsal or superior to the fourth ventricle. The facial and vestibulocochlear nerves (cranial nerves VII and VIII) are seen exiting from the pons. Other structures seen in this section include the nasal septum, lateral nasal cartilage, ethmoid labyrinth, temporalis muscle, internal carotid artery, confluence of sinuses, greater wing of the sphenoid bone, zygomatic bone, and bone marrow of the sphenoid bone.

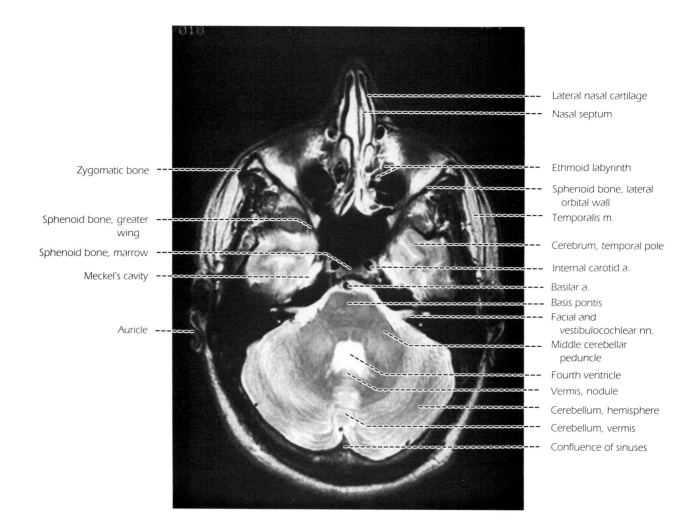

Axial T2-weighted image through the cerebellum and medulla oblongata. The vertebral arteries are seen beneath and lateral to the medulla oblongata. Within the medulla, the medullary pyramids are seen. Within the cerebellum, the cerebellar vermis and cerebellar hemispheres are identified. The fourth ventricle is located between the medulla oblongata and cerebellum. Non-neural structures found in this section include the lateral nasal cartilage, septal nasal cartilage, maxillary sinus, masseter muscle, internal carotid artery, auricle, occipital bone, petrosal part of the temporal bone, basiocciput, sphenoid sinus, middle nasal concha, and condylar process of the mandible.

Figure 1-70

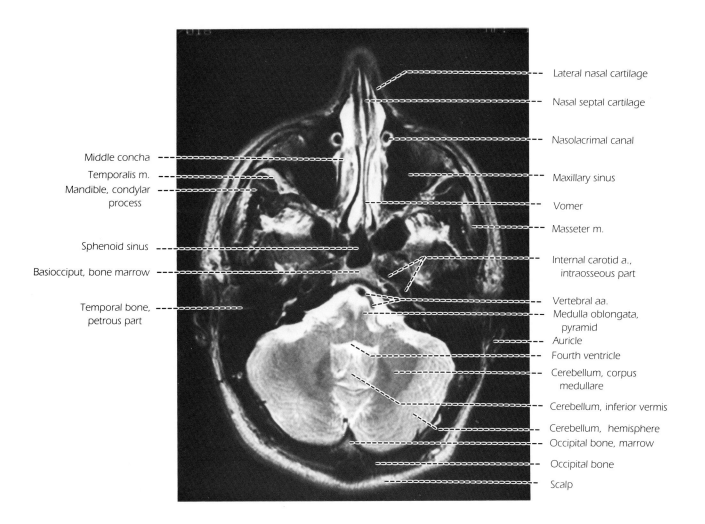

Lateral nasal cartilage

Nasal septal cartilage

Nasolacrimal canal

Middle concha

Temporalis m.

Mandible, condylar process

Maxillary sinus

Vomer

Masseter m.

Sphenoid sinus

Basiocciput, bone marrow

Internal carotid a., intraosseous part

Temporal bone, petrous part

Vertebral aa.

Medulla oblongata, pyramid

Auricle

Fourth ventricle

Cerebellum, corpus medullare

Cerebellum, inferior vermis

Cerebellum, hemisphere

Occipital bone, marrow

Occipital bone

Scalp

## Figure 1-71

Axial T2-weighted image through the medulla oblongata and cerebellum. Within the medulla oblongata the pyramids and inferior cerebellar peduncle (restiform body) are seen. The vertebral artery is inferior and lateral to the medulla oblongata. The fourth ventricle is located between the medulla oblongata and cerebellum. Within the cerebellum, the cerebellar tonsils, cerebellar hemispheres, and vermis are seen. Non-neural structures found in this section include the nasal cartilages, zygomatic process of the temporal bone, superficial temporal artery, condylar process of the mandible, internal carotid artery, mastoid process of the temporal bone, and bone marrow within the basiocciput.

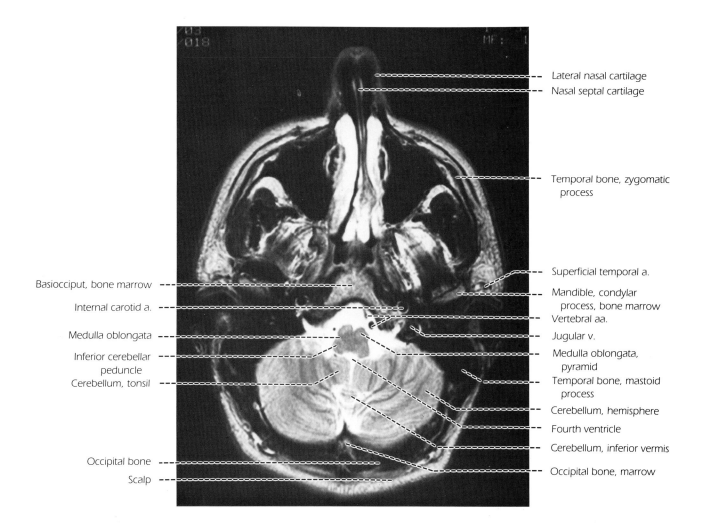

Axial T2-weighted image through the lower medulla and pons. The vertebral arteries are ventral to the medulla oblongata. The fourth ventricle is located between the medulla and cerebellum. Within the cerebellum, the cerebellar hemispheres and the tonsil are seen. Caudal to the cerebellum is the cisterna magna. Non-neural structures found in this section include the nasal septum, vomer bone, lateral fissure of the nasopharynx (Rosenmüller's fossa), parotid gland, bone marrow of the condylar process of the mandible, internal carotid artery, internal jugular vein, mastoid process, lateral and medial pterygoid muscles, masseter and temporalis muscles, and coronoid process of the mandible.

# Figure 1-72

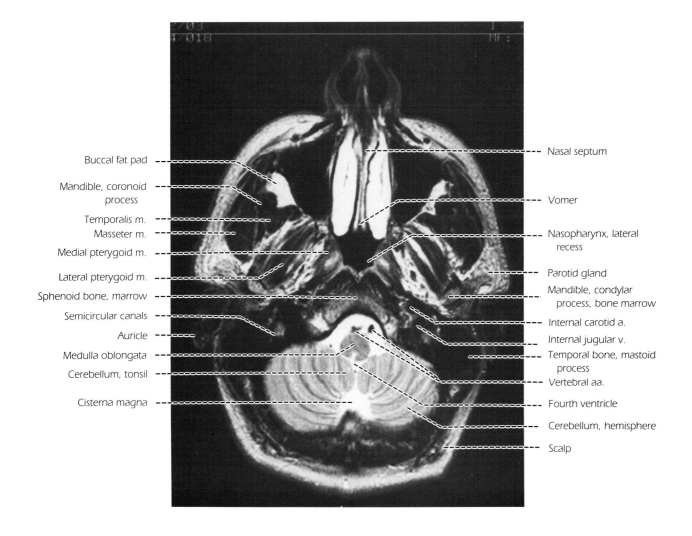

Buccal fat pad

Mandible, coronoid process

Temporalis m.
Masseter m.

Medial pterygoid m.

Lateral pterygoid m.

Sphenoid bone, marrow

Semicircular canals

Auricle

Medulla oblongata

Cerebellum, tonsil

Cisterna magna

Nasal septum

Vomer

Nasopharynx, lateral recess

Parotid gland

Mandible, condylar process, bone marrow

Internal carotid a.

Internal jugular v.

Temporal bone, mastoid process

Vertebral aa.

Fourth ventricle

Cerebellum, hemisphere

Scalp

## Figure 1-73

Axial T2-weighted image through the lower medulla. The vertebral arteries are inferior and lateral to the medulla oblongata within the subarachnoid space. The cerebellar hemispheres are seen dorsal to the medulla oblongata. Several skeletal muscles are seen in this section including the temporalis, masseter, and medial and lateral pterygoids. Other structures seen in this section include the maxillary sinus, vomer bone, inferior concha, mandible, parotid gland, condylar process of the mandible, internal carotid artery, internal jugular vein, nasopharynx, and coronoid process of the mandible.

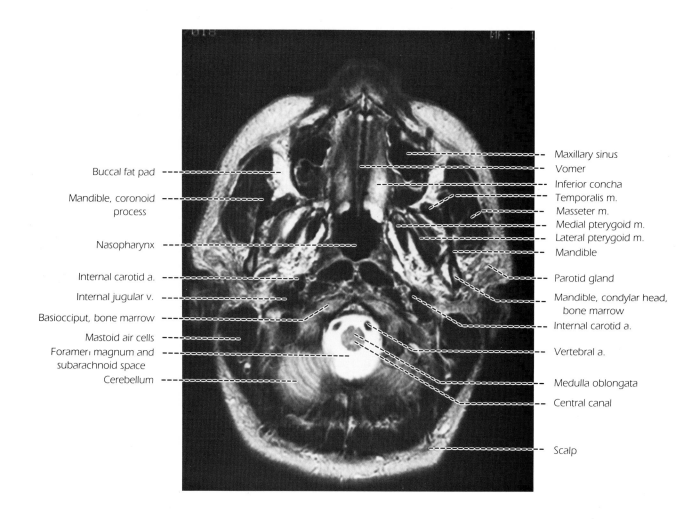

Buccal fat pad

Mandible, coronoid process

Nasopharynx

Internal carotid a.

Internal jugular v.

Basiocciput, bone marrow

Mastoid air cells

Foramen magnum and subarachnoid space

Cerebellum

Maxillary sinus

Vomer

Inferior concha

Temporalis m.

Masseter m.

Medial pterygoid m.

Lateral pterygoid m.

Mandible

Parotid gland

Mandible, condylar head, bone marrow

Internal carotid a.

Vertebral a.

Medulla oblongata

Central canal

Scalp

Axial T2-weighted image through the base of the skull and upper cervical spinal cord. The spinal cord is surrounded by subarachnoid space, containing cerebrospinal fluid. Several muscles are seen in this section including the masseter, lateral and medial pterygoids, longus capitis, rectus capitis anterior, rectus capitis lateralis, sternocleidomastoid, rectus capitis posterior major, and digastric (posterior belly) muscles. Other structures seen in this section include the hard palate, parotid gland, ligamentum nuchae, nasopharynx, mandible, and alveolar recess of the maxilla.

## Figure 1-74

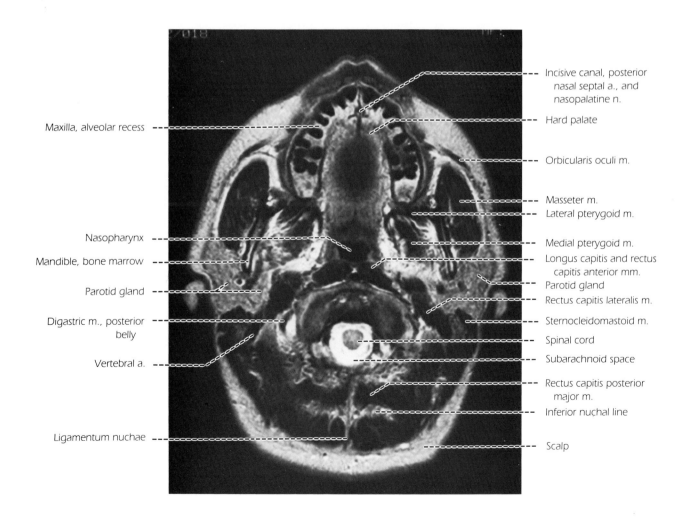

Maxilla, alveolar recess

Nasopharynx

Mandible, bone marrow

Parotid gland

Digastric m., posterior belly

Vertebral a.

Ligamentum nuchae

Incisive canal, posterior nasal septal a., and nasopalatine n.

Hard palate

Orbicularis oculi m.

Masseter m.

Lateral pterygoid m.

Medial pterygoid m.

Longus capitis and rectus capitis anterior mm.

Parotid gland

Rectus capitis lateralis m.

Sternocleidomastoid m.

Spinal cord

Subarachnoid space

Rectus capitis posterior major m.

Inferior nuchal line

Scalp

# Figure 1-75

Axial T2-weighted image through the upper spinal cord. The spinal cord is surrounded by subarachnoid space containing cerebrospinal fluid. All other structures in this section are non-neural and include the alveolar process of the maxilla, hard palate, and masseter, medial pterygoid, and sternocleidomastoid muscles. Other structures include the nasopharynx, anterior arch of the atlas, internal carotid artery, internal jugular vein, odontoid process of the axis, posterior arch of the atlas, scalp, inferior nuchal line, and parotid gland.

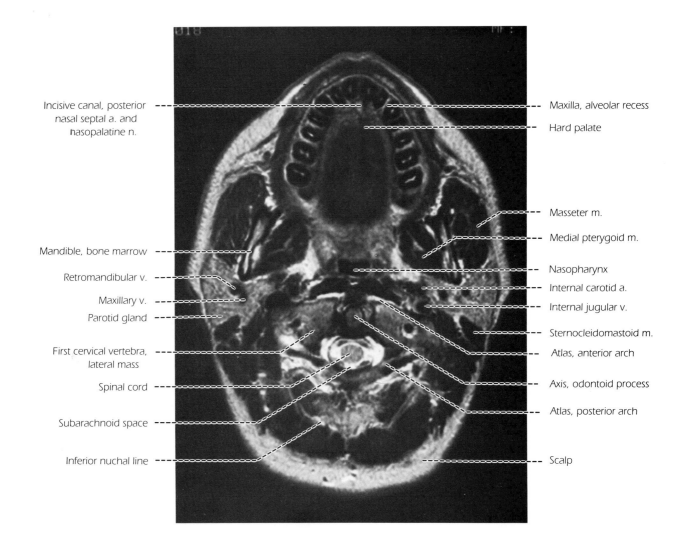

Incisive canal, posterior nasal septal a. and nasopalatine n.

Maxilla, alveolar recess

Hard palate

Masseter m.

Medial pterygoid m.

Mandible, bone marrow

Retromandibular v.

Maxillary v.

Parotid gland

First cervical vertebra, lateral mass

Spinal cord

Subarachnoid space

Inferior nuchal line

Nasopharynx

Internal carotid a.

Internal jugular v.

Sternocleidomastoid m.

Atlas, anterior arch

Axis, odontoid process

Atlas, posterior arch

Scalp

# CORONAL VIEWS

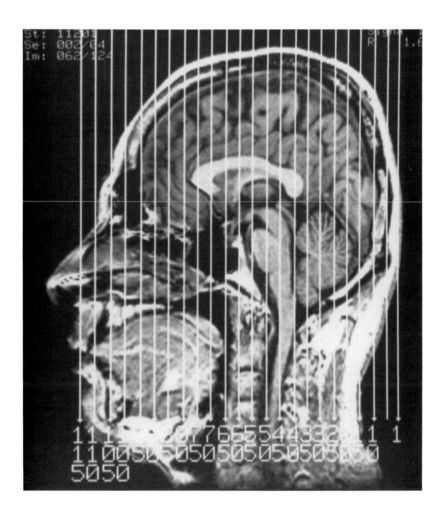

Key to the coronal planes of inspection for T1-weighted images.

## Figure 1-76

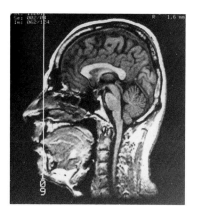

Coronal T1-weighted image through the nose showing the nasion, nasal septum, and incisive teeth.

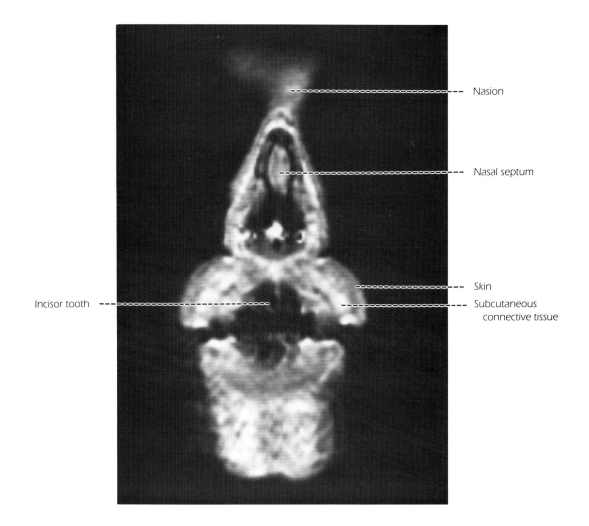

Coronal T1-weighted image through the nose and tongue. Within the nasal cavity, the nasal septum is seen in the midline. The inferior turbinate bone (concha) is located in the lateral wall of the nose. The tongue and teeth are caudal to the nose. The bone marrow is shown in the alveolar process of the maxilla.

## Figure 1-77

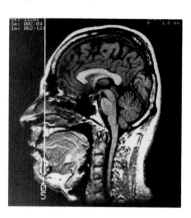

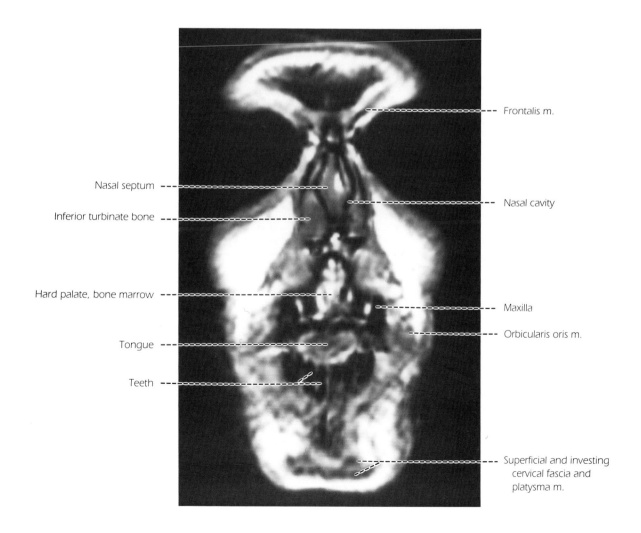

Frontalis m.

Nasal septum

Nasal cavity

Inferior turbinate bone

Hard palate, bone marrow

Maxilla

Orbicularis oris m.

Tongue

Teeth

Superficial and investing cervical fascia and platysma m.

# Figure I-78

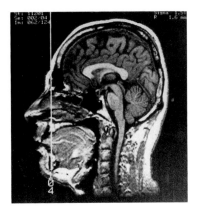

Coronal T1-weighted image through the nose and tongue. The nasal septum is in the midline of the nasal cavity. The inferior turbinate bone (concha) is in the lateral wall of the nose. The tongue, mandible, and maxilla are seen caudal to the nose.

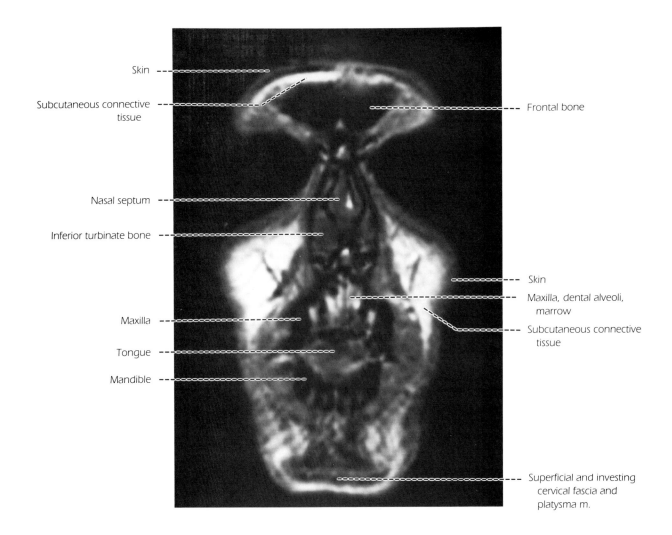

Coronal T1-weighted image through the tongue and mandible. The frontal, ethmoid, and maxillary sinuses are seen. The lens of the eyeball is shown to one side. The tongue and mandible are caudally located. The orbital plate of the frontal bone is seen anteriorly.

## Figure 1-79

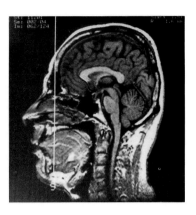

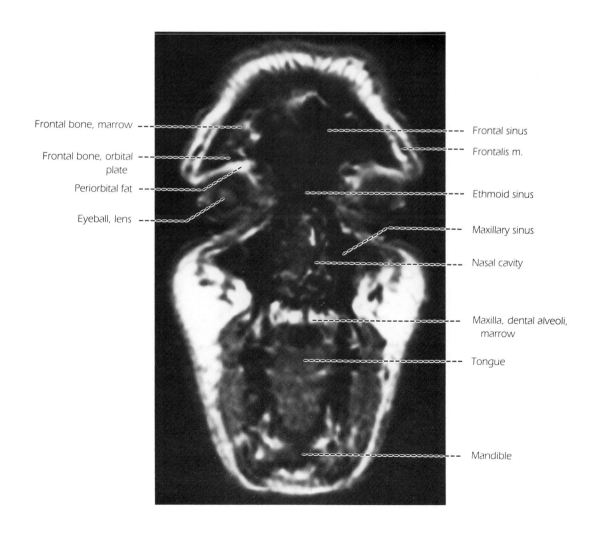

Frontal bone, marrow

Frontal bone, orbital plate

Periorbital fat

Eyeball, lens

Frontal sinus

Frontalis m.

Ethmoid sinus

Maxillary sinus

Nasal cavity

Maxilla, dental alveoli, marrow

Tongue

Mandible

# Figure 1-80

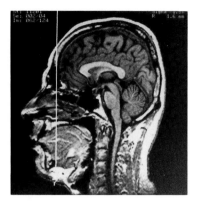

Coronal T1-weighted image through the eyeball. The superior oblique muscle and ethmoid and maxillary sinuses are seen. The nasal cavity is in the midline. The hard palate is dorsal to the tongue, and the mandible is inferior to the tongue.

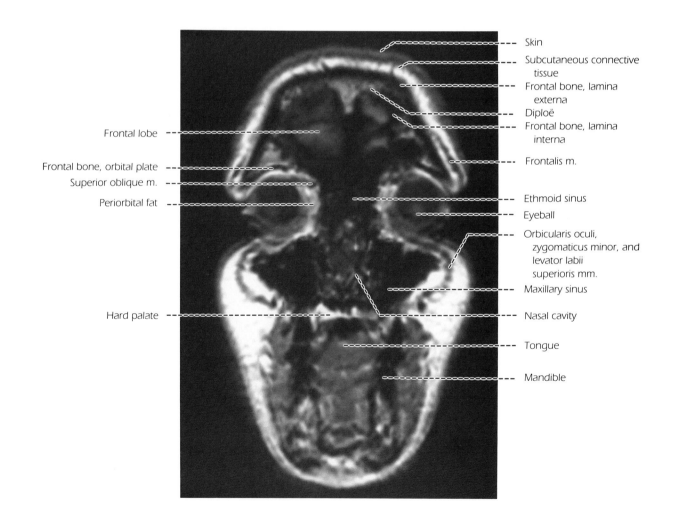

Skin

Subcutaneous connective tissue

Frontal bone, lamina externa

Diploë

Frontal bone, lamina interna

Frontal lobe

Frontalis m.

Frontal bone, orbital plate

Superior oblique m.

Ethmoid sinus

Periorbital fat

Eyeball

Orbicularis oculi, zygomaticus minor, and levator labii superioris mm.

Maxillary sinus

Hard palate

Nasal cavity

Tongue

Mandible

Coronal T1-weighted image through the frontal pole. The falx cerebri separates the two frontal poles. The eyeball is surrounded by periorbital fat. The superior oblique muscle is dorsal to the eyeball. The orbital plate of the frontal bone is superior to the orbit. The middle concha is in the wall of the nose. The maxillary sinus is seen lateral to the nose. The tongue is in the midline. The maxilla is dorsal and lateral to the tongue, whereas the mandible is ventral to the tongue.

Figure 1-81

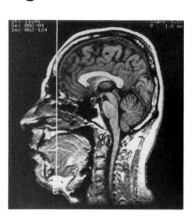

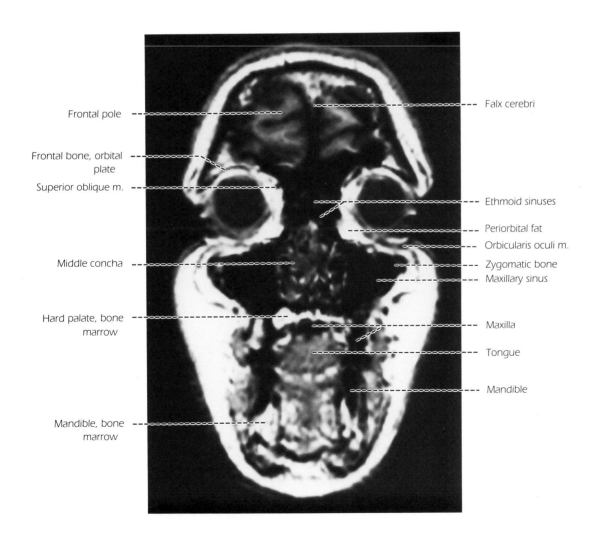

# Figure 1-82

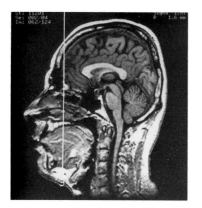

Coronal T1-weighted image through the frontal lobe. The falx cerebri separates the two frontal lobes. The dura mater caps the frontal lobe superiorly. The eyeball is seen on each side of the midline surrounded by periorbital fat. Several muscles of extraocular movement are seen including the superior oblique, medial rectus, lateral rectus, and inferior rectus. The crista galli and the cribriform plate of the ethmoid are seen in the midline. The tongue is inferior to the maxilla. Inferior and lateral to the tongue is the mandible. The sublingual gland is ventral to the tongue.

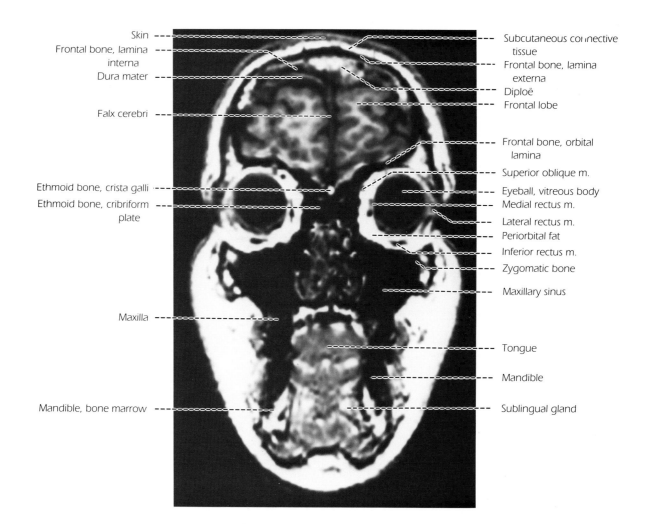

Coronal T1-weighted image through the frontal lobe. The longitudinal cerebral fissure separates the two cerebral hemispheres. The superior sagittal sinus is found between the two hemispheres dorsally. Within the frontal lobe, the superior frontal sulcus separates the superior and middle frontal gyri. On the ventral surface of the frontal lobe, the gyrus rectus is located medially, and the orbital gyri are located laterally. The ethmoid sinuses are on each side of the midline. The globe is lateral to the ethmoid sinuses, surrounded by periorbital fat. The following muscles of extraocular movement are seen: the superior rectus, medial rectus, lateral rectus, and superior oblique. The middle and inferior turbinate bones (conchae) are seen within the nasal cavity. The nasal septum is seen in the midline. The tongue is inferior to the nasal septum and dorsal to the mandible. Beneath the tongue is the sublingual gland. The orbital plate of the frontal bone separates the frontal lobe from the eyeball.

## Figure 1-83

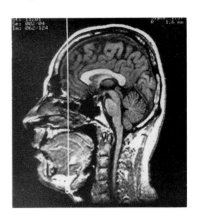

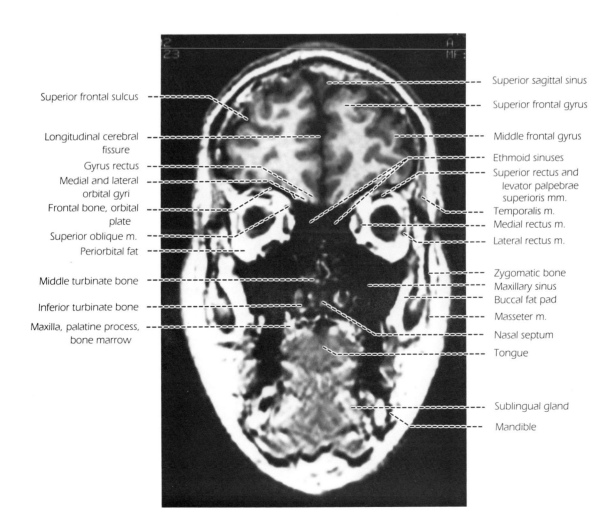

# Figure 1-84

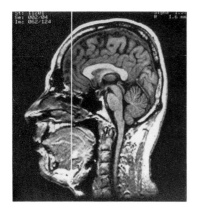

Coronal T1-weighted image through the frontal lobe. The superior sagittal sinus is seen between the two hemispheres. The superior and middle frontal gyri are separated by the superior frontal sulcus. On the ventral surface of the frontal lobe, the gyrus rectus is located medially, and the orbital gyri are located laterally. The orbital plate of the frontal bone separates the frontal lobe from the eyeball. The eyeball is surrounded by periorbital fat. Surrounding the eyeball are muscles of extraocular movement including superior rectus, medial rectus, lateral rectus, inferior rectus, and superior oblique muscles. In the midline are the nasal septum and the middle and inferior turbinate bones (conchae). The tongue is seen beneath the nose. The sublingual gland is inferior to the tongue. The ethmoid sinuses are identified.

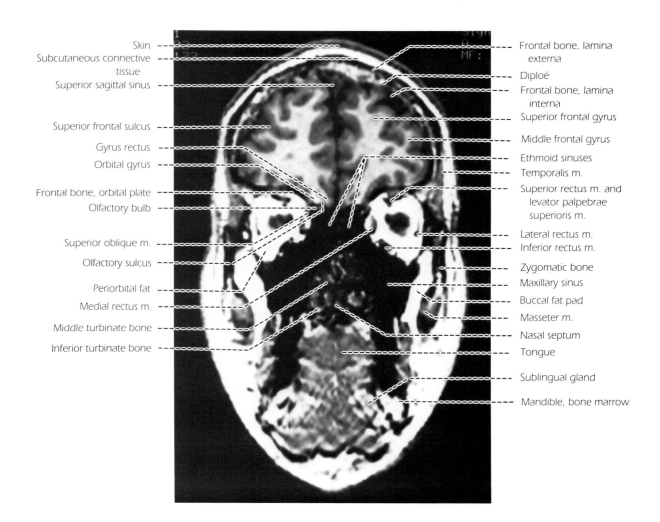

Coronal T1-weighted image through the frontal lobe. The superior, middle, and inferior frontal gyri are seen. The first two are separated by the superior frontal sulcus. Ventrally in the frontal lobe are seen the gyrus rectus and the lateral and medial orbital gyri. In the white matter core of the frontal lobe is the frontal radiation and the superior longitudinal fasciculus (long association bundle). The eyeball, surrounded by periorbital fat, is inferior to the frontal lobe. Several muscles of extraocular movement surround the eyeball, including the superior rectus, superior oblique, lateral rectus, medial rectus, and inferior rectus. In the midline below the eyeball is the nasal cavity, which contains the nasal septum as well as the middle and inferior turbinate bones (conchae). Inferior to the nasal cavity is the tongue. The sublingual gland is inferior to the tongue. The superior sagittal sinus is located dorsally between the two frontal lobes.

## Figure 1-85

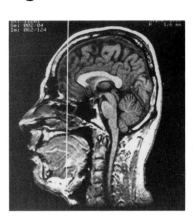

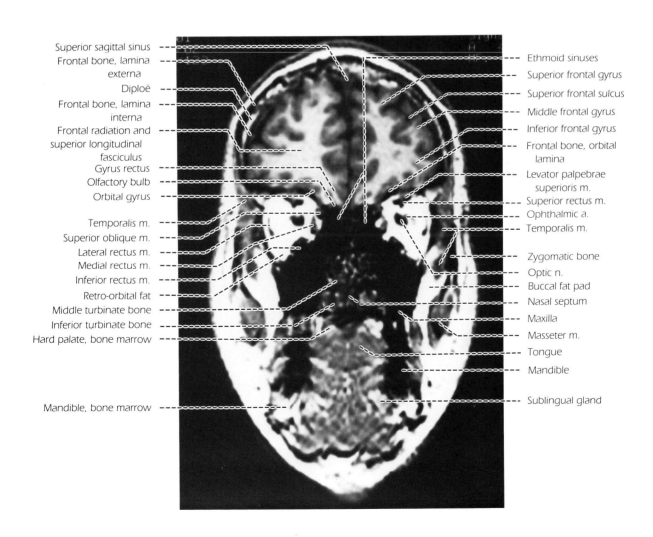

## Figure 1-86

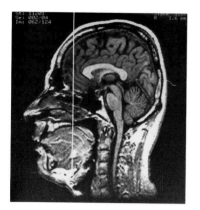

Coronal T1-weighted image through the frontal lobe. The falx cerebri separates the two hemispheres. The superior sagittal sinus is seen dorsally between the two hemispheres. Within the frontal lobe, the superior and middle frontal gyri are separated by the superior frontal sulcus. The inferior frontal sulcus separates the middle and inferior frontal gyri. On the ventral surface of the frontal lobe are the gyrus rectus and medial orbital gyrus separated by the olfactory sulcus. Inferior to the frontal lobe and separated from it by the orbital plate of the frontal bone is the eyeball, surrounded by periorbital fat. The optic nerve is in the center of the eyeball. Muscles of extraocular movement in this section include the superior rectus. medial rectus, lateral rectus, and inferior rectus. The maxillary and ethmoid sinuses are seen. In the midline is the nasal septum as well as the middle and inferior conchae. The tongue is inferior to the nasal cavity. Ventral and lateral to the tongue is the mandible.

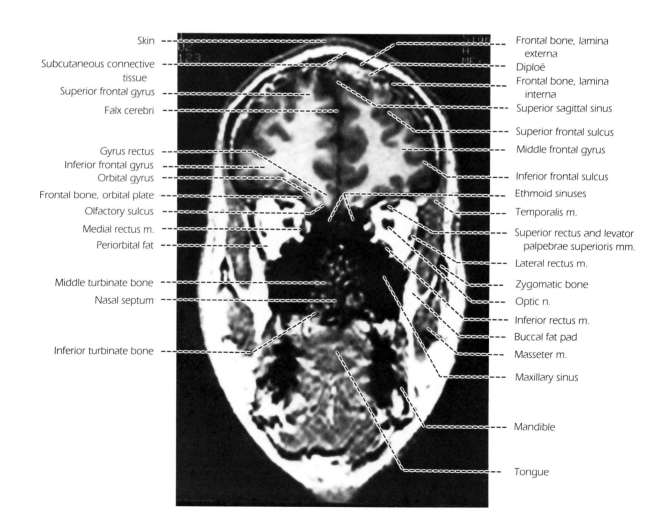

Coronal T1-weighted image through the frontal lobe. The superior frontal sulcus separates the superior and middle frontal gyri. The inferior frontal gyrus is inferior to the inferior frontal sulcus. The orbital plate of the frontal bone separates the frontal lobe from the orbit. In the ventral surface of the frontal lobe are the gyrus rectus and the medial and lateral orbital gyri. In the deep white matter core of the frontal lobe is the frontal radiation and the superior longitudinal fasciculus (long association bundle). Surrounding the eyeball is periorbital fat. The optic nerve is found in the center of the eyeball. Muscles of extraocular movement in this section include the superior rectus, lateral rectus, medial rectus, inferior rectus, and superior oblique. The ophthalmic artery is close to the optic nerve. In the midline is the nasal septum, as well as the superior, middle, and inferior turbinate bones (conchae). Ventral to the nasal cavity is the tongue. The mandible occupies a ventral and lateral position compared with that of the tongue.

## Figure 1-87

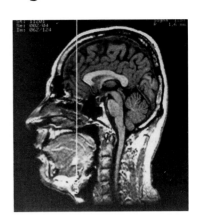

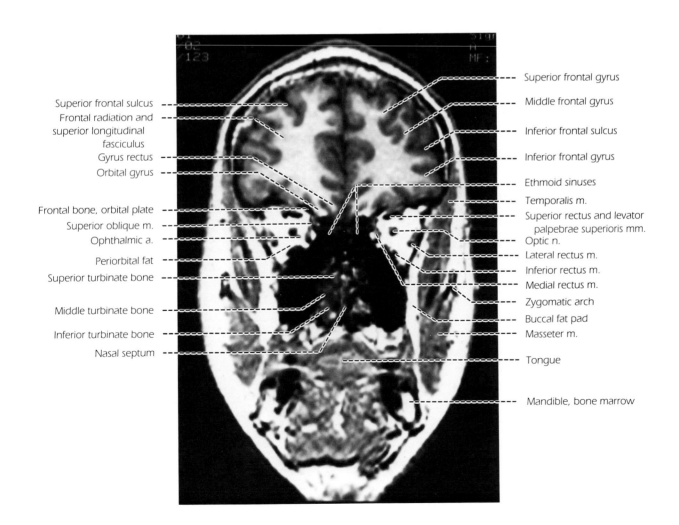

Superior frontal sulcus

Frontal radiation and superior longitudinal fasciculus

Gyrus rectus

Orbital gyrus

Frontal bone, orbital plate

Superior oblique m.

Ophthalmic a.

Periorbital fat

Superior turbinate bone

Middle turbinate bone

Inferior turbinate bone

Nasal septum

Superior frontal gyrus

Middle frontal gyrus

Inferior frontal sulcus

Inferior frontal gyrus

Ethmoid sinuses

Temporalis m.

Superior rectus and levator palpebrae superioris mm.

Optic n.

Lateral rectus m.

Inferior rectus m.

Medial rectus m.

Zygomatic arch

Buccal fat pad

Masseter m.

Tongue

Mandible, bone marrow

## Figure 1-88

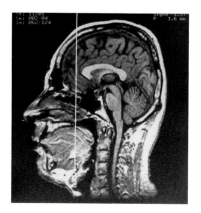

Coronal T1-weighted image through the frontal lobe. The falx cerebri separates the two frontal lobes. The superior sagittal sinus is in the falx cerebri dorsal to the frontal lobes. Within the frontal lobes, the superior frontal sulcus separates the superior and middle frontal gyri. The inferior frontal sulcus separates the middle and inferior frontal gyri. On each side of the falx cerebri is the cingulate gyrus. The cingulate sulcus is dorsal to the cingulate gyrus. In the inferior aspect of the frontal lobe are the gyrus rectus medially and the medial and lateral orbital gyri laterally. The gyrus rectus and the orbital gyri are separated by the olfactory sulcus. The orbital lamina of the frontal bone separates the frontal lobe from the orbit. The eyeball is surrounded by periorbital fat. The optic nerve is in the center of the eyeball. Muscles of extraocular movement in this section include the superior rectus, lateral rectus, medial rectus, and inferior rectus. The nasal septum and the middle and inferior conchae are in the midline. On each side of the nasal cavity is the maxillary sinus. The hard palate is dorsal to the tongue. The lingual septum is in the midline.

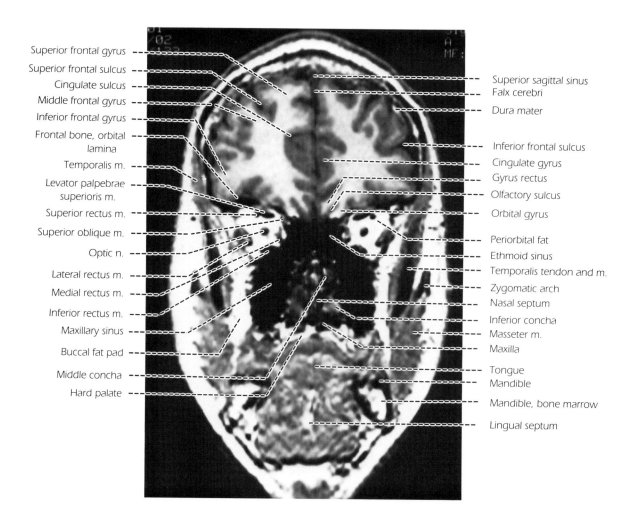

Coronal T1-weighted image through the frontal lobe. The superior sagittal sinus is dorsal to the frontal lobes. Extending from the superior sagittal sinus and separating the two hemispheres is the falx cerebri. The dura mater is seen lateral to the frontal lobe. Within the frontal lobe, the middle and superior frontal gyri are separated by the superior frontal sulcus. The inferior frontal sulcus separates the middle and inferior frontal gyri. The cingulate gyrus is located on each side of the midline. The cingulate sulcus delineates the dorsal boundary of the cingulate gyrus. On the inferior surface of the frontal lobe are the gyrus rectus and the medial orbital gyrus. The two are separated by the olfactory sulcus. The orbital lamina of the frontal bone separates the frontal lobe from the orbit. Within the orbit is the retro-orbital fat. The optic nerve is seen in the center of the globe. Muscles of extraocular movement in this section include the superior rectus, lateral rectus, medial rectus, and inferior rectus. In the midline are the nasal septum and the middle and inferior conchae. Other important structures include the temporalis muscle, zygomatic arch, masseter muscle, mandible, and tongue.

## Figure 1-89

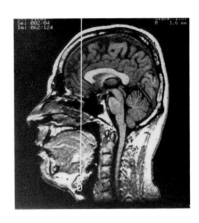

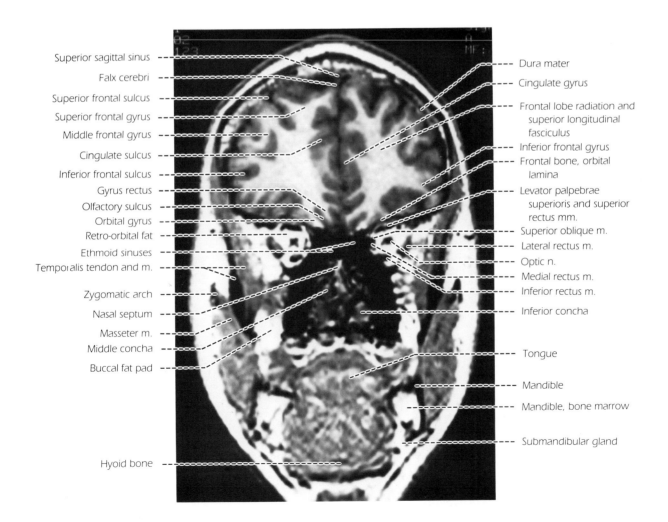

Superior sagittal sinus
Falx cerebri
Superior frontal sulcus
Superior frontal gyrus
Middle frontal gyrus
Cingulate sulcus
Inferior frontal sulcus
Gyrus rectus
Olfactory sulcus
Orbital gyrus
Retro-orbital fat
Ethmoid sinuses
Temporalis tendon and m.
Zygomatic arch
Nasal septum
Masseter m.
Middle concha
Buccal fat pad

Hyoid bone

Dura mater
Cingulate gyrus
Frontal lobe radiation and superior longitudinal fasciculus
Inferior frontal gyrus
Frontal bone, orbital lamina
Levator palpebrae superioris and superior rectus mm.
Superior oblique m.
Lateral rectus m.
Optic n.
Medial rectus m.
Inferior rectus m.
Inferior concha

Tongue

Mandible
Mandible, bone marrow

Submandibular gland

## Figure 1-90

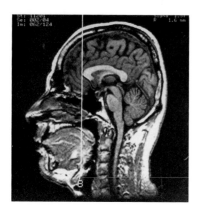

Coronal T1-weighted image through the frontal lobe. The falx cerebri separates the two frontal lobes. The superior sagittal sinus is dorsal to the falx cerebri. Within the frontal lobe, the superior and middle frontal gyri are seen. The cingulate gyrus is located on each side of the falx cerebri. The cingulum is the white matter core of the cingulate gyrus. The cingulate sulcus delineates the dorsal boundary of the cingulate gyrus. On the inferior surface of the frontal lobe are the gyrus rectus medially and the orbital gyrus laterally. The two are separated by the olfactory sulcus. Inferior to the frontal lobe is the orbit. The optic nerve is surrounded by periorbital fat. Muscles of extraocular movement include the superior rectus, superior oblique, medial rectus, inferior rectus, and lateral rectus. The inferior concha is seen in the wall of the nose. The maxillary sinus is lateral to the nasal cavity. Other important structures include the ethmoid sinuses, lesser wing of the sphenoid bone, temporalis muscle and tendon, greater wing of the sphenoid bone, maxillary sinus, maxilla, parotid duct, tongue, and mandible.

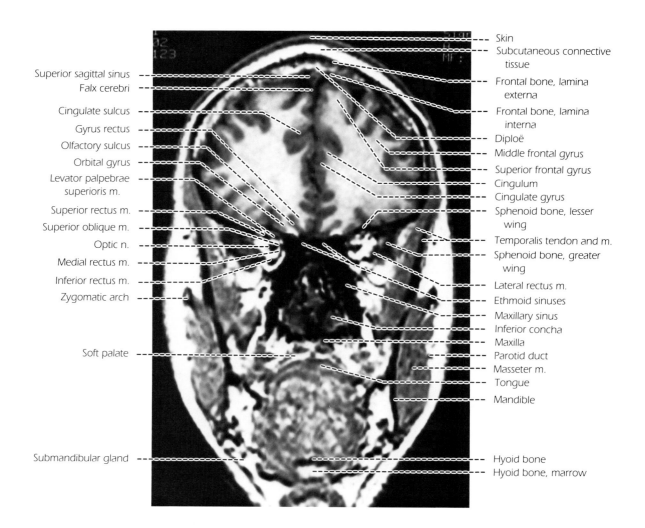

Coronal T1-weighted image through the frontal lobe and a small part of the temporal lobe. The falx cerebri separates the two cerebral hemispheres. The superior sagittal sinus is dorsal to the falx cerebri. The cingulate gyrus is found on each side of the midline. The cingulum forms the deep white matter core of the cingulate gyrus. The cingulate sulcus delineates the cingulate gyrus dorsally. The corpus callosum connects the two hemispheres. Dorsal and ventral to the corpus callosum are branches of the anterior cerebral artery. On the ventral surface of the frontal lobe are the gyrus rectus and the medial orbital gyrus. In the ventral surface of the gyrus rectus is the olfactory tract. The superior and middle frontal gyri are separated by the superior frontal sulcus. Periorbital fat surrounds the optic nerve. Muscles of extraocular movement include the superior, medial, and inferior rectus muscles. Other important structures include the lesser and greater wings of the sphenoid bone, frontal branch of the superficial temporal artery, temporalis tendon and muscle, nasal septum, soft palate, tongue, hyoid bone, mandible, parotid duct, masseter muscle, middle and inferior conchae, zygomatic arch, and ethmoid sinuses.

## Figure 1-91

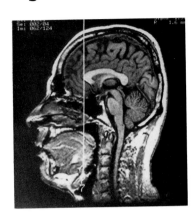

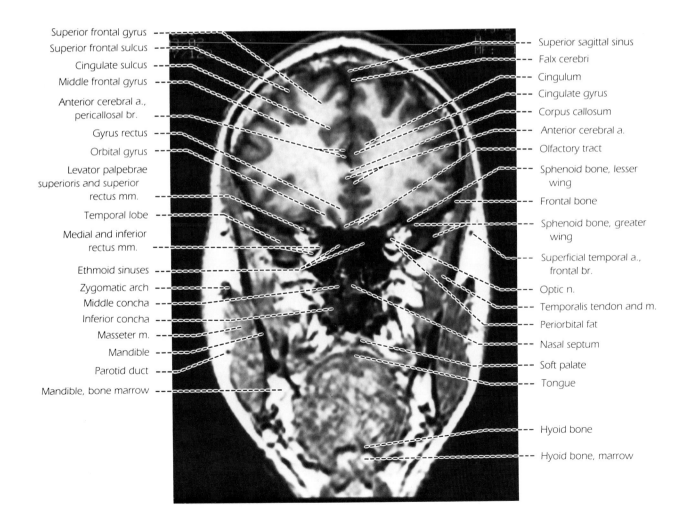

## Figure 1-92

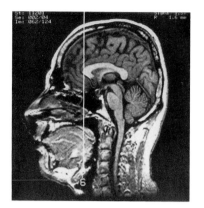

Coronal T1-weighted image through the anterior part of the corpus callosum. The corpus callosum connects the two hemispheres. Dorsal and ventral to the corpus callosum are branches of the anterior cerebral artery. The falx cerebri separates the two frontal lobes. The superior sagittal sinus is dorsal to the falx cerebri. Within the frontal lobe, the superior and middle frontal gyri are separated by the superior frontal sulcus. The inferior frontal lobule is also seen. On the inferior surface of the frontal lobe are the gyrus rectus and medial orbital gyrus. The two are separated by the olfactory sulcus. Ventral to the gyrus rectus is the olfactory tract. Beneath the frontal lobe is periorbital fat. Muscles of extraocular movement include the superior rectus, lateral rectus, and inferior rectus muscles. The optic nerve is found within the periorbital fat. The anterior horn of the lateral ventricle is located on each side of the corpus callosum. Other important structures include the dura mater surrounding the frontal lobe, lesser and greater wings of the sphenoid bone, a portion of the temporal lobe, nasal septum, mandible, soft palate, tongue, submandibular gland, hyoid bone, parotid duct, masseter muscle, zygomatic arch, temporalis tendon and muscle, and ethmoid sinuses.

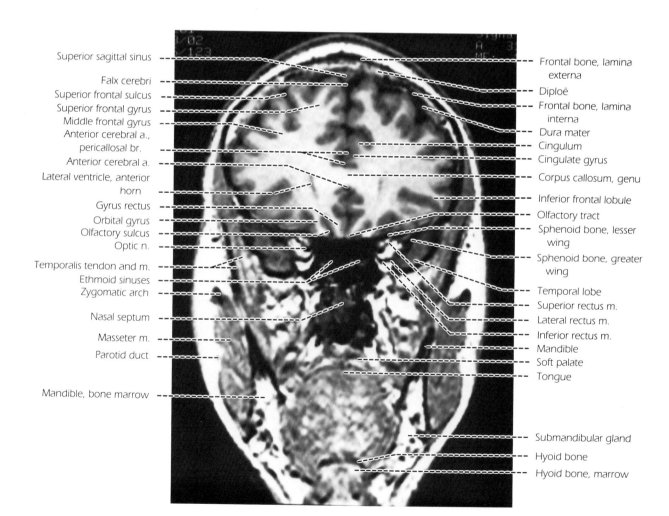

Coronal T1-weighted image of the frontal and temporal lobes. The corpus callosum connects the two frontal lobes. The superior sagittal sinus is dorsal to the frontal lobes. Within the frontal lobe, the superior and middle frontal gyri are separated by the superior frontal sulcus. The cingulate gyrus is dorsal to the corpus callosum. The cingulate sulcus delineates the dorsal boundary of the cingulate gyrus. The cingulum is the white matter core of the cingulate gyrus. Dorsal and ventral to the corpus callosum are branches of the anterior cerebral artery. The anterior horn of the lateral ventricle is seen on each side of the corpus callosum. The head of the caudate nucleus is located in the lateral wall of the lateral ventricle. In the ventral aspect of the frontal lobe are the gyrus rectus and orbital gyrus. Other important structures in this section include the lesser wing of the sphenoid bone, temporal lobe, greater wing of the sphenoid bone, soft palate, tongue, hyoid bone, medial and lateral pterygoid muscles, parotid duct, masseter muscle, zygomatic arch, common tendinous ring (Zinn's ring), frontal branches of the superficial temporal artery, and temporalis tendon and muscle.

## Figure 1-93

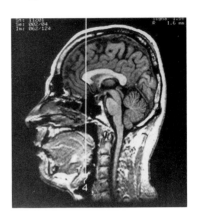

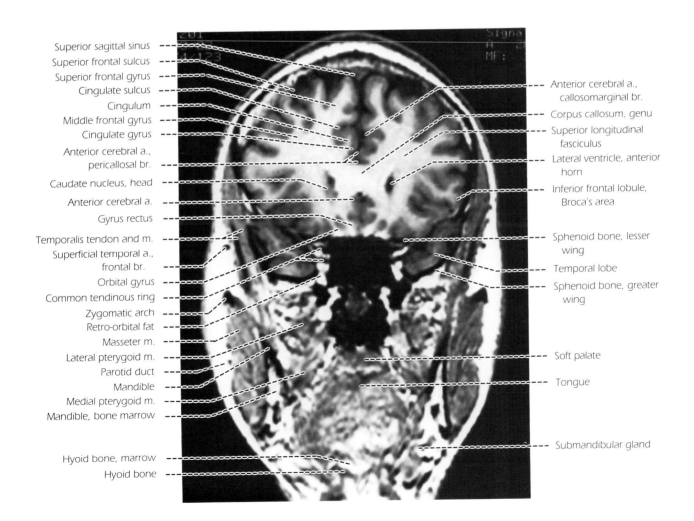

## Figure 1-94

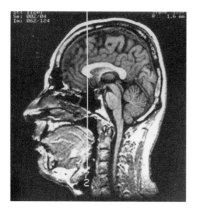

Coronal T1-weighted image of the frontal and temporal lobes. The lateral (sylvian) fissure separates the frontal and temporal lobes. The superior sagittal sinus is dorsal to the frontal lobes. Within the frontal lobes, the superior and middle frontal gyri are seen. The cingulate sulcus is on each side of the midline delineating the dorsal boundary of the cingulate gyrus. The corpus callosum connects the two frontal lobes. Both the genu and rostrum of the corpus callosum are seen. Lateral to the corpus callosum is the anterior horn of the lateral ventricle. The head of the caudate nucleus is in the lateral wall of the lateral ventricle. The subcallosal gyrus is beneath the rostrum of the corpus callosum. In the ventral aspect of the frontal lobe, the rectus and orbital gyri are seen. The olfactory tract is ventral to the gyrus rectus. The sphenoid air sinus is located in the midline. The lesser and greater wings of the sphenoid bone are seen. Other important structures in this section include the common tendinous ring (Zinn's ring), nasopharynx, parapharyngeal fat, soft palate, tongue, facial artery, medial and lateral pterygoid muscles, masseter muscle, zygomatic arch, and hyoid bone.

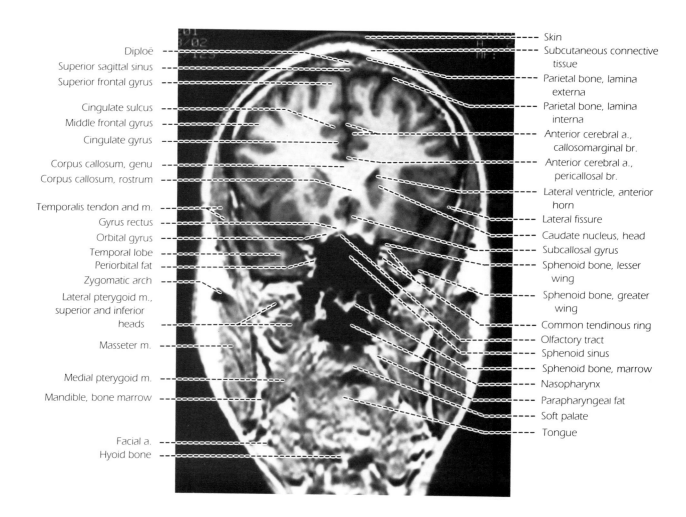

Coronal T1-weighted image of the frontal and temporal lobes at the level of the body of the corpus callosum. The corpus callosum connects the two frontal lobes. The lateral ventricle is located ventral to the corpus callosum. Separating the two ventricular cavities is the septum pellucidum. Within the septum pellucidum is a cavity (cavum septi pellucidi). The caudate nucleus occupies a position in the lateral wall of the lateral ventricle. The anterior limb of the internal capsule separates the caudate nucleus from the putamen. Lateral to the putamen is the external capsule. The claustrum is lateral to the external capsule. The lateral (sylvian) fissure separates the frontal and temporal lobes. Deep within the lateral fissure is the insular cortex. The insular cortex is surrounded by the limen insulae. The olfactory tract is ventral to the frontal lobe. Other structures in this section include the sphenoid sinus, zygomatic arch, sphenoid bone, nasopharynx, lateral and medial pterygoid muscles, masseter muscle, ramus of the mandible, facial artery, soft palate, and anterior cerebral artery.

## Figure 1-95

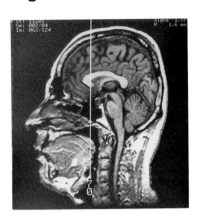

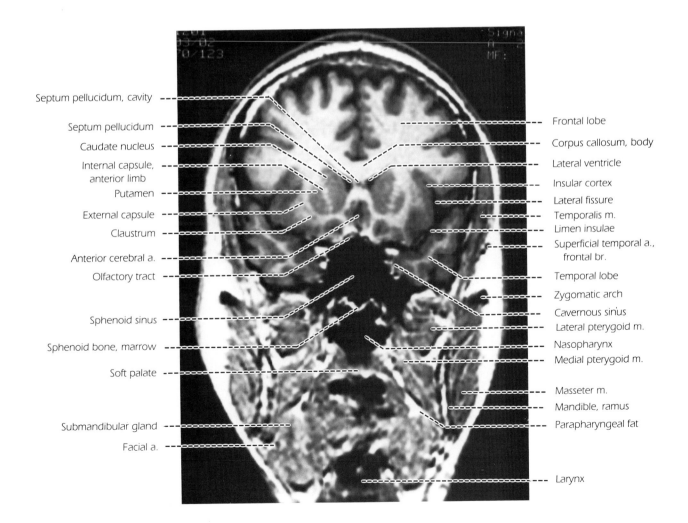

- Septum pellucidum, cavity
- Septum pellucidum
- Caudate nucleus
- Internal capsule, anterior limb
- Putamen
- External capsule
- Claustrum
- Anterior cerebral a.
- Olfactory tract
- Sphenoid sinus
- Sphenoid bone, marrow
- Soft palate
- Submandibular gland
- Facial a.

- Frontal lobe
- Corpus callosum, body
- Lateral ventricle
- Insular cortex
- Lateral fissure
- Temporalis m.
- Limen insulae
- Superficial temporal a., frontal br.
- Temporal lobe
- Zygomatic arch
- Cavernous sinus
- Lateral pterygoid m.
- Nasopharynx
- Medial pterygoid m.
- Masseter m.
- Mandible, ramus
- Parapharyngeal fat
- Larynx

## Figure 1-96

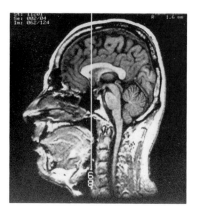

Coronal T1-weighted image through the striatum. The caudate and putamen nuclei are separated by the anterior limb of the internal capsule. Lateral to the putamen is the external capsule. Between the external and the extreme capsules is the claustrum. The insular cortex (island of Reil) is deep within the lateral fissure. The corpus callosum connects the two hemispheres. Dorsal to the corpus callosum are pericallosal branches of the anterior cerebral artery and the cingulate gyrus. The cingulum is the white matter core of the cingulate gyrus. The superior and middle frontal gyri are separated by the superior frontal sulcus. The corona radiata forms the white matter core of the hemispheres. The septal area is medial to the caudate nucleus and putamen. The olfactory tract is located ventral to the gyrus rectus of the frontal lobe. The limen insulae surrounds the insular cortex. Other important structures include the frontal branches of the superficial temporal artery and vein, zygomatic arch, sphenoid sinus, eustachian tube, nasopharynx, oropharynx, ramus of the mandible, parapharyngeal fat, epiglottis, pharyngeal constrictor muscle, medial pterygoid muscle, lateral pterygoid muscle, and anterior commissure.

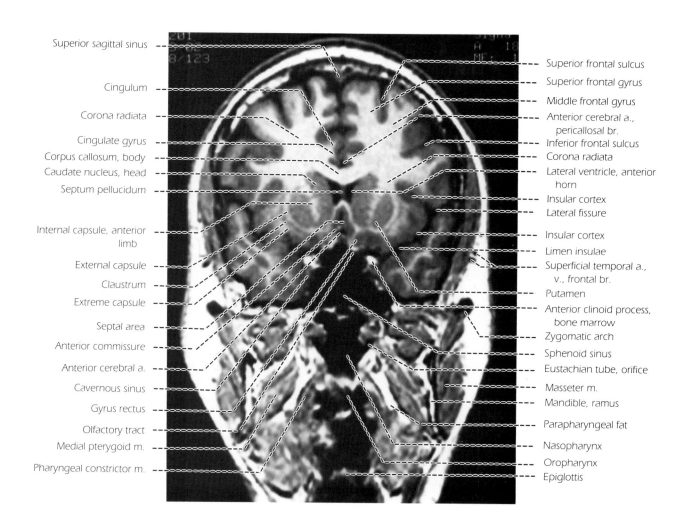

Coronal T1-weighted image through the frontal and temporal lobes. The corpus callosum connects the two hemispheres. Dorsal to the corpus callosum are branches of the anterior cerebral artery and cingulate gyrus. The cingulate sulcus delineates the dorsal boundary of the cingulate gyrus. The cingulum is the white matter core of the cingulate gyrus. The corona radiata is the deep white matter core of the hemisphere. Ventral to the corpus callosum are the cavities of the lateral ventricle separated by the septum pellucidum. The caudate nucleus occupies a position in the lateral wall of the lateral ventricle. The anterior limb of the internal capsule separates the caudate nucleus from the putamen. Ventral to the septum pellucidum is the septal area. Lateral to the putamen is the external capsule. The claustrum is located between the external and extreme capsules. The lateral fissure separates the frontal and temporal lobes. Deep within the lateral fissure is the insular cortex (island of Reil). The gyrus rectus is found in the ventral aspect of the frontal lobe. The superior and middle temporal gyri are seen within the temporal lobe. Branches of the anterior cerebral artery are dorsal to the corpus callosum and ventral to the septal area. Other structures in this section include the zygomatic arch, superficial temporal artery and vein (frontal branches), sphenoid sinus, nasopharynx, masseter muscle, ramus of the mandible, parapharyngeal fat, epiglottis, glossoepiglottic fold, facial artery, soft palate, lateral pterygoid muscle, temporalis muscle, and superior sagittal sinus.

# Figure 1-97

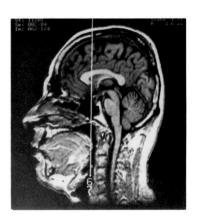

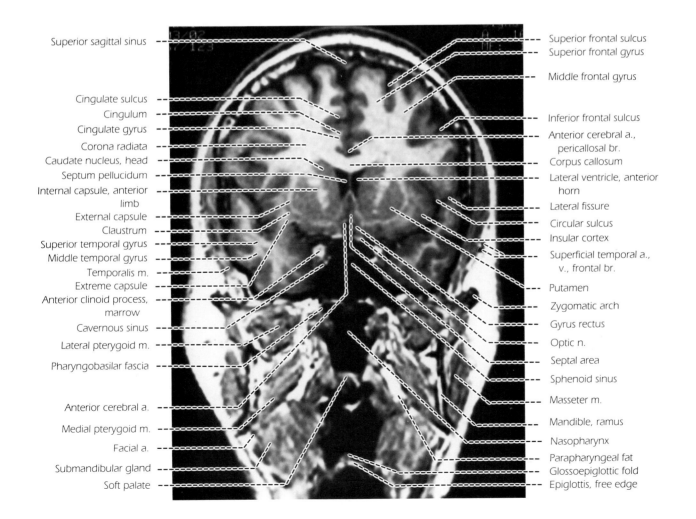

# Figure 1-98

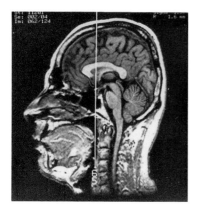

Coronal T1-weighted image through the frontal and temporal lobes. The corpus callosum connects the two frontal lobes. The superior frontal gyrus is located dorsally in the frontal lobe. The cingulate gyrus is dorsal to the corpus callosum. The cingulum forms the deep white matter core of the cingulate gyrus. Inferior to the corpus callosum are the cavities of the lateral ventricle separated by the septum pellucidum. The caudate nucleus is located in the lateral wall of the lateral ventricle. The anterior limb of the internal capsule separates the caudate nucleus from the putamen. Medial to the putamen is the globus pallidus. The external capsule delineates the lateral boundary of the putamen. The claustrum is lateral to the external capsule. The nucleus accumbens septi is medial to the globus pallidus. The insular cortex (island of Reil) is deep within the lateral fissure. The optic chiasm is a bright signal intensity dorsal to the suprasellar cistern. The hypophysis is another bright signal intensity ventral to the suprasellar cistern. The amygdaloid nucleus is in the medial part of the temporal lobe. Other structures in this section include the sphenoid sinus, temporal bone, zygomatic process, lateral pterygoid muscle, torus tubarius, nasopharynx, ramus of the mandible, masseter muscle, medial pterygoid muscle, free edge of the epiglottis with the pharyngoepiglottic fold, and parotid gland. The superior occipitofrontal fasciculus occupies a characteristic location dorsal to the caudate nucleus.

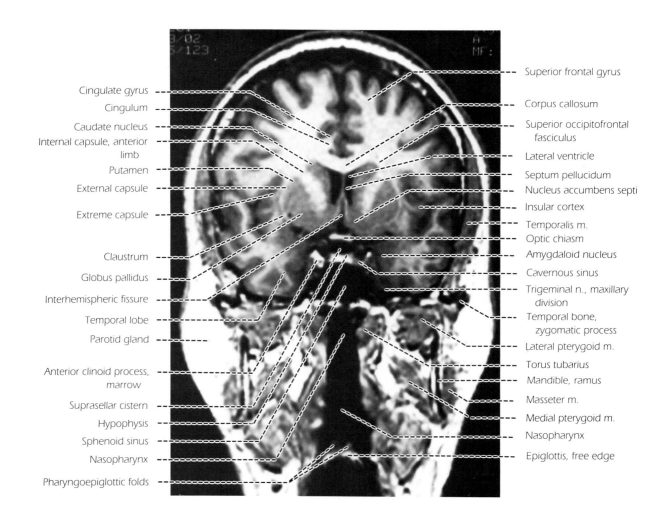

Coronal T1-weighted image through the frontal and temporal lobes. The corpus callosum connects the two hemispheres. Dorsal to the corpus callosum are branches of the anterior cerebral artery and cingulate gyrus. The superior frontal gyrus is also seen in the frontal lobe. The septum pellucidum separates the two cavities of the lateral ventricle. The caudate nucleus occupies a position in the lateral wall of the lateral ventricle. The superior occipitofrontal fasciculus, one of the long association bundles, occupies a characteristic location dorsal to the caudate nucleus. The anterior limb of the internal capsule separates the caudate nucleus from the putamen. Lateral to the putamen is the external capsule and the claustrum. Ventral to the septum are the septal nuclei. The lateral fissure separates the frontal and temporal lobes. The insular cortex is found deep within the lateral fissure. The amygdaloid nucleus is located in the medial part of the temporal lobe. The suprasellar cistern separates the optic chiasm dorsally and the hypophysis ventrally. Other important structures in this section include the sphenoid sinus, zygomatic process of the temporal bone, lateral and medial pterygoid muscles, torus tubarius, masseter muscle, pharyngeal constrictor muscle, pharynx, parapharyngeal fat, parotid gland, and eustachian tube.

## Figure 1-99

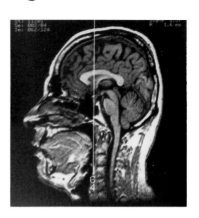

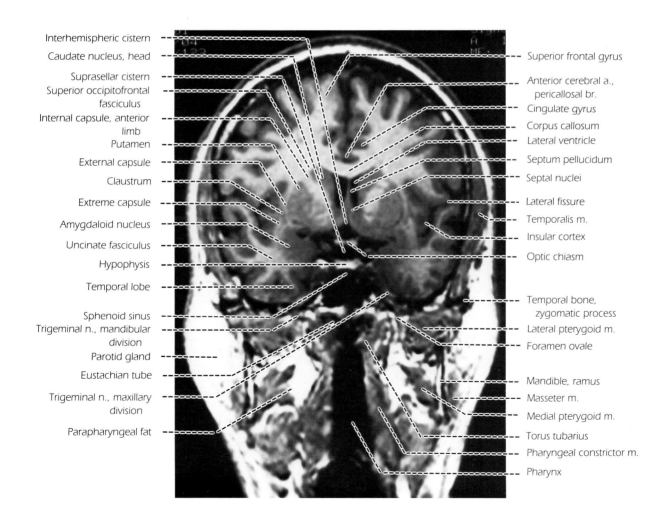

Interhemispheric cistern
Caudate nucleus, head
Suprasellar cistern
Superior occipitofrontal fasciculus
Internal capsule, anterior limb
Putamen
External capsule
Claustrum
Extreme capsule
Amygdaloid nucleus
Uncinate fasciculus
Hypophysis
Temporal lobe
Sphenoid sinus
Trigeminal n., mandibular division
Parotid gland
Eustachian tube
Trigeminal n., maxillary division
Parapharyngeal fat

Superior frontal gyrus
Anterior cerebral a., pericallosal br.
Cingulate gyrus
Corpus callosum
Lateral ventricle
Septum pellucidum
Septal nuclei
Lateral fissure
Temporalis m.
Insular cortex
Optic chiasm
Temporal bone, zygomatic process
Lateral pterygoid m.
Foramen ovale
Mandible, ramus
Masseter m.
Medial pterygoid m.
Torus tubarius
Pharyngeal constrictor m.
Pharynx

## Figure 1-100

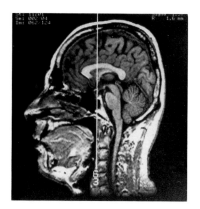

Coronal T1-weighted image through the frontal and temporal lobes. The falx cerebri separates the two frontal lobes. Within the frontal lobe, the superior, middle, and inferior frontal gyri are seen. The corpus callosum connects the two hemispheres. Dorsal to the corpus callosum are anterior cerebral artery branches and the cingulate gyrus. The septum pellucidum separates the two cavities of the lateral ventricle. The caudate nucleus occupies a position in the lateral wall of the lateral ventricle. The anterior limb of the internal capsule separates the caudate nucleus from the putamen. Medial to the putamen is the globus pallidus. Ventral to the globus pallidus is the anterior commissure. Lateral to the putamen is the external capsule and the claustrum. The lateral fissure separates the temporal and frontal lobes. In the depth of the lateral fissure is the insular cortex. The optic chiasm is a bright signal intensity separated from the hypophysis by the suprasellar cistern. The inferior temporal gyrus, middle temporal gyrus, superior temporal gyrus, and the amygdala are seen within the temporal lobe. Other structures found in this section include the sphenoid sinus, zygomatic process of the temporal bone, nasopharynx, lateral and medial pterygoid muscles, torus tubarius, ramus of the mandible, parotid gland, middle cerebral artery, and superior sagittal sinus.

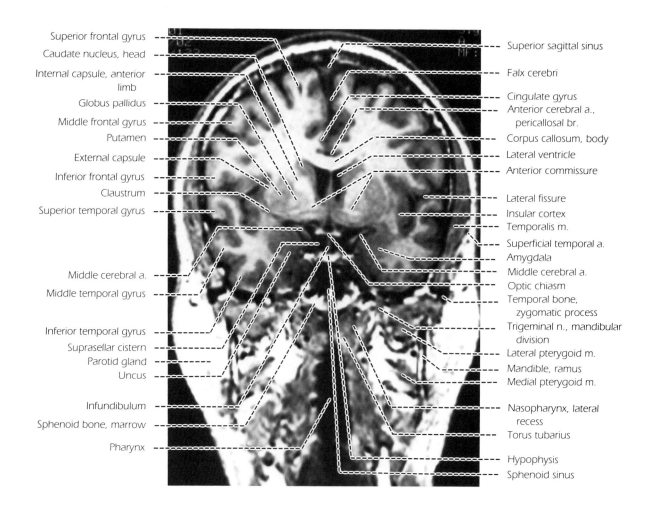

Coronal T1-weighted image through the frontal and temporal lobes. The section also shows the basal ganglia. The corpus callosum connects the two cerebral hemispheres. The falx cerebri separates the two hemispheres. The superior sagittal sinus is located in the dorsal part of the falx cerebri. The two components of the lentiform nucleus are seen in this section: the putamen laterally and globus pallidus medially. The corona radiata forms the white matter core of the cerebral hemisphere. Two long association fiber bundles are seen in this section, the superior and inferior occipitofrontal fasciculi. The third ventricle is seen below the fornix. The optic tract is a bright signal intensity below the third ventricle. The amygdala is on the medial surface of the temporal lobe. Dorsal to the hypophysis is the infundibulum. Also dorsal to the hypophysis is the suprasellar cistern. Branches of the anterior cerebral artery are seen dorsal to the corpus callosum. Other important structures in this section include the temporalis muscle, sphenoid sinus, zygomatic process of the temporal bone, lateral and medial pterygoid muscles, ramus of the mandible, pharynx, parotid gland, and sphenoid bone.

# Figure 1-101

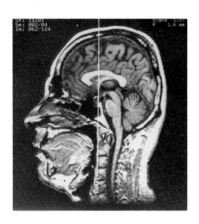

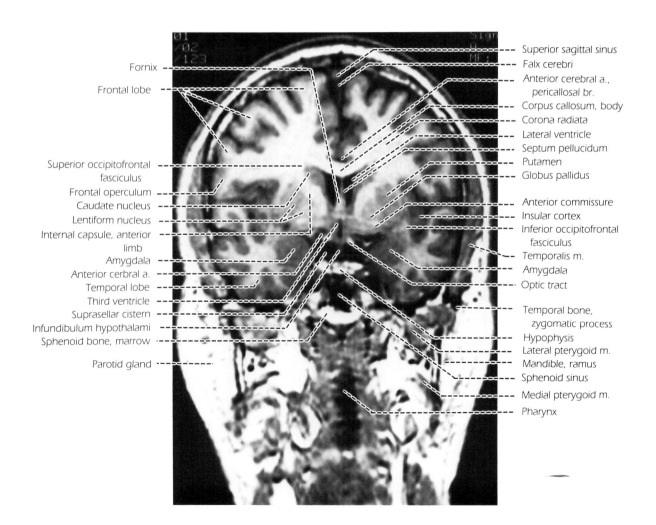

# Figure 1-102

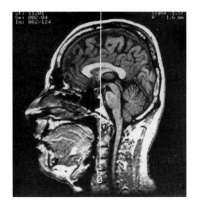

Coronal T1-weighted image through the frontal and temporal lobes. The basal ganglia and hypothalamus are also present. The falx cerebri separates the two cerebral hemispheres. The superior sagittal sinus is dorsal to the falx cerebri. The corpus callosum connects the two cerebral hemispheres. The lateral ventricle is found beneath the corpus callosum. The crus of the fornix is located in the midline between the two ventricles. The third ventricle is ventral to the fornix. The anterior limb of the internal capsule separates the caudate nucleus from the putamen. Medial to the putamen is the globus pallidus. Laminae separating the globus pallidus from the putamen and external part of the globus pallidus from its internal parts are seen. The lateral fissure separates the frontal and temporal lobes. The insular cortex is deep within the lateral fissure. In the medial part of the temporal lobe is the amygdala. Dorsal to the hypophysis is the suprasellar cistern. The external capsule is lateral to the putamen. Other important structures in this section include the sphenoid bone, lateral pterygoid muscle, ramus of the mandible, internal jugular vein, parotid gland, condylar head of the mandible, external auditory meatus, and internal carotid artery.

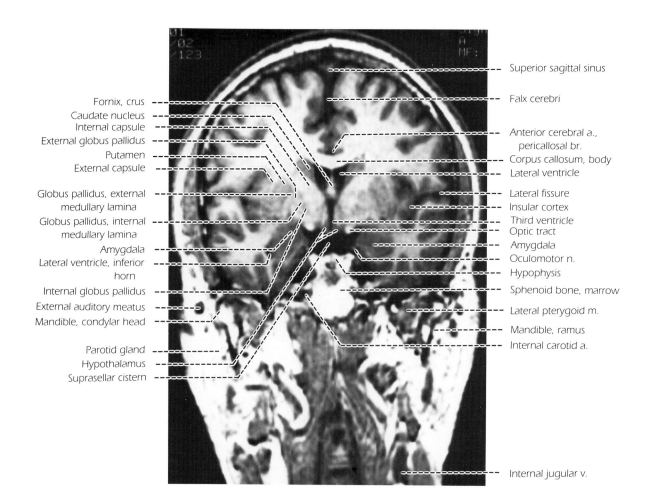

Coronal T1-weighted image through the frontal and temporal lobes. This section also shows the basal ganglia and hypothalamus. The corpus callosum connects the two cerebral hemispheres. The two cerebral hemispheres are separated by the interhemispheric fissure. The superior sagittal sinus is located dorsal to the interhemispheric fissure. The cavities of the lateral ventricle are found beneath the corpus callosum. The caudate nucleus is located in the lateral wall of the lateral ventricle. The lateral and third ventricles are connected by the interventricular foramen (foramen of Monro). The fornix is seen above the third ventricle. The putamen and globus pallidus are separated by the external medullary lamina of the globus pallidus. The internal medullary lamina of the globus pallidus separates the outer from the inner components of the globus pallidus. Lateral to the putamen is the external capsule. On each side of the third ventricle is the hypothalamus. Within the hypothalamus is the column of the fornix. The amygdala is seen on the medial surface of the temporal lobe. Adjacent to the amygdala is the hippocampus. Branches of the anterior cerebral artery are dorsal to the corpus callosum within the interhemispheric fissure. Other structures in this section include the optic tract, lateral pterygoid muscle, sphenoid bone, internal jugular vein, common carotid artery, parotid gland, condylar head of the mandible, external auditory meatus, and lateral (sylvian) fissure.

## Figure 1-103

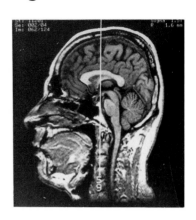

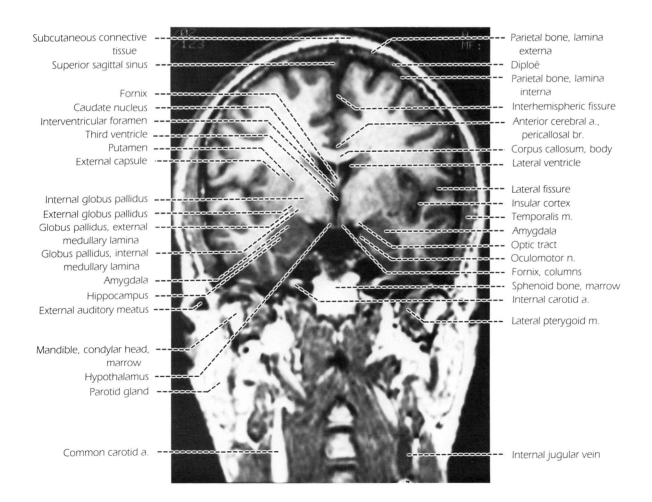

# Figure 1-104

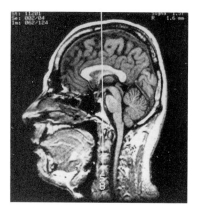

Coronal T1-weighted image through the thalamus and third ventricle. The falx cerebri is located between the two cerebral hemispheres. The superior sagittal sinus is seen as a fold of dura mater dorsal to the falx cerebri. On each side of the interhemispheric fissure is the cingulate gyrus. The cingulate sulcus delineates the dorsal boundary of the cingulate gyrus. The cingulum is the white matter core of the cingulate gyrus. Within the interhemispheric fissure and dorsal to the corpus callosum are branches of the anterior cerebral artery. The two cavities of the lateral ventricle are separated by the septum pellucidum. Ventral to the septum pellucidum is the body of the fornix. The interventricular foramen connects the lateral ventricle with the third ventricle. On each side of the third ventricle are the hypothalamus and thalamus. In the ventral part of the hypothalamus is the mamillary body. The caudate nucleus is located in the lateral wall of the lateral ventricle. The internal capsule separates the thalamus from the putamen and globus pallidus. The external medullary lamina of the globus pallidus separates the putamen and globus pallidus. The lateral fissure separates the frontal and temporal lobes. Within the temporal lobe, the amygdala is seen. The parahippocampal gyrus is seen. Lateral to the putamen is the external capsule and claustrum. Other structures in this section include the optic tract, temporalis muscle, basiocciput, atlas, internal jugular vein, and external auditory meatus.

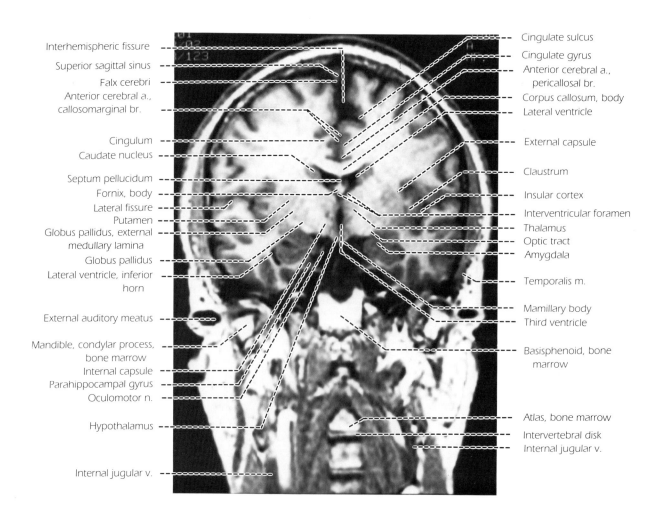

Coronal T1-weighted image of the thalamus and third ventricle. The corpus callosum connects the two cerebral hemispheres. Dorsal to the corpus callosum is the cingulate gyrus. The cingulum forms the white matter core of the cingulate gyrus. Also dorsal to the corpus callosum are branches of the anterior cerebral artery. The septum pellucidum separates the two lateral ventricles. The fornix is seen ventral to the septum pellucidum. The interventricular foramen (foramen of Monro) connects each lateral ventricle with the third ventricle. On each side of the third ventricle is the thalamus. The caudate nucleus occupies a position in the lateral wall of the lateral ventricle. The internal capsule separates the thalamus from the globus pallidus and putamen. Lateral to the putamen is the external capsule and claustrum. The extreme capsule separates the claustrum from the insular cortex. The insular cortex is deep within the lateral fissure. Within the temporal lobe, the hippocampus, parahippocampal gyrus, and occipitotemporal gyrus are seen. The subcallosal bundle (superior occipitofrontal fasciculus) is in its characteristic location dorsolateral to the caudate nucleus. Other structures in this section include the optic tract, posterior cerebral artery, oculomotor nerve, basiocciput, internal jugular vein, parotid gland, and external auditory meatus.

## Figure 1-105

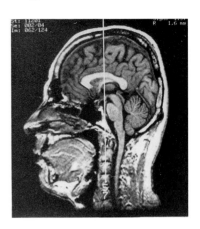

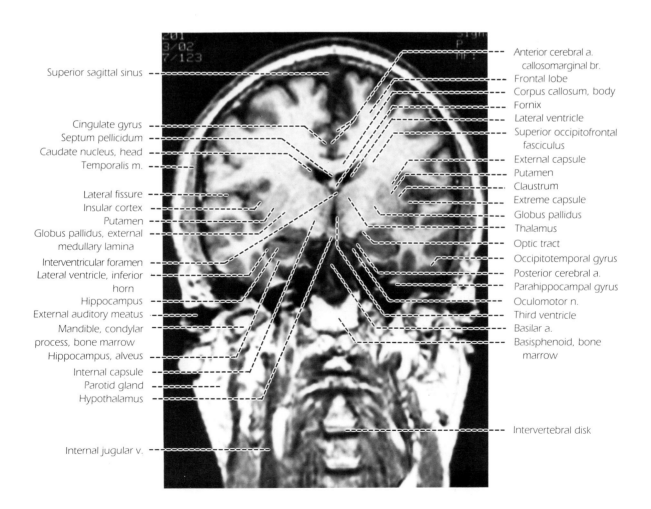

## Figure 1-106

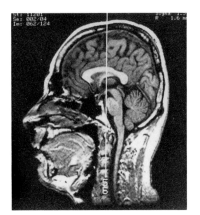

Coronal T1-weighted image through the third ventricle and thalamus. The corpus callosum connects the two cerebral hemispheres. Ventral to the corpus callosum and separating the two ventricular cavities is the septum pellucidum. Ventral to the septum pellucidum is the fornix. The third ventricle is in the midline between the two thalami. Ventral to the thalamus are the midbrain and pons. Within the midbrain is the substantia nigra and cerebral peduncle. The interpeduncular cistern is seen between the two cerebral peduncles. Dorsal to the substantia nigra is the subthalamic nucleus. The caudate nucleus occupies a position in the lateral wall of the third ventricle. The internal capsule separates the thalamus from the globus pallidus and putamen. The external medullary lamina of the globus pallidus separates the putamen from the globus pallidus. The hippocampus, alveus of hippocampus, and fimbria are seen in the medial part of the temporal lobe. The mamillothalamic tract is seen coursing through the thalamus. Dorsal to the corpus callosum is the cingulate gyrus. In the cavity between the two cerebral hemispheres are branches of the anterior cerebral artery. The ambient and prepontine cisterns are seen related to the midbrain and pons. The insular cortex is located deep within the lateral fissure. Other structures in this section include the basiocciput, internal jugular vein, axis, common carotid artery, parotid gland, and external auditory meatus. The basilar artery is seen ventral to the pons.

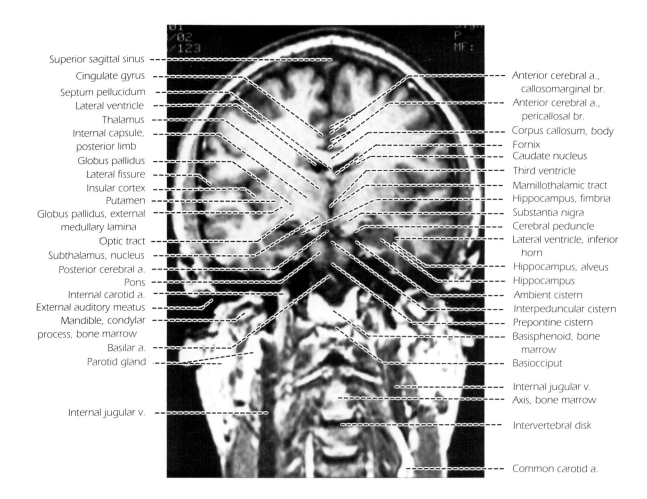

Coronal T1-weighted image through the thalamus and brain stem. The corpus callosum connects the two cerebral hemispheres. Dorsal to the corpus callosum, within the inter-hemispheric fissure, are branches of the anterior cerebral artery. The third ventricle separates the two thalami. The two thalami are connected in the midline through the massa intermedia, interthalamic adhesion. One of the thalamic nuclei, the anterior thalamic nucleus, is located dorsally within the thalamus. The two cavities of the lateral ventricle are separated by the septum pellucidum. Ventral to the septum pellucidum is the fornix. Parts of the midbrain and pons are seen ventral to the thalamus. Within the midbrain, the cerebral peduncle and the substantia nigra are seen. The interpeduncular cistern separates the two cerebral peduncles. Dorsal to the substantia nigra is the subthalamic nucleus. Within the temporal lobe, the hippocampus and fimbria are seen. The inferior horn of the lateral ventricle is also seen close to the hippocampus. The posterior limb of the internal capsule separates the thalamus from the putamen. Lateral to the putamen is the external capsule and claustrum. Lateral to the claustrum is the extreme capsule. Other structures seen in this section include the optic tract, pons, internal carotid artery, and ambient cistern. The optic radiation is seen coursing ventral to the putamen.

## Figure 1-107

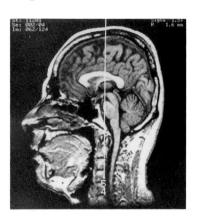

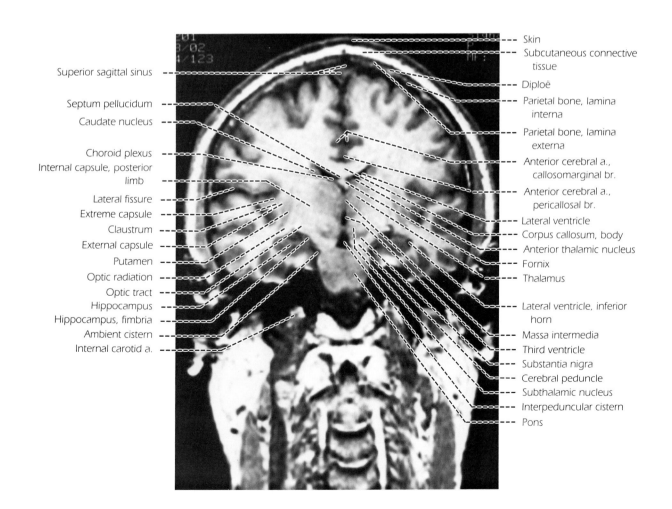

## Figure 1-108

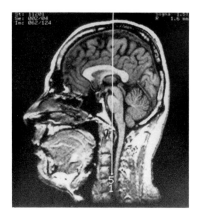

Coronal T1-weighted image through the thalamus and brain stem. The corpus callosum connects the two cerebral hemispheres. The corona radiata is seen within the white matter core of the cerebral hemisphere. Dorsal to the corpus callosum is the cingulate gyrus. The cingulate sulcus delineates the dorsal boundary of the cingulate gyrus. Also dorsal to the corpus callosum are branches of the anterior cerebral artery. The caudate nucleus is located in the lateral wall of the lateral ventricle. The fornix is ventral to the corpus callosum. On each side of the third ventricle is the thalamus. The stria medullaris thalami is found dorsal and medial to the thalamus. Lateral to the thalamus is the putamen nucleus, separated from the claustrum by the external capsule. The extreme capsule is lateral to the claustrum. The red nucleus and substantia nigra are seen within the midbrain. The interpeduncular cistern is located between the two cerebral peduncles. The pons is ventral to the interpeduncular cistern. Within the temporal lobe, the hippocampus and parahippocampal gyrus are seen. The inferior horn of the lateral ventricle is in close proximity to the hippocampus. The superior temporal gyrus is dorsal to the superior temporal sulcus. The posterior limb of the internal capsule separates the thalamus from the putamen. Other structures seen in this section include the temporal bone, internal carotid artery, and ambient cistern.

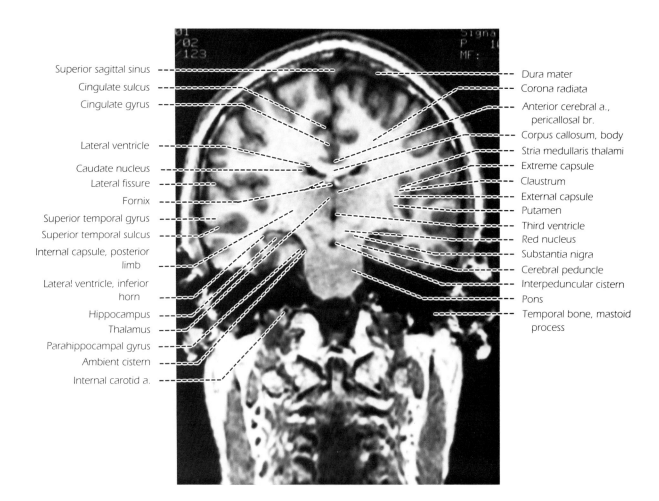

HEAD • CORONAL VIEWS 113

Coronal T1-weighted image through the thalamus and brain stem. The corpus callosum connects the two cerebral hemispheres. Dorsal to the corpus callosum is the cingulate gyrus and branches of the anterior cerebral artery. The cingulate sulcus delineates the dorsal boundary of the cingulate gyrus. Also dorsal to the cingulate gyrus are branches of the anterior cerebral artery. The cingulum, a long association fiber bundle, is the deep white matter core of the cingulate gyrus. Within the frontal lobe is the precentral gyrus (primary motor cortex). Ventral to the corpus callosum is the fornix. The caudate nucleus is seen in the lateral wall of the lateral ventricle. The third ventricle separates the two thalami. Within the temporal lobe, the hippocampus and parahippocampal gyrus are seen. The alveus of the hippocampus is in close proximity to the hippocampus, in the wall of the inferior horn of the lateral ventricle. The ambient cistern is seen around the pons. Ventral to the pons is the pyramid of the medulla oblongata. The vertebral arteries are seen ventral to the medulla oblongata. The facial and vestibulocochlear nerves (cranial nerves VII and VIII) are seen emanating from the pons. Also within the temporal lobe is the middle temporal gyrus. The superior temporal sulcus separates the middle temporal gyrus from the superior temporal gyrus, site of the auditory association cortex. The superior and inferior cerebellar pontine cisterns are seen.

## Figure 1-109

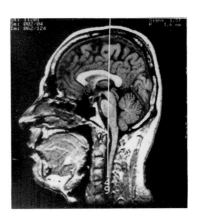

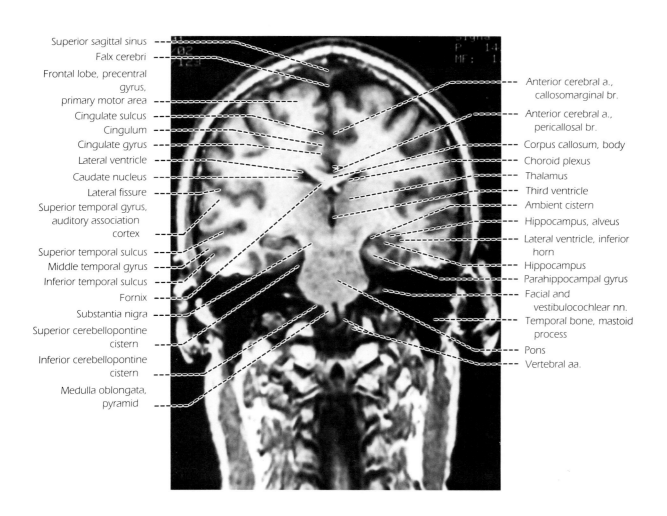

## Figure 1-110

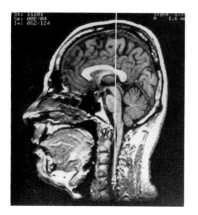

Coronal T1-weighted image through the thalamus and the brain stem. The corpus callosum connects the two cerebral hemispheres. Dorsal to the corpus callosum are branches of the anterior cerebral artery and cingulate gyrus. Dorsal to the cingulate gyrus is the cingulate sulcus. Within the parietal lobe, the postcentral gyrus, site of the primary somesthetic cortex, is seen. The fornix is inferior to the corpus callosum. The caudate nucleus is in the lateral wall of the lateral ventricle. The third ventricle separates the two thalami. The stria medullaris thalami is seen as a bright signal intensity on the medial surface of the thalamus. The cerebral aqueduct (aqueduct of Sylvius) and posterior commissure are seen caudal to the thalamus. The pons and medulla oblongata are located inferior to the thalamus. Within the temporal lobe, the superior temporal gyrus, site of the auditory association cortex, and the inferior temporal gyrus are seen. The parahippocampal gyrus is in close association with the hippocampus. The alveus of the hippocampus is seen in the wall of the inferior horn of the lateral ventricle. A portion of the cerebellum is seen close to the pons. Other structures in this section include the mastoid process of the temporal bone, vertebral arteries, and cerebellar pontine cisterns.

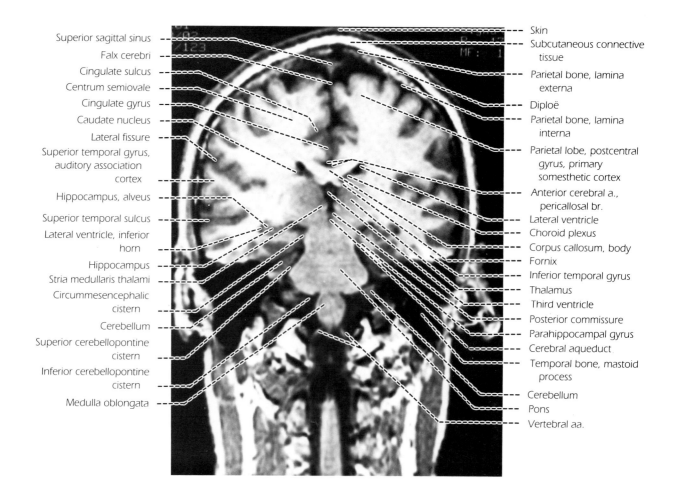

Superior sagittal sinus
Falx cerebri
Cingulate sulcus
Centrum semiovale
Cingulate gyrus
Caudate nucleus
Lateral fissure
Superior temporal gyrus, auditory association cortex
Hippocampus, alveus
Superior temporal sulcus
Lateral ventricle, inferior horn
Hippocampus
Stria medullaris thalami
Circummesencephalic cistern
Cerebellum
Superior cerebellopontine cistern
Inferior cerebellopontine cistern
Medulla oblongata

Skin
Subcutaneous connective tissue
Parietal bone, lamina externa
Diploë
Parietal bone, lamina interna
Parietal lobe, postcentral gyrus, primary somesthetic cortex
Anterior cerebral a., pericallosal br.
Lateral ventricle
Choroid plexus
Corpus callosum, body
Fornix
Inferior temporal gyrus
Thalamus
Third ventricle
Posterior commissure
Parahippocampal gyrus
Cerebral aqueduct
Temporal bone, mastoid process
Cerebellum
Pons
Vertebral aa.

Coronal T1-weighted image through the thalamus and brain stem. The corpus callosum connects the two cerebral hemispheres. Dorsal to the corpus callosum are branches of the anterior cerebral arteries and cingulate gyrus. The cingulate sulcus delineates the dorsal boundary of the cingulate gyrus. The falx cerebri separates the two cerebral hemispheres. Dorsal to the falx cerebri is the superior sagittal sinus. Within the parietal lobe, the postcentral gyrus, site of the primary somesthetic cortex, is seen. Inferior to the corpus callosum is the crus of the fornix. The caudate nucleus is located in the lateral wall of the lateral ventricle. The pineal gland is seen dorsal to the posterior commissure. The cerebral aqueduct (aqueduct of Sylvius) is located ventral to the posterior commissure. Ventrolateral, within the thalamus, is the lateral geniculate nucleus. The parahippocampal gyrus, hippocampus, alveus, and inferior horn of the lateral ventricle are seen in the temporal lobe. The pons is seen dorsal to the medulla oblongata. Other structures in this section include the vertebral artery, mastoid process of the temporal bone, inferior cerebellar pontine cistern, cerebellum, superior cerebellar pontine cistern, and ambient cistern.

## Figure 1-111

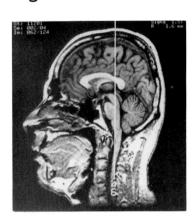

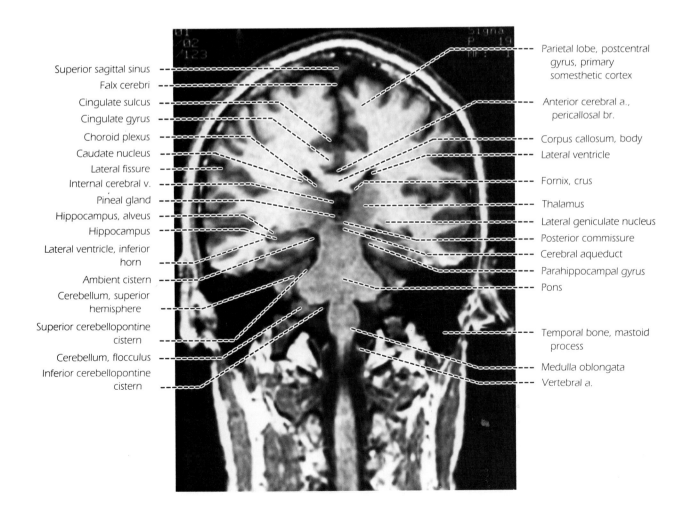

## Figure 1-112

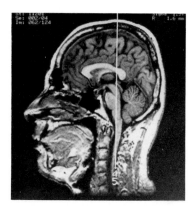

Coronal T1-weighted image through the thalamus and brain stem. The corpus callosum connects the two cerebral hemispheres. Dorsal to the corpus callosum are branches of the anterior cerebral artery and cingulate gyrus. Within the cingulate gyrus is the cingulum, one of the long association fiber bundles. The cingulate sulcus delineates the dorsal boundary of the cingulate gyrus. The falx cerebri is seen between the two cerebral hemispheres. Dorsal to the falx cerebri is the superior sagittal sinus. The thalamus is located on each side of the midline. The caudate nucleus is in the lateral wall of the lateral ventricle. The fornix is inferior to the corpus callosum. The pineal gland is found dorsal to the posterior commissure. Ventral to the posterior commissure is the cerebral aqueduct. On each side of the cerebral aqueduct is the periaqueductal gray matter. The middle cerebellar peduncle (brachium pontis) extends from the pons to the cerebellum. Ventral to the pons is the medulla oblongata. The spinal cord is seen as an extension of the medulla oblongata. The superior and inferior cerebellar pontine cisterns are seen. The hippocampus, alveus, and inferior horn of the lateral ventricle are in close proximity to each other. The inferior temporal gyrus is seen in the ventral part of the temporal lobe.

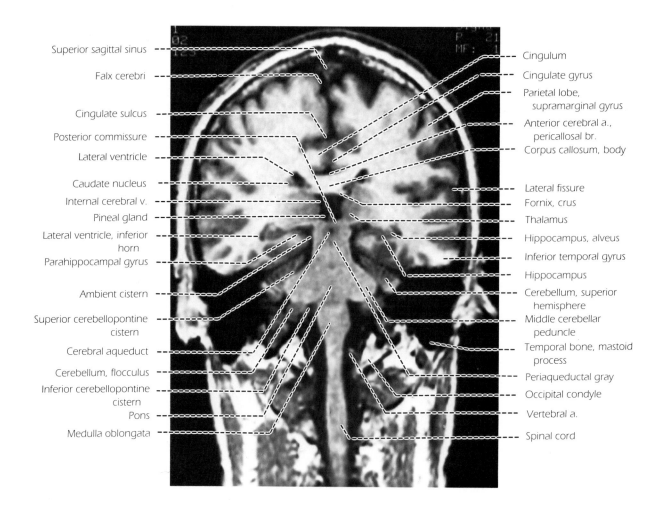

Coronal T1-weighted image through the splenium of the corpus callosum and brain stem. The splenium connects the two cerebral hemispheres. Dorsal to the splenium is the cingulate gyrus and branches of the anterior cerebral artery. The cingulate sulcus delineates the dorsal boundary of the cingulate gyrus. The cingulum, one of the long association fiber bundles, is seen within the cingulate gyrus. Ventral to the splenium of the corpus callosum is the crus of the fornix. Within the thalamus, the pulvinar nucleus is seen. The superior and inferior colliculi are seen in the midbrain. The superior colliculus receives fibers from the retina and cerebral cortex, and the inferior colliculus is a component of the central auditory pathway. Dorsal to the superior colliculus are the quadrigeminal cistern and pineal gland. The cerebral aqueduct is seen in the midline within the superior and inferior colliculi. The middle cerebellar peduncle connects the pons with the cerebellum. The medulla oblongata and part of the spinal cord are seen caudal to the pons. Within the temporal lobe, the hippocampus and inferior horn of the lateral ventricle are seen. Close to the splenium of the corpus callosum is the cavity of the trigone of the lateral ventricle containing choroid plexus. The caudate nucleus is seen in the wall of the trigone.

## Figure 1-113

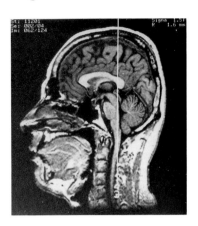

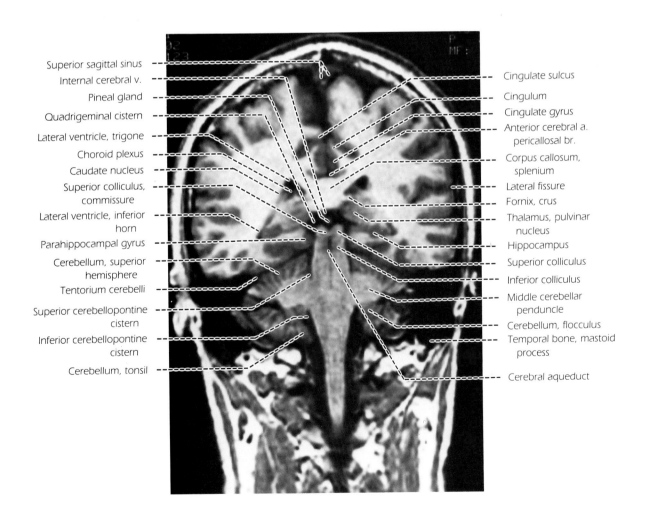

Superior sagittal sinus
Internal cerebral v.
Pineal gland
Quadrigeminal cistern
Lateral ventricle, trigone
Choroid plexus
Caudate nucleus
Superior colliculus, commissure
Lateral ventricle, inferior horn
Parahippocampal gyrus
Cerebellum, superior hemisphere
Tentorium cerebelli
Superior cerebellopontine cistern
Inferior cerebellopontine cistern
Cerebellum, tonsil

Cingulate sulcus
Cingulum
Cingulate gyrus
Anterior cerebral a. pericallosal br.
Corpus callosum, splenium
Lateral fissure
Fornix, crus
Thalamus, pulvinar nucleus
Hippocampus
Superior colliculus
Inferior colliculus
Middle cerebellar penduncle
Cerebellum, flocculus
Temporal bone, mastoid process
Cerebral aqueduct

# Figure 1-114

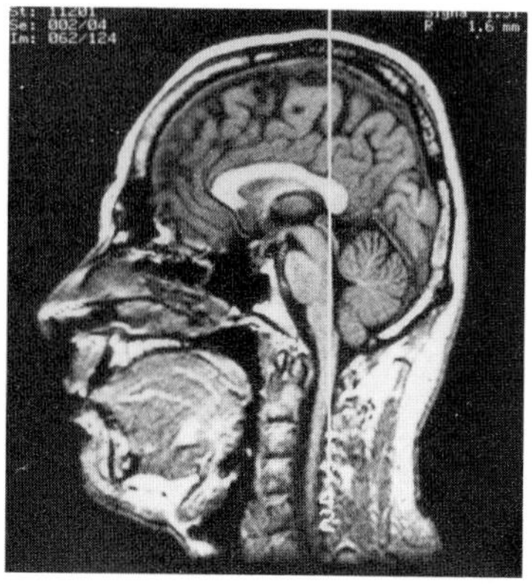

Coronal T1-weighted image through the splenium of the corpus callosum. The splenium connects the two cerebral hemispheres. Dorsal to the splenium are branches of the anterior cerebral artery and cingulate gyrus. The cingulum is seen within the white matter core of the cingulate gyrus. The cingulate sulcus delineates the dorsal boundary of the cingulate gyrus. Within the parietal lobe, the supramarginal gyrus is located dorsal to the lateral fissure. Ventral to the splenium of the corpus callosum is the crus of the fornix. Also ventral to the splenium in the midline are the internal cerebral veins. Ventral and lateral to the splenium is the subsplenial gyrus. The caudate nucleus occupies a position in the lateral wall of the trigone of the lateral ventricle. The superior colliculus is seen on each side of the midbrain. Dorsal to the superior colliculi are the pineal gland and quadrigeminal cistern. The cerebral aqueduct is seen in the midline within the superior colliculus. The middle cerebellar peduncle connects the pons with the cerebellum. The medulla oblongata and spinal cord are caudal to the pons. Within the temporal lobe, the hippocampus, fimbria fornix, and inferior horn of the lateral ventricle are seen. The inferior and superior cerebellar pontine cisterns are identified. The floor of the fourth ventricle is formed by the pons and medulla oblongata.

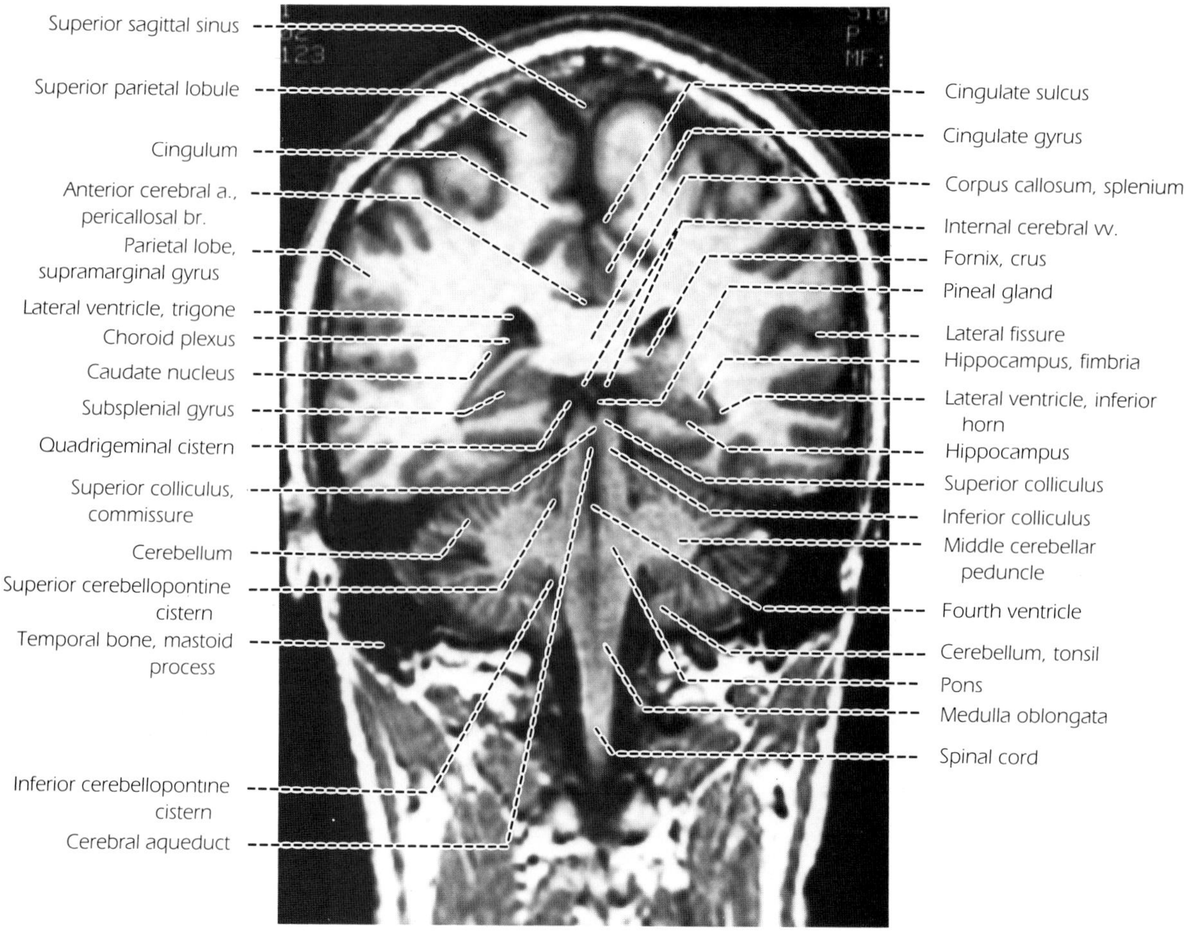
Superior sagittal sinus
Superior parietal lobule
Cingulum
Anterior cerebral a., pericallosal br.
Parietal lobe, supramarginal gyrus
Lateral ventricle, trigone
Choroid plexus
Caudate nucleus
Subsplenial gyrus
Quadrigeminal cistern
Superior colliculus, commissure
Cerebellum
Superior cerebellopontine cistern
Temporal bone, mastoid process
Inferior cerebellopontine cistern
Cerebral aqueduct
Cingulate sulcus
Cingulate gyrus
Corpus callosum, splenium
Internal cerebral vv.
Fornix, crus
Pineal gland
Lateral fissure
Hippocampus, fimbria
Lateral ventricle, inferior horn
Hippocampus
Superior colliculus
Inferior colliculus
Middle cerebellar peduncle
Fourth ventricle
Cerebellum, tonsil
Pons
Medulla oblongata
Spinal cord

Coronal T1-weighted image through the splenium of the corpus callosum. The splenium connects the two cerebral hemispheres. Dorsal to the splenium are branches of the anterior cerebral artery and the cingulate gyrus. Within the cingulate gyrus is the cingulum, one of the long association fiber bundles. The cingulate sulcus is the dorsal boundary of the cingulate gyrus. Callosomarginal branches of the anterior cerebral artery are found dorsal to the cingulate gyrus. The caudate nucleus is in the lateral wall of the trigone of the lateral ventricle. In the white matter of the hemisphere, lateral to the trigone, is the visual radiation. The quadrigeminal cistern is dorsal to the inferior colliculi. The middle cerebellar peduncle connects the pons and cerebellum. The superior cerebellar peduncle (brachium conjunctivum) connects the cerebellum with the midbrain. The area postrema is seen rostrally in the medulla oblongata. The floor of the fourth ventricle is formed by the pons and medulla oblongata. The spinal cord extends from the medulla oblongata downward. The superior cerebellar hemisphere and cerebellar tonsils are seen. The close proximity of the cerebellar tonsils and medulla oblongata is evident. In the parietal lobe, the supramarginal gyrus is seen.

## Figure 1-115

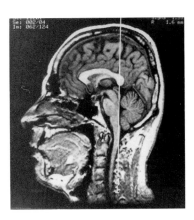

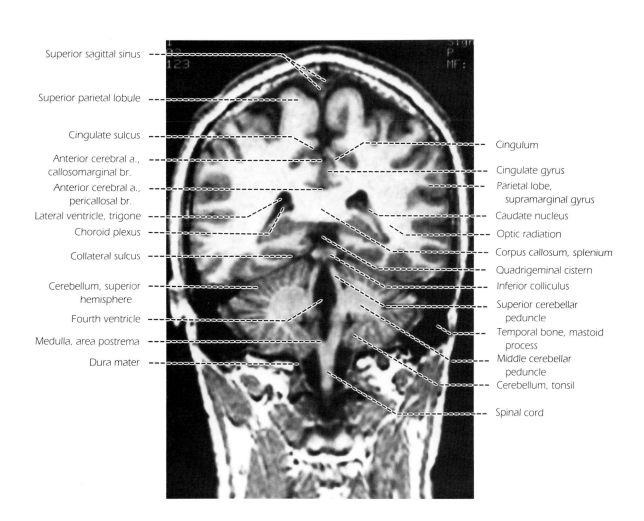

Superior sagittal sinus

Superior parietal lobule

Cingulate sulcus

Anterior cerebral a., callosomarginal br.

Anterior cerebral a., pericallosal br.

Lateral ventricle, trigone

Choroid plexus

Collateral sulcus

Cerebellum, superior hemisphere

Fourth ventricle

Medulla, area postrema

Dura mater

Cingulum

Cingulate gyrus

Parietal lobe, supramarginal gyrus

Caudate nucleus

Optic radiation

Corpus callosum, splenium

Quadrigeminal cistern

Inferior colliculus

Superior cerebellar peduncle

Temporal bone, mastoid process

Middle cerebellar peduncle

Cerebellum, tonsil

Spinal cord

# Figure 1-116

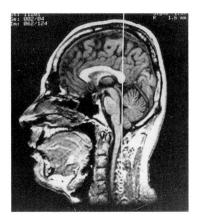

Coronal T1-weighted image through the splenium of the corpus callosum. The splenium connects the two cerebral hemispheres. Dorsal to the splenium are branches of the anterior cerebral artery and the cingulate gyrus. Dorsal to the cingulate gyrus is the cingulate sulcus. The cingulum forms the deep white matter core of the cingulate gyrus. The trigone of the lateral ventricle is seen lateral to the splenium. The choroid plexus is seen within the trigone. Within the parietal lobe, the supramarginal gyrus is seen. Ventral to the splenium are the internal cerebral veins. Lateral to the trigone of the lateral ventricle, within the white matter core of the cerebral hemisphere, is the optic radiation. The cerebellum is seen inferior to the cerebral hemispheres. The superior and middle cerebellar peduncles are seen within the white matter core of the cerebellum. The superior cerebellar peduncle is rostral to the middle cerebellar peduncle. The cisterna magna is located caudal to the cerebellum. The fourth ventricular cavity is seen between the two cerebellar hemispheres.

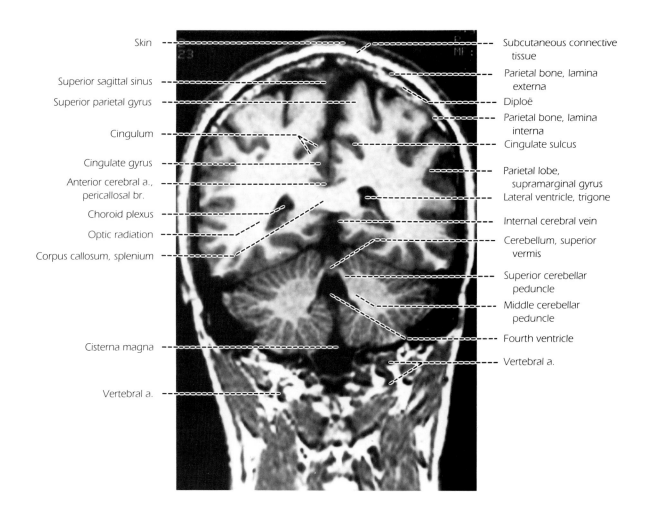

Coronal T1-weighted image through the splenium of the corpus callosum. The splenium connects the two cerebral hemispheres. Dorsal to the splenium is the cingulate gyrus. The cingulum forms the white matter core of the cingulate gyrus. The cingulate sulcus delineates the dorsal boundary of the cingulate gyrus. Dorsal to the cingulate sulcus is the precuneus. Ventral and lateral to the precuneus is the angular gyrus of the parietal lobe. The trigone of the lateral ventricle is seen lateral to the splenium of the corpus callosum. Lateral to the trigone, within the white matter core of the cerebral hemisphere, is the optic radiation. Ventral to the splenium are the internal cerebral veins. Within the cerebellum, the cerebellar vermis and cerebellar hemispheres are seen. The superior medullary velum is also seen. The superior cerebellar peduncle, connecting the cerebellum with the midbrain, is in close proximity to the superior medullary velum. Caudal to the cerebellum is the cisterna magna.

## Figure 1-117

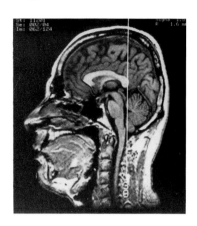

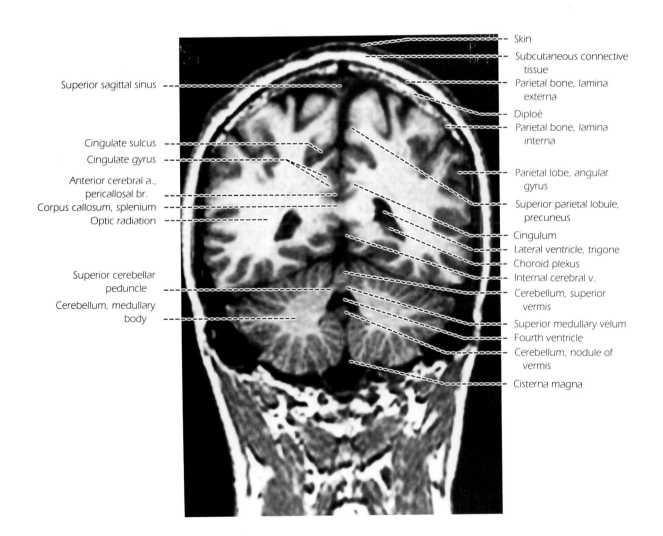

# Figure 1-118

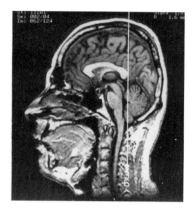

Coronal T1-weighted image through the trigone of the lateral ventricle. The interhemispheric fissure separates the two cerebral hemispheres. Within the parietal lobe, the precuneus is seen as part of the superior parietal lobule. The intraparietal sulcus separates the superior and inferior parietal lobules. Within the inferior parietal lobule is the angular gyrus. The trigone of the lateral ventricle is seen. Within the cerebellum, the superior vermis, superior medullary velum, and corpus medullare are seen. Caudal to the cerebellum is the cisterna magna. Lateral to the trigone of the lateral ventricle is the optic radiation.

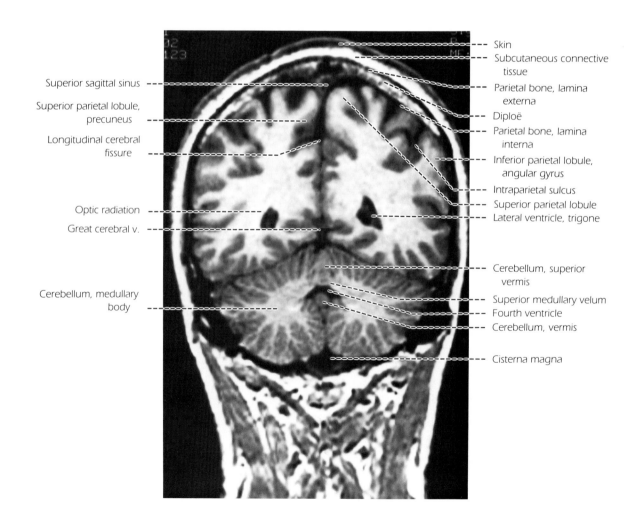

Coronal T1-weighted image through the parietal lobe. Within the parietal lobe, the superior and inferior parietal lobules are separated by the intraparietal sulcus. On the medial surface of the parietal lobe is the precuneus. The angular gyrus is seen within the inferior parietal lobule. The optic radiation is located in the deep white matter lateral to the ventricle. The tentorium cerebelli separates the cerebral hemispheres and cerebellum. Within the cerebellum, the vermis and cerebellar hemispheres are seen. Within the deep white matter core of the cerebellum is the dentate nucleus. The longitudinal cerebral fissure separates the two cerebral hemispheres.

## Figure 1-119

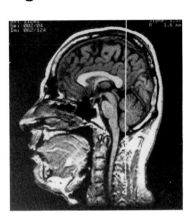

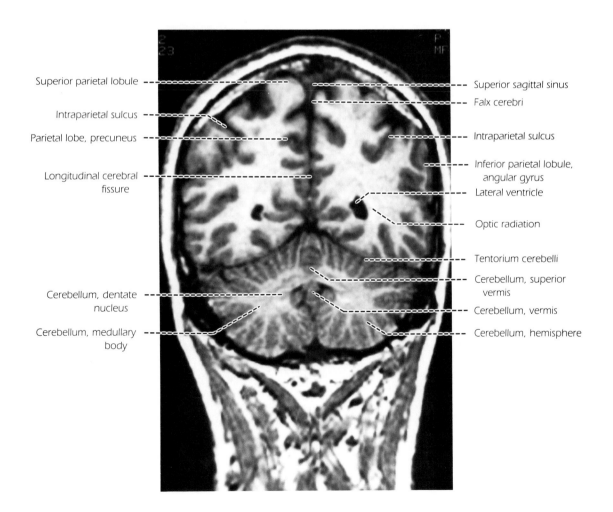

## Figure 1-120

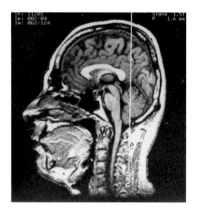

Coronal T1-weighted image through the parietal lobe. Within the parietal lobe, the superior parietal lobule is separated from the inferior parietal lobule by the intraparietal sulcus. Within the parietal lobe medially is the precuneus. The tentorium cerebelli separates the cerebrum from the cerebellum. Within the cerebellum, the corpus medullare is located deep within the cerebellum. The dentate nucleus is located within the corpus medullare. The transverse sinus is located laterally in relation to the tentorium cerebelli.

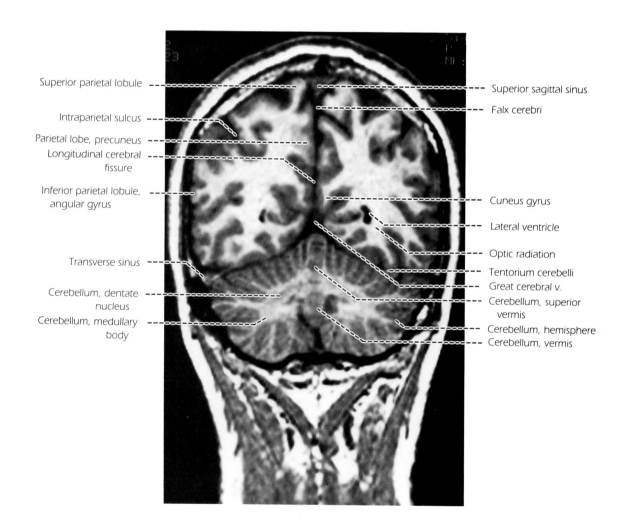

Coronal T1-weighted image through the parietal lobe and cerebellum. The longitudinal cerebral fissure separates the two cerebral hemispheres. The falx cerebri is located within the cerebral fissure. The superior sagittal sinus is located dorsal to the falx cerebri. The intraparietal sulcus separates the parietal lobe into superior and inferior parietal lobules. The angular gyrus is in the inferior parietal lobule. Within the parietal lobe, the precuneus is seen on each side of the longitudinal cerebral fissure. The visual radiation is found in the white matter core of the cerebral hemisphere lateral to the posterior horn of the lateral ventricle. The tentorium cerebelli separates the cerebral hemisphere from the cerebellum. The dentate nucleus is seen in the white matter core of the cerebellum.

## Figure 1-121

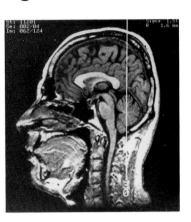

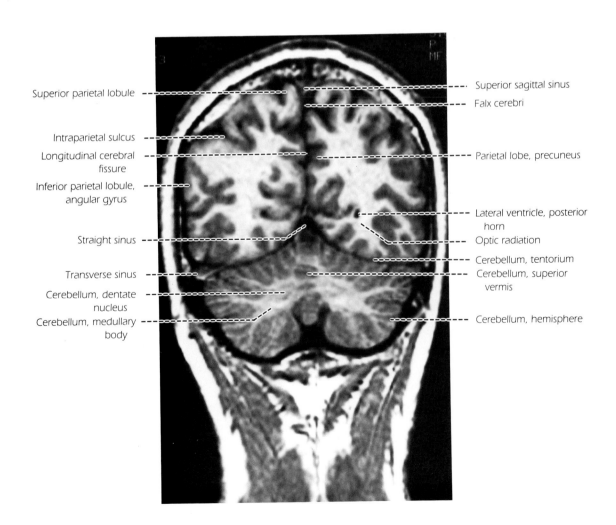

# Figure 1-122

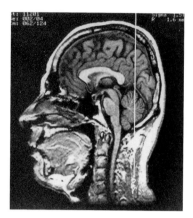

Coronal T1-weighted image through the parietal and occipital lobes and cerebellum. The longitudinal cerebral fissure separates the two hemispheres. The falx cerebri is located within the longitudinal cerebral fissure. The superior sagittal sinus is dorsal to the falx. The intraparietal sulcus separates the parietal lobe into superior and inferior parietal lobules. Within the inferior parietal lobule is the angular gyrus. The calcarine fissure separates the cuneus and lingual gyri. The visual radiation is seen within the white matter core of the occipital lobe. The tentorium cerebelli separates the cerebral hemisphere from the cerebellum. The dentate nucleus is found in the white matter core of the cerebellum.

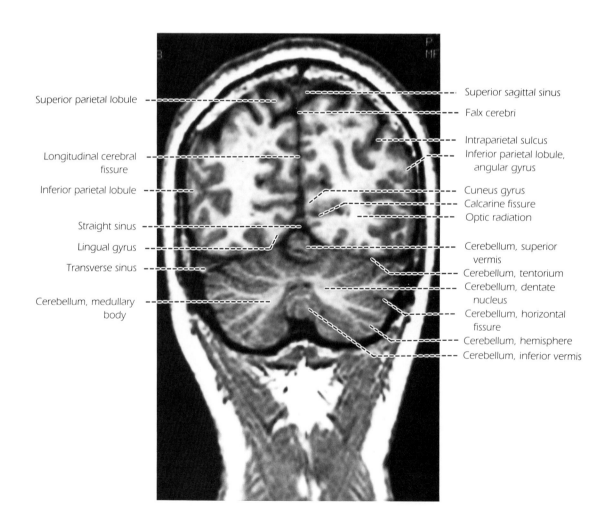

Coronal T1-weighted image through the posterior part of the cerebral hemisphere and cerebellum. The interhemispheric fissure separates the two cerebral hemispheres. The falx cerebri is located within the cerebral fissure. The superior sagittal sinus is dorsal to the falx cerebri. The calcarine fissure separates the cuneus and lingual gyri. Within the cerebellum, the corpus medullare, horizontal fissure, inferior vermis, and cerebellar hemispheres are seen.

## Figure 1-123

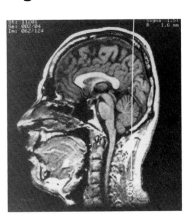

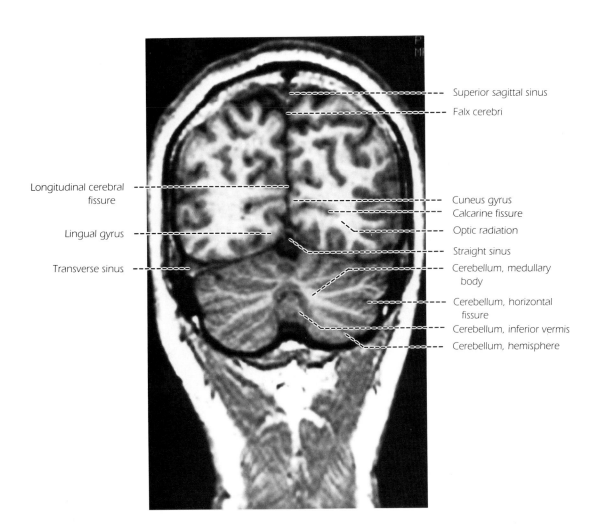

## Figure 1-124

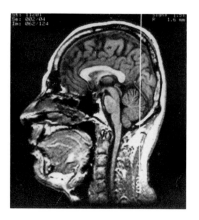

Coronal T1-weighted image through the occipital lobes and cerebellum. The longitudinal cerebral fissure separates the two cerebral hemispheres. The calcarine fissure separates the cuneus and lingual gyri. Within the cerebellum, the vermis is seen in the midline, and the cerebellar hemispheres are more laterally placed.

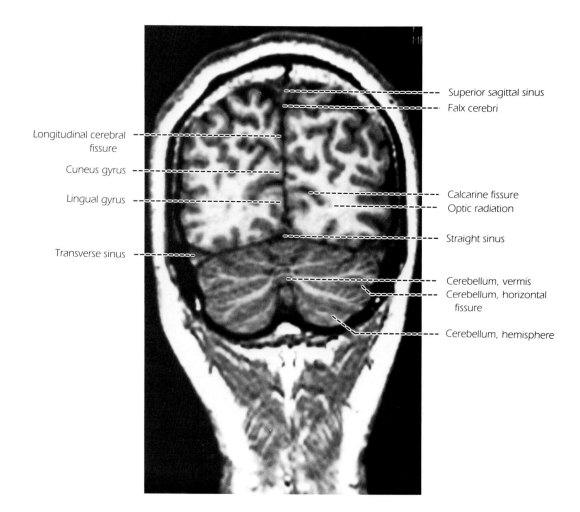

Coronal T1-weighted image through the occipital lobes and cerebellum. The longitudinal cerebral fissure separates the two cerebral hemispheres. The falx cerebri is seen within the longitudinal cerebral fissure. The calcarine fissure separates the cuneus and lingual gyri. Within the cerebellum, the cerebellar vermis and cerebellar hemispheres are seen. The tentorium cerebelli separates the cerebral hemispheres from the cerebellum.

## Figure 1-125

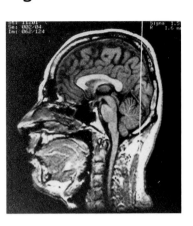

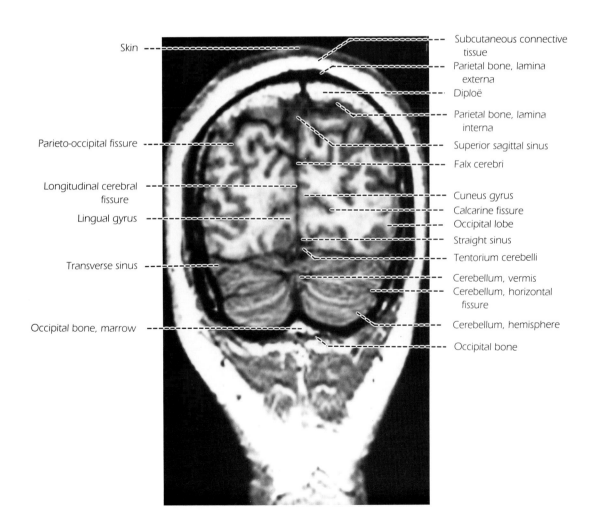

Skin
Subcutaneous connective tissue
Parietal bone, lamina externa
Diploë
Parietal bone, lamina interna
Parieto-occipital fissure
Superior sagittal sinus
Falx cerebri
Longitudinal cerebral fissure
Cuneus gyrus
Calcarine fissure
Lingual gyrus
Occipital lobe
Straight sinus
Tentorium cerebelli
Transverse sinus
Cerebellum, vermis
Cerebellum, horizontal fissure
Cerebellum, hemisphere
Occipital bone, marrow
Occipital bone

## Figure 1-126

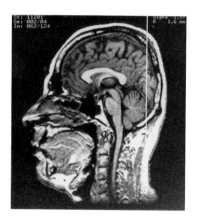

Coronal T1-weighted image through the occipital lobes and cerebellum. The longitudinal cerebral fissure separates the two hemispheres. The calcarine fissure separates the cuneus and lingual gyri. The tentorium cerebelli separates the occipital lobes from the cerebellum.

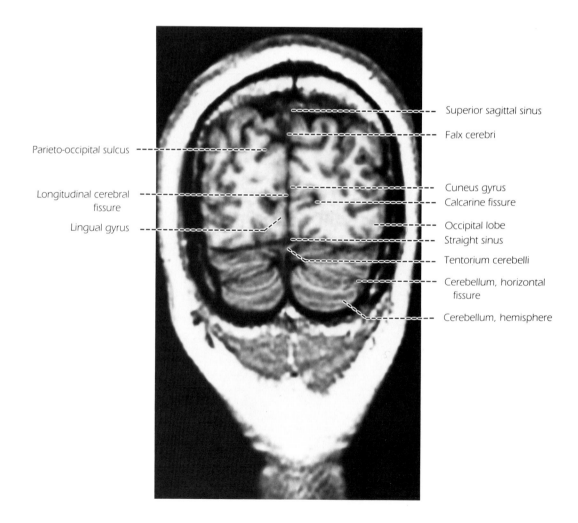

Coronal T1-weighted image through the occipital lobes and cerebellum. The calcarine sulcus is seen within the occipital lobe. The horizontal fissure of the cerebellum separates the cerebellum into dorsal and ventral surfaces.

## Figure 1-127

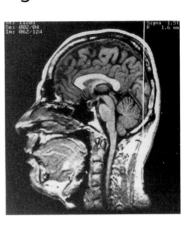

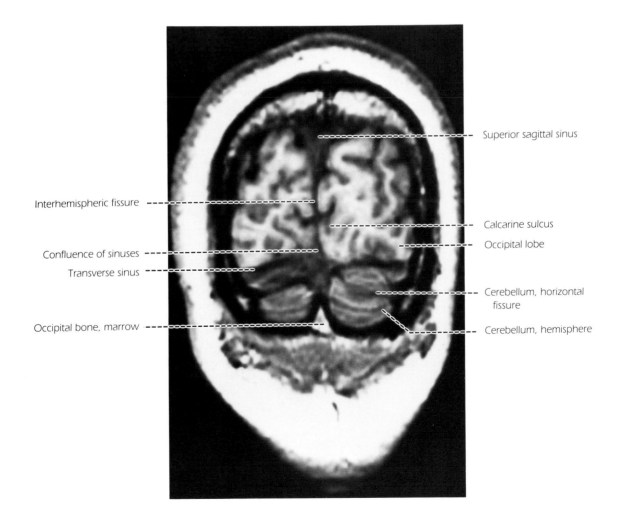

Interhemispheric fissure

Confluence of sinuses

Transverse sinus

Occipital bone, marrow

Superior sagittal sinus

Calcarine sulcus

Occipital lobe

Cerebellum, horizontal fissure

Cerebellum, hemisphere

# Figure 1-128

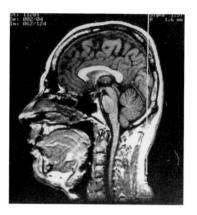

Coronal T1-weighted image through the occipital lobes and cerebellum. Within the occipital lobe, the calcarine sulcus separates the cuneus and lingual gyri. The confluence of sinuses is seen inferior to the occipital lobes. The horizontal fissure of the cerebellum separates the cerebellum into dorsal and ventral surfaces.

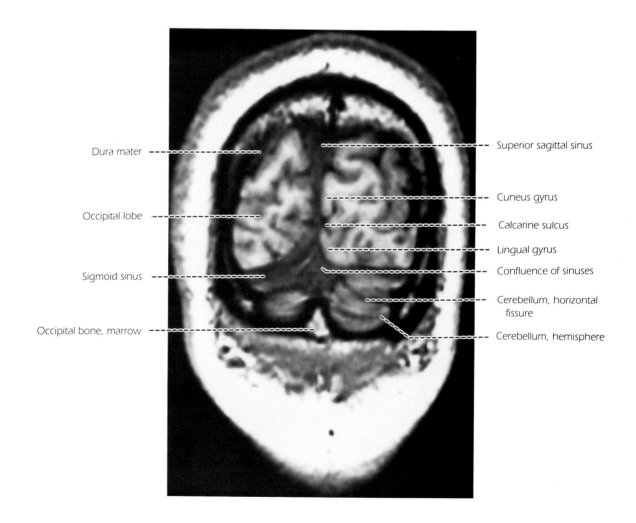

Dura mater

Occipital lobe

Sigmoid sinus

Occipital bone, marrow

Superior sagittal sinus

Cuneus gyrus

Calcarine sulcus

Lingual gyrus

Confluence of sinuses

Cerebellum, horizontal fissure

Cerebellum, hemisphere

Coronal T1-weighted image through the occipital pole. A small part of the cerebellar hemisphere is seen. The superior sagittal sinus is located between the two occipital lobes.

## Figure 1-129

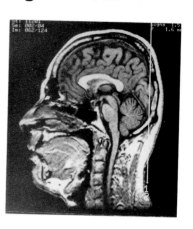

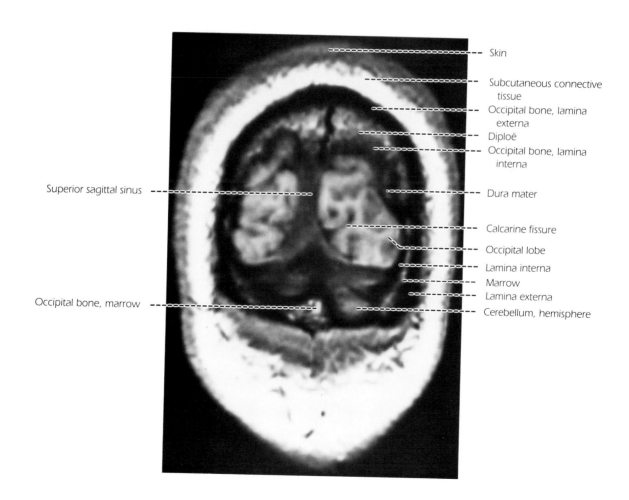

Skin

Subcutaneous connective tissue

Occipital bone, lamina externa

Diploë

Occipital bone, lamina interna

Dura mater

Calcarine fissure

Occipital lobe

Lamina interna

Marrow

Lamina externa

Cerebellum, hemisphere

Superior sagittal sinus

Occipital bone, marrow

## Figure 1-130

Coronal T1-weighted image through the occipital pole. The falx cerebri is seen between the two occipital poles.

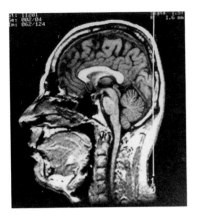

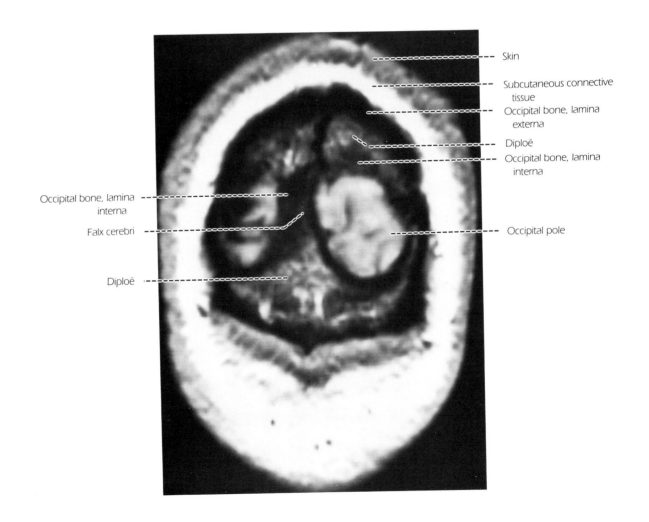

Coronal T1-weighted image through the occipital pole.

## Figure 1-131

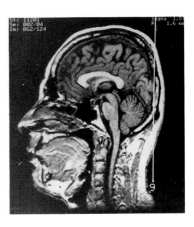

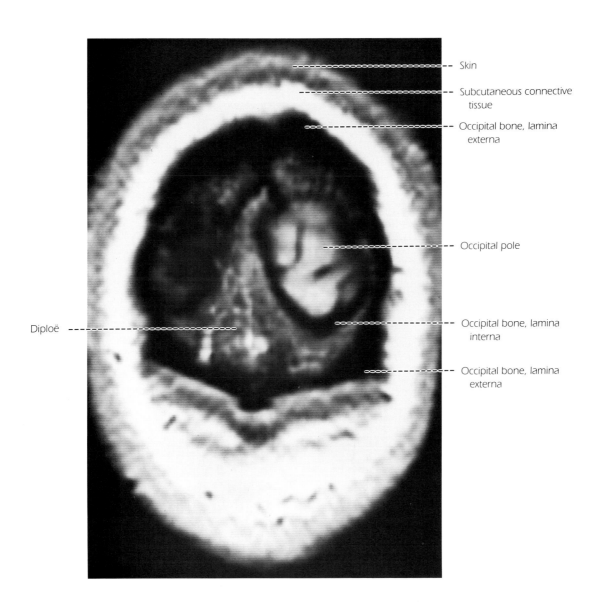

Skin

Subcutaneous connective tissue

Occipital bone, lamina externa

Occipital pole

Diploë

Occipital bone, lamina interna

Occipital bone, lamina externa

## Figure 1-132

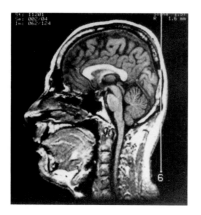

Coronal T1-weighted image through the occipital bone. No neural tissue is seen in this section. The lamina externa of the occipital bone and diploë are seen.

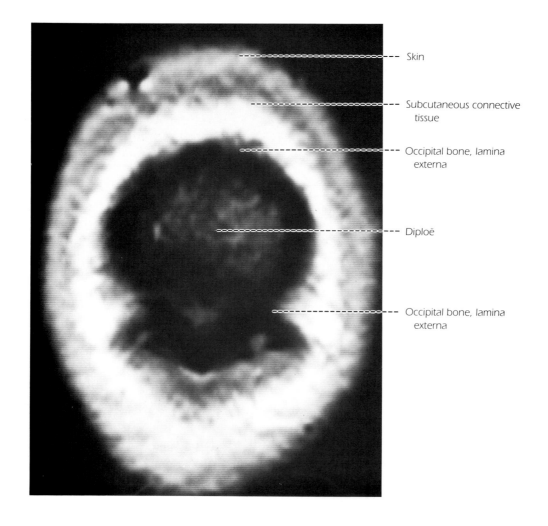

Coronal T2-weighted image of the frontal pole. The interhemispheric fissure (longitudinal cerebral fissure) separates the two hemispheres. The falx cerebri is found within the interhemispheric fissure. The superior sagittal sinus is within the falx cerebri. The crista galli is seen in the midline. The cribriform plate of the ethmoid is on each side of the crista galli. The muscles of extraocular movement include the inferior rectus, medial rectus, lateral rectus, and superior oblique muscles and are seen surrounding the eyeball. The levator palpebrae superioris of the eyelid is also seen. Other important structures seen in this section include the maxillary sinus, nasal septum, and inferior and middle turbinate bones (conchae).

Figure 1-133

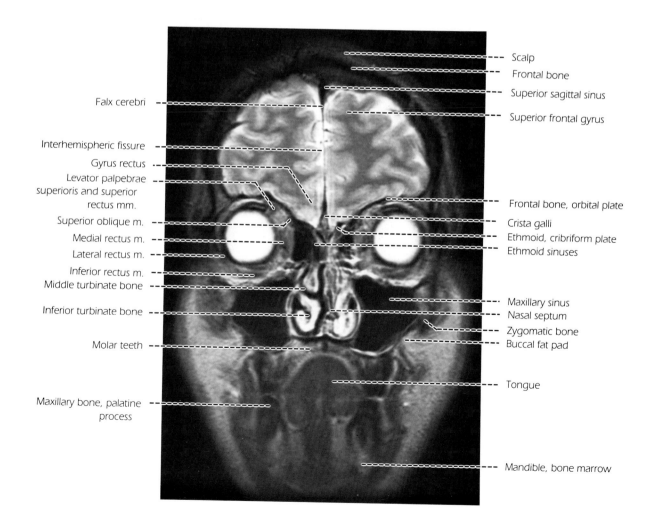

Falx cerebri

Interhemispheric fissure

Gyrus rectus

Levator palpebrae superioris and superior rectus mm.

Superior oblique m.

Medial rectus m.

Lateral rectus m.

Inferior rectus m.

Middle turbinate bone

Inferior turbinate bone

Molar teeth

Maxillary bone, palatine process

Scalp

Frontal bone

Superior sagittal sinus

Superior frontal gyrus

Frontal bone, orbital plate

Crista galli

Ethmoid, cribriform plate

Ethmoid sinuses

Maxillary sinus

Nasal septum

Zygomatic bone

Buccal fat pad

Tongue

Mandible, bone marrow

Figure 1-134

Coronal T2-weighted image through the frontal lobes. The superior frontal sulcus separates the superior and middle frontal gyri. The gyrus rectus is medial to the orbital gyrus in the floor of the frontal lobe. The crista galli and cribriform plate of the ethmoid are in the anterior midline. The inferior and middle conchae are seen in the wall of the nose. Several muscles of extraocular movement are seen including the superior oblique, lateral rectus, medial rectus, and inferior rectus muscles. Other muscles seen in this section include the levator palpebrae superioris, temporalis, and masseter muscles. Other important structures include the hard palate, tongue, mandible, alveolar process of the maxilla, and optic nerve.

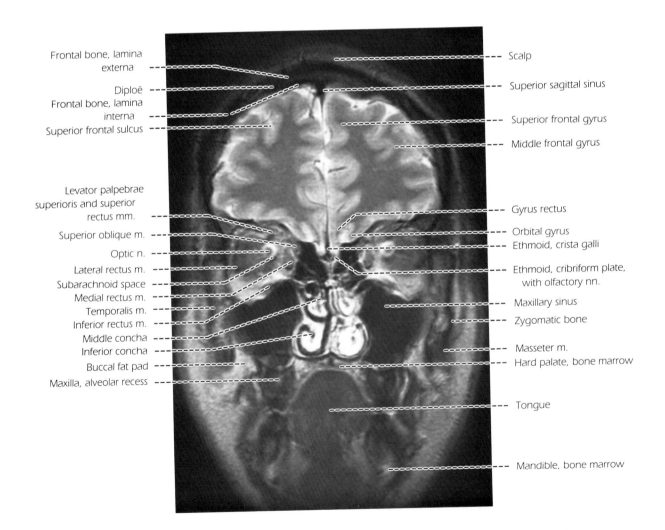

Frontal bone, lamina externa
Diploë
Frontal bone, lamina interna
Superior frontal sulcus

Levator palpebrae superioris and superior rectus mm.
Superior oblique m.
Optic n.
Lateral rectus m.
Subarachnoid space
Medial rectus m.
Temporalis m.
Inferior rectus m.
Middle concha
Inferior concha
Buccal fat pad
Maxilla, alveolar recess

Scalp
Superior sagittal sinus
Superior frontal gyrus
Middle frontal gyrus

Gyrus rectus
Orbital gyrus
Ethmoid, crista galli
Ethmoid, cribriform plate, with olfactory nn.
Maxillary sinus
Zygomatic bone
Masseter m.
Hard palate, bone marrow

Tongue

Mandible, bone marrow

Coronal T2-weighted image through the frontal lobes. The superior and middle frontal gyri are separated by the superior frontal sulcus. Inferiorly in the frontal lobe, the gyrus rectus is medial to the orbital gyrus. The anterior cerebral artery is seen between the two hemispheres. The superior sagittal sinus is seen dorsal to the cerebral hemisphere within the dura mater. Several of the muscles of extraocular movement are seen including the superior rectus, lateral rectus, medial rectus, and inferior rectus muscles. The levator palpebrae superioris muscle of the eyelid is also present. The optic nerve is seen within the periorbital fat. The superior, medial, and inferior conchae are seen in the wall of the nose. The nasal septum is seen separating the two nasal cavities. Other structures seen include the frontal bone, ethmoid sinus, frontal branch of the superficial temporal artery, zygomatic arch, soft palate, tongue, masseter muscle, and mandible.

Figure 1-135

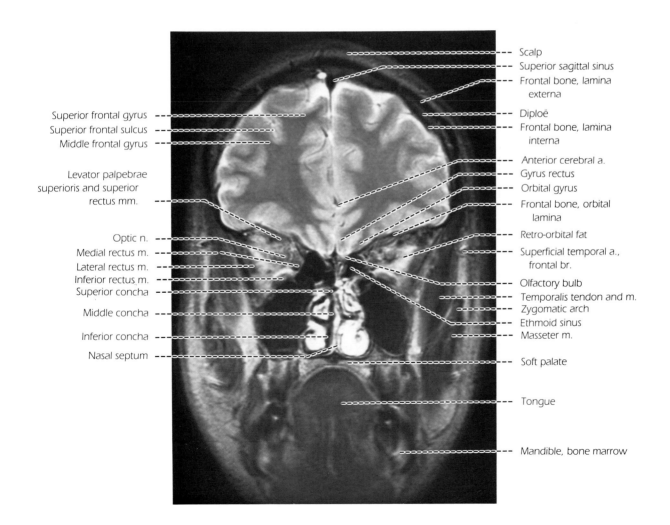

## Figure 1-136

Coronal T2-weighted image through the frontal lobe. The genu of the corpus callosum is seen connecting the two cerebral hemispheres. The most anterior part of the frontal horn of the lateral ventricle is seen. Dorsal to the corpus callosum is the cingulate gyrus. The cingulum is the white matter core of the cingulate gyrus. Anterior cerebral artery branches are seen dorsal and ventral to the genu of the corpus callosum. The superior frontal sulcus separates the superior and middle frontal gyri. The inferior frontal lobule is seen in the ventral part of the frontal lobe. A portion of the temporal lobe is seen beneath the frontal lobe. The superior sagittal sinus is seen within the dura mater dorsal to the cerebral hemisphere. Muscles in this section include temporalis, medial and lateral pterygoid, and masseter muscles. Other important structures include the lesser and greater wings of the sphenoid bone, common tendinous ring (Zinn's ring), nasal septum, inferior and middle conchae, parotid duct, mandible, lingual septum of the tongue, submandibular gland, soft palate, and zygomatic arch.

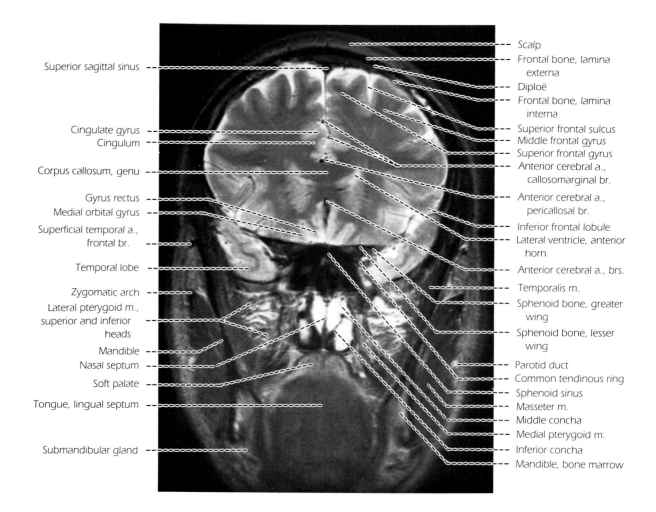

Coronal T2-weighted image through the frontal lobes and basal ganglia. The falx cerebri separates the two cerebral hemispheres. The superior sagittal sinus is located dorsally within the falx cerebri. The superior and middle frontal gyri are separated by the superior frontal sulcus. The corpus callosum is seen dorsal to the anterior horn of the lateral ventricle. Branches of the anterior cerebral artery are seen dorsal and ventral to the corpus callosum. The cingulate gyrus is also dorsal to the corpus callosum. The gyrus rectus is seen medially in the inferior part of the frontal lobe. The temporal lobe is seen inferior to the frontal lobe. The anterior limb of the internal capsule separates the head of the caudate nucleus from the adjacent putamen. External to the putamen is the external capsule. Other important structures include the optic canal, sphenoid sinus, temporalis muscle, zygomatic arch, lateral recess of the nasopharynx, eustachian tube orifice, nasopharynx, masseter muscle, soft palate, tongue, facial artery and vein, medial and lateral pterygoid muscles, and olfactory tracts.

# Figure 1-137

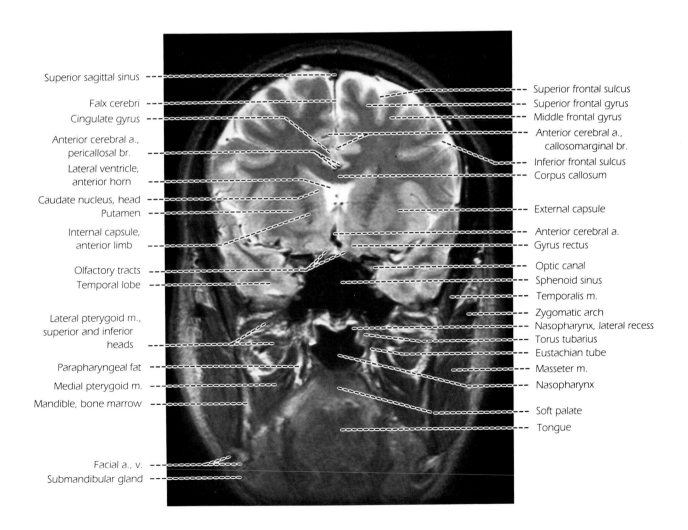

## Figure 1-138

Coronal T2-weighted image through the frontal lobes and striatum. The superior sagittal sinus is seen dorsal to the cerebral hemisphere. The corpus callosum connects the two cerebral hemispheres. Dorsal to the corpus callosum are anterior cerebral artery branches in the interhemispheric fissure. Ventral to the corpus callosum is the anterior (frontal) horn of the lateral ventricle. The two ventricular cavities are separated by the septum pellucidum. Ventral to the ventricular cavities is the fornix. The caudate nucleus bulges into the frontal horn of the lateral ventricle. The anterior limb of the internal capsule separates the caudate nucleus from the putamen nucleus. The hypophysis is in the midline ventrally. The internal carotid artery is seen close to the hypophysis. The optic chiasm is dorsal to the hypophysis. Close to the optic chiasm are branches of the anterior cerebral artery. The insular cortex is seen in the depth of the lateral fissure. The superficial temporal artery is lateral to the temporalis muscle. The cavernous sinus is medial to the temporal lobe and lateral to the hypophysis. Other structures seen in this section include the eustachian tube, uvula, the oropharynx and nasopharynx, mandible, torus tubarius, and parotid gland.

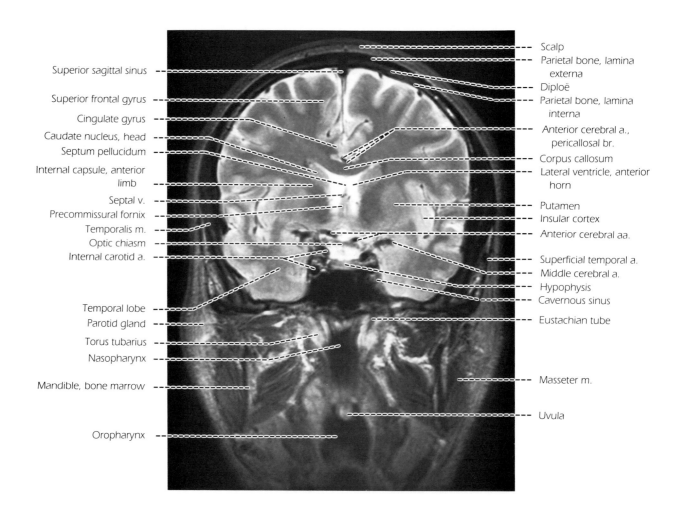

Figure 1-139

Coronal T2-weighted image through the frontal and temporal lobes showing the basal ganglia. The corpus callosum connects the two cerebral hemispheres. Dorsal to the corpus callosum is the cingulate gyrus. The pericallosal branches of the anterior cerebral artery are seen in the interhemispheric fissure. The falx cerebri and superior sagittal sinus are located between the two cerebral hemispheres. The lateral fissure separates the frontal and temporal lobes. Branches of the middle cerebral artery are seen deep within the lateral fissure. The septum pellucidum separates the two cavities of the lateral ventricle. Ventral to the septum pellucidum are the columns of the fornix. The anterior limb of the internal capsule separates the putamen and caudate nuclei. Medial to the putamen is the globus pallidus. The putamen and globus pallidus are referred to as the lentiform nucleus. On each side of the hypophysis are the internal carotid arteries. Other important structures include the eustachian tube, ramus of the mandible, parotid gland, and temporalis muscle.

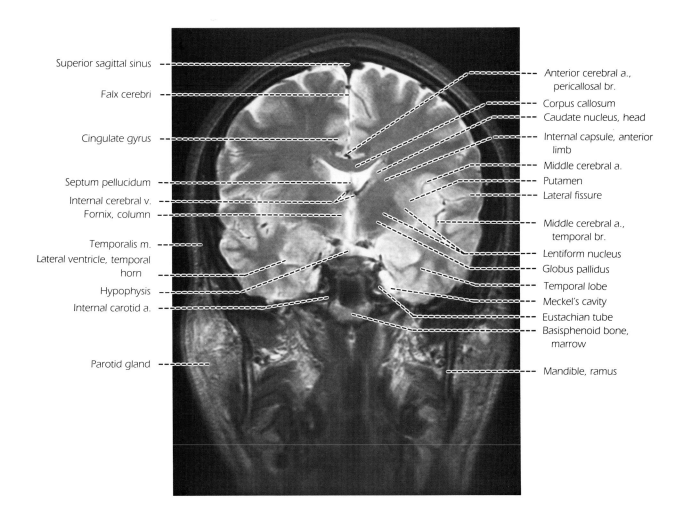

## Figure 1-140

Coronal T2-weighted image through the thalamus and third ventricle. The corpus callosum is seen connecting the two cerebral hemispheres. Dorsal to the corpus callosum are pericallosal branches of the anterior cerebral artery. The interhemispheric fissure separates the two hemispheres. Superficial to the hemispheres are the superior cerebral veins. The third ventricle separates the two thalami. Dorsal to the third ventricle are the internal cerebral veins. The caudate nucleus is located in the lateral wall of the lateral ventricle. Deep within the lateral fissure is the insular cortex. Branches of the middle cerebral artery are in the lateral fissure. The inferior horn of the lateral ventricle is found in the temporal lobe. The hippocampus is seen close to the inferior horn of the lateral ventricle. The basilar artery and the two posterior cerebral arteries are seen dorsal to the basiocciput.

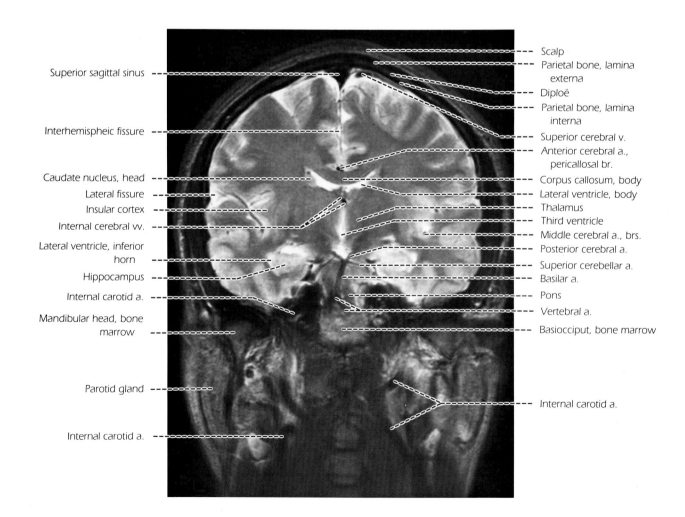

Superior sagittal sinus

Interhemispheic fissure

Caudate nucleus, head
Lateral fissure
Insular cortex
Internal cerebral vv.
Lateral ventricle, inferior horn
Hippocampus
Internal carotid a.
Mandibular head, bone marrow

Parotid gland

Internal carotid a.

Scalp
Parietal bone, lamina externa
Diploë
Parietal bone, lamina interna
Superior cerebral v.
Anterior cerebral a., pericallosal br.
Corpus callosum, body
Lateral ventricle, body
Thalamus
Third ventricle
Middle cerebral a., brs.
Posterior cerebral a.
Superior cerebellar a.
Basilar a.
Pons
Vertebral a.
Basiocciput, bone marrow

Internal carotid a.

Coronal T2-weighted image through the thalamus and third ventricle. The corpus callosum connects the two cerebral hemispheres. Dorsal to the corpus callosum is the cingulate gyrus. The pericallosal branches of the internal cerebral artery are also dorsal to the corpus callosum within the interhemispheric fissure. The falx cerebri is located in the interhemispheric fissure. The superior sagittal sinus is a fold of the falx cerebri. Superficial to the hemisphere are the superior cerebral veins. The head of the caudate nucleus is seen bulging into the lateral ventricle. Ventral to the ventricles are the columns of the fornix. The third ventricle separates the two thalami. Dorsal to the third ventricle are the internal cerebral veins. The lateral fissure separates the frontal and temporal lobes. Branches of the middle cerebral artery are deep within the lateral fissure. Within the temporal lobe, the hippocampus is seen in close proximity to the inferior horn of the lateral ventricle. The parahippocampal gyrus is inferior to the hippocampus. The interpeduncular cistern is seen between the two halves of the midbrain. Within the midbrain, the cerebral peduncle, substantia nigra, and red nucleus are seen. Ventral to the midbrain is the pons. The vertebral arteries are visualized ventral to the pons. Other important structures include the cochlea, internal jugular vein, internal carotid artery, atlanto-occipital joint, and occipital condyle.

# Figure 1-141

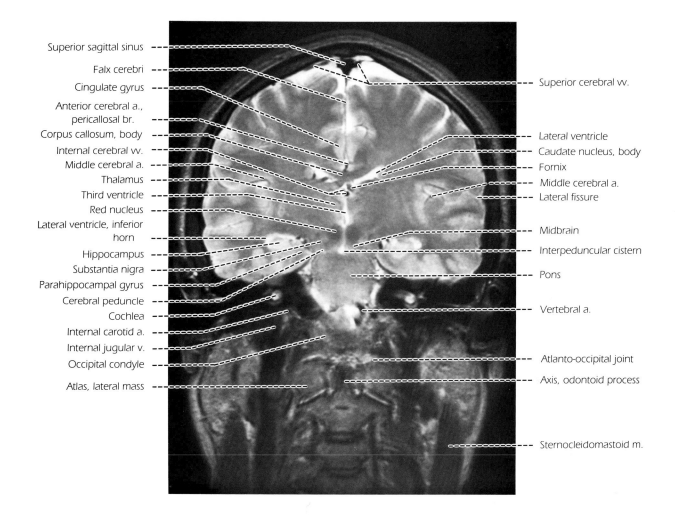

## Figure 1-142

Coronal T2-weighted image through the third ventricle, thalamus, and brain stem. The corpus callosum connects the two cerebral hemispheres. Beneath the corpus callosum is the fornix. The lateral ventricles are seen beneath the corpus callosum. Dorsal to the corpus callosum is the cingulate gyrus and pericallosal branches of the internal cerebral artery. The falx cerebri separates the two hemispheres. The superior sagittal sinus occupies a fold within the falx cerebri. The third ventricle separates the two thalami. The internal cerebral veins are found dorsal to the third ventricle. Ventral to the thalamus and the third ventricle is the red nucleus within the midbrain. The pons is surrounded by the superior and inferior cerebellar pontine cisterns. The ambient cistern (cisterna ambiens) surrounds the midbrain. The vertebral arteries are seen inferior to the medulla oblongata. The cochlea and semicircular canals are shown. In the temporal lobe, the parahippocampal gyrus is medial and ventral to the hippocampus. Close to the hippocampus is the inferior horn of the lateral ventricle. Other structures seen in this section include the odontoid process, transverse arch of the atlas, and occipital condyle.

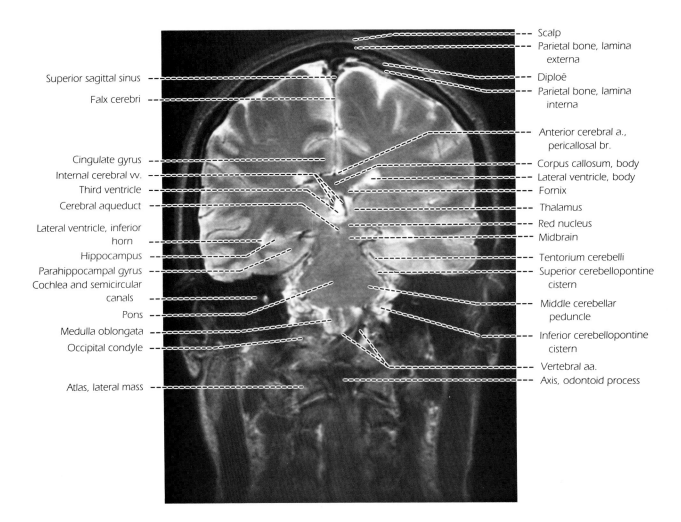

Coronal T2-weighted image through the cerebral hemispheres and brain stem. The corpus callosum connects the two cerebral hemispheres. Ventral to the corpus callosum are the lateral ventricles. Dorsal to the corpus callosum is the cingulate gyrus. The falx cerebri separates the two hemispheres. The superior cerebral veins are seen dorsal to the cerebral hemispheres. Dorsal to the superior and inferior colliculi are the internal cerebral veins. The inferior horn of the lateral ventricle is found in close proximity to the hippocampus. The middle cerebellar peduncle (brachium pontis) is seen connecting the pons with the cerebellum. The median sulcus of the floor of the fourth ventricle is seen in the midline. The inferior cerebellar pontine cistern is located between the pons and cerebellum. The spinal cord extends from the medulla downward. Other structures include the mastoid process of the temporal bone, foramen magnum, transverse arch of the atlas, and branches of the middle cerebral artery.

# Figure 1-143

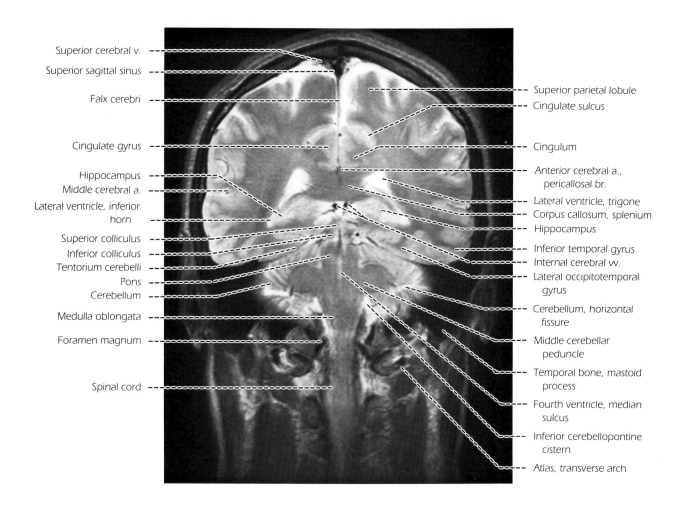

## Figure 1-144

Coronal T2-weighted image through the parietal and temporal lobes. The superior sagittal sinus is located between the two parietal lobes. Within the temporal lobe, the inferior temporal and lateral occipitotemporal gyri are found. The tentorium cerebelli separates the cerebral hemisphere from the cerebellum. Deep within the cerebellum is the corpus medullare, the white matter core of the cerebellum. The fourth ventricle is seen with the bright signal intensity of cerebrospinal fluid within it. The cisterna magna is caudal to the cerebellum. The horizontal fissure of the cerebellum divides it into dorsal and ventral surfaces. The optic radiation is seen as a decreased signal intensity lateral to the trigone of the lateral ventricle.

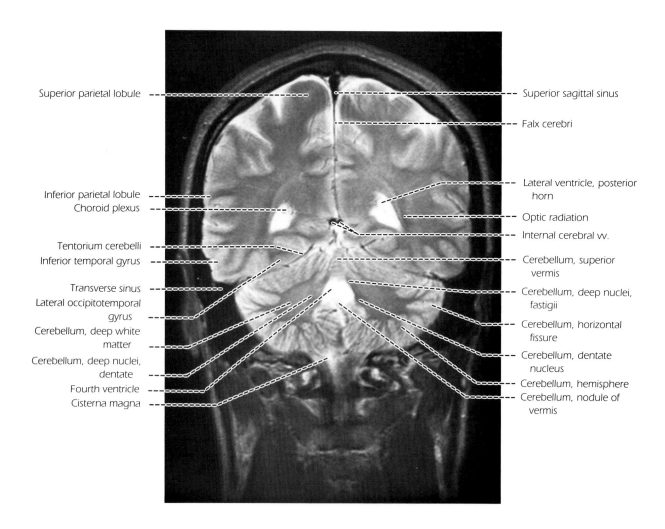

Superior parietal lobule

Inferior parietal lobule
Choroid plexus

Tentorium cerebelli
Inferior temporal gyrus

Transverse sinus
Lateral occipitotemporal gyrus
Cerebellum, deep white matter
Cerebellum, deep nuclei, dentate
Fourth ventricle
Cisterna magna

Superior sagittal sinus

Falx cerebri

Lateral ventricle, posterior horn

Optic radiation

Internal cerebral vv.

Cerebellum, superior vermis

Cerebellum, deep nuclei, fastigii

Cerebellum, horizontal fissure

Cerebellum, dentate nucleus

Cerebellum, hemisphere
Cerebellum, nodule of vermis

Coronal T2-weighted image of the parietal and occipital lobes. The superior sagittal sinus is seen between the two hemispheres. In the parietal lobe, the superior and inferior parietal lobules are seen. The optic radiation is found lateral to the lateral ventricle. The occipitotemporal gyrus of the temporal lobe is identified. The lingual gyrus is seen. Within the deep white matter core of the cerebellum, two of the deep cerebellar nuclei are found, the dentate more laterally and fastigi more medially. The superior cerebellar vermis is seen in the midline. The cerebellar hemispheres are seen laterally. Laterally located is the transverse sinus.

## Figure 1-145

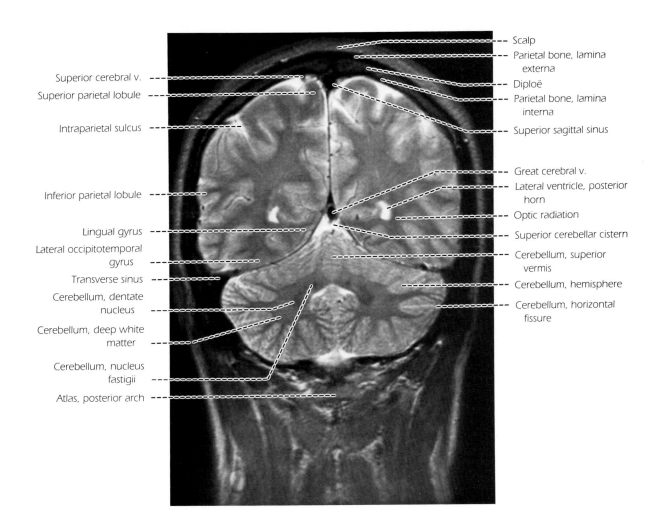

Scalp

Parietal bone, lamina externa

Superior cerebral v.

Diploë

Superior parietal lobule

Parietal bone, lamina interna

Intraparietal sulcus

Superior sagittal sinus

Great cerebral v.

Lateral ventricle, posterior horn

Inferior parietal lobule

Optic radiation

Lingual gyrus

Superior cerebellar cistern

Lateral occipitotemporal gyrus

Cerebellum, superior vermis

Transverse sinus

Cerebellum, hemisphere

Cerebellum, dentate nucleus

Cerebellum, horizontal fissure

Cerebellum, deep white matter

Cerebellum, nucleus fastigii

Atlas, posterior arch

# Figure 1-146

Coronal T2-weighted image through the occipital lobe and cerebellum. The lingual gyrus is seen ventral to the calcarine sulcus. The straight sinus is located between the two hemispheres ventrally, and the superior sagittal sinus is found between the two hemispheres dorsally. The superior cerebellar cistern is found dorsal to the cerebellum. In the cerebellum, the vermis and cerebellar hemisphere are seen.

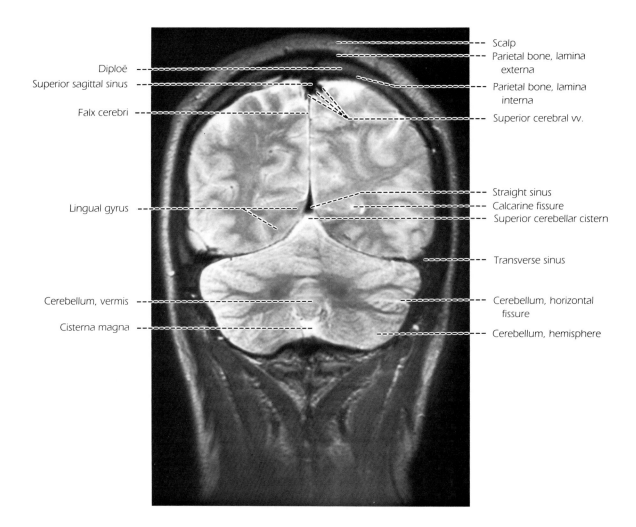

Coronal T2-weighted image through the occipital pole and cerebellum. The falx cerebri separates the two occipital lobes. The superior sagittal sinus is in the interhemispheric fissure. Superior cerebral veins are seen dorsal to the occipital lobe. The lingual gyrus is inferior to the calcarine fissure. The tentorium cerebelli separates the occipital lobe from the cerebellum. Within the cerebellum, the horizontal fissure separates the cerebellum into dorsal and ventral surfaces. The cerebellar vermis is located in the midline, and the cerebellar hemispheres are more laterally located. The transverse sinus is seen dorsal and lateral to the cerebellum.

## Figure 1-147

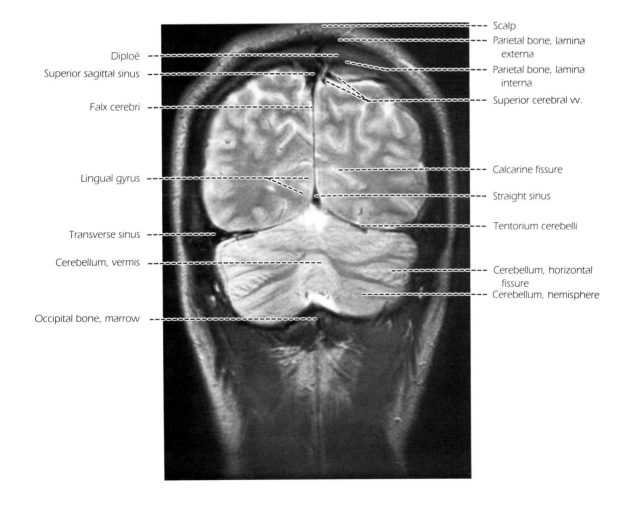

Scalp

Parietal bone, lamina externa

Diploë

Parietal bone, lamina interna

Superior sagittal sinus

Superior cerebral vv.

Falx cerebri

Lingual gyrus

Calcarine fissure

Straight sinus

Transverse sinus

Tentorium cerebelli

Cerebellum, vermis

Cerebellum, horizontal fissure

Cerebellum, hemisphere

Occipital bone, marrow

# SAGITTAL VIEWS

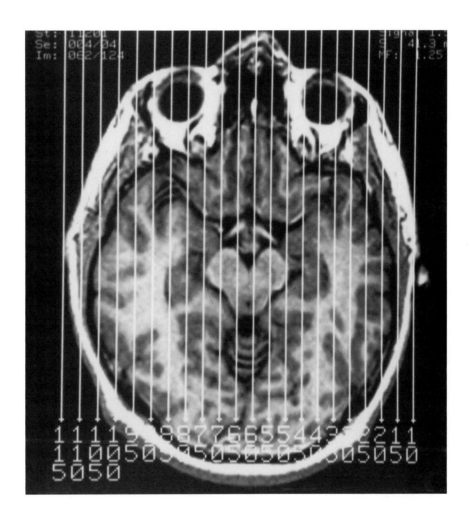

Key to the sagittal planes of inspection for T1-weighted images.

# Figure 1-148

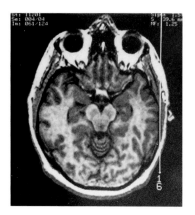

Superficial parasagittal T1-weighted image on the left side showing subcutaneous connective tissue, skin, and diploë.

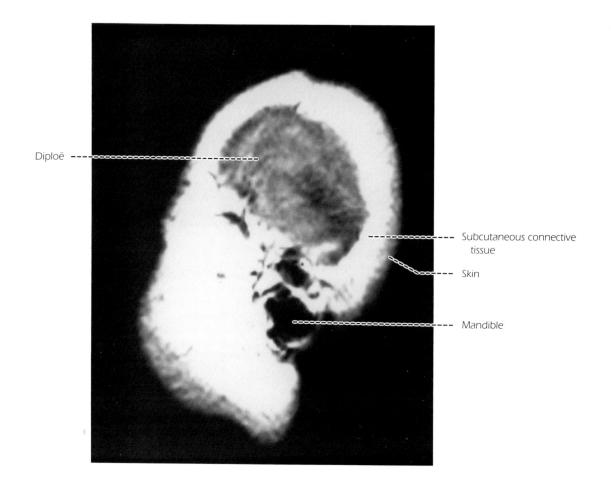

Superficial parasagittal T1-weighted image through the left temporal lobe showing the superior and middle temporal gyri. Bony and subcutaneous elements and skin are also seen.

Figure 1-149

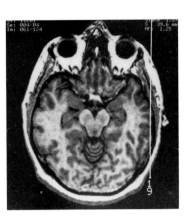

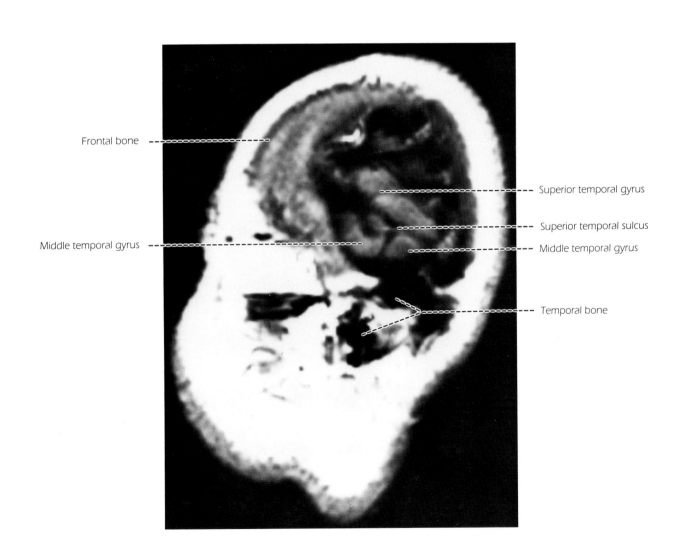

## Figure 1-150

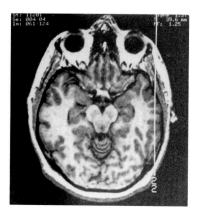

Parasagittal T1-weighted image through the left temporal lobe showing the lateral (sylvian) fissure and the superior and middle temporal gyri. The beginning of the inferior temporal gyrus is also seen. The mastoid process and zygomatic arch are shown. The fat component of the parotid gland is also demonstrated.

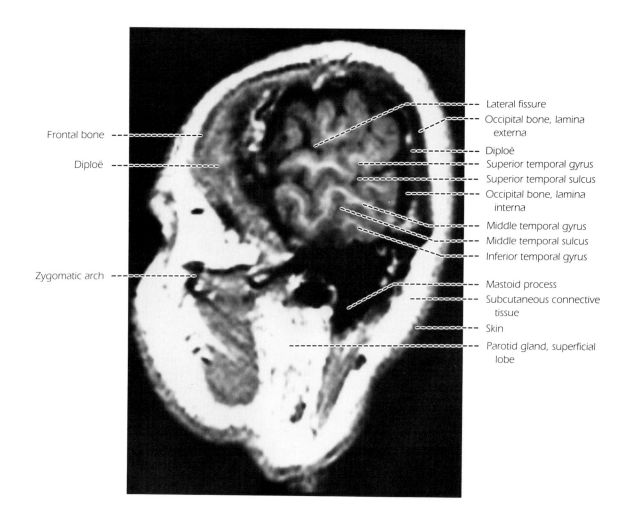

Parasagittal T1-weighted image through the left frontal, parietal, and temporal lobes. The dura mater covering the frontal lobe is seen. The lateral (sylvian) fissure is shown separating the temporal lobe from the frontal and parietal lobes. Within the temporal lobe, the superior temporal sulcus is shown separating the superior and middle temporal gyri. The middle temporal sulcus is also shown separating the middle and inferior temporal gyri. The bright signal intensity of fat within the parotid gland is seen. Other structures apparent in this section include the articular tubercle of the temporal bone, condylar process of the mandible, mastoid process, ramus of the mandible, and coronoid process of the mandible. The masseter and lateral pterygoid muscles are also seen.

## Figure 1-151

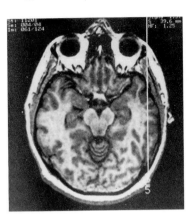

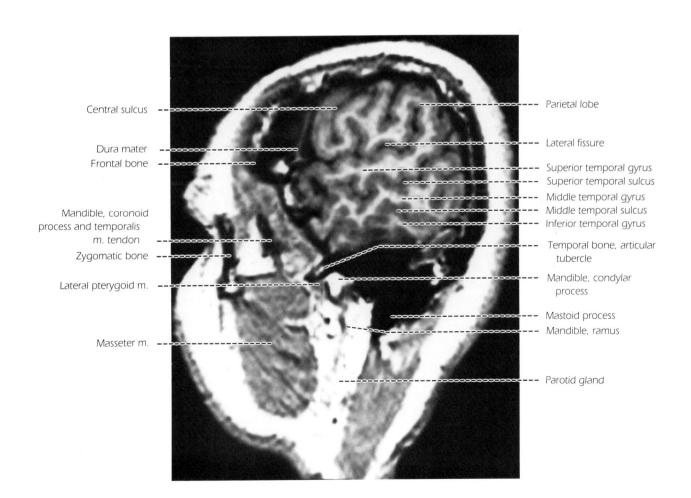

Central sulcus

Dura mater
Frontal bone

Mandible, coronoid process and temporalis m. tendon
Zygomatic bone

Lateral pterygoid m.

Masseter m.

Parietal lobe

Lateral fissure

Superior temporal gyrus
Superior temporal sulcus
Middle temporal gyrus
Middle temporal sulcus
Inferior temporal gyrus

Temporal bone, articular tubercle

Mandible, condylar process

Mastoid process
Mandible, ramus

Parotid gland

## Figure 1-152

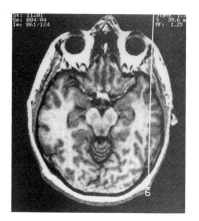

Parasagittal T1-weighted image of the left cerebral hemisphere showing the frontal, parietal, and temporal lobes. The lateral fissure is shown separating the frontal and parietal lobes from the temporal lobe. The supramarginal gyrus of the parietal lobe is shown capping the upper limit of the lateral fissure. In the temporal lobe, the superior, middle, and inferior temporal gyri are shown. They are separated by the superior and inferior temporal sulci. The angular gyrus of the parietal lobe is shown capping the upper end of the superior temporal sulcus. The bright signal intensity of fat within the parotid gland is seen. The sternocleidomastoid, masseter, lateral pterygoid, and temporalis muscles are shown. Bony landmarks include the occipital bone, articular tubercle of the temporal bone, mastoid process, condylar process of the mandible, ramus of the mandible, coronoid process of the mandible, and zygomatic bone.

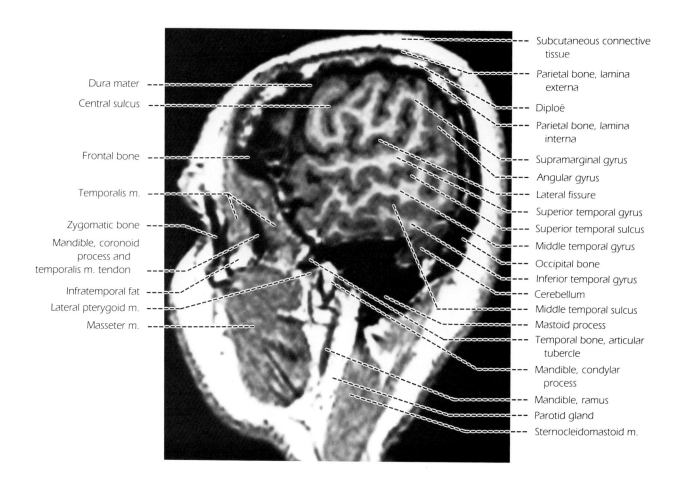

Parasagittal T1-weighted image through the left hemisphere showing the frontal, parietal, and temporal lobes. The lateral (sylvian) fissure is shown separating the frontal and parietal lobes from the temporal lobe. The dura mater is shown superficial to the frontal and parietal lobes. The central (rolandic) sulcus separates the pre- and postcentral gyri. The postcentral sulcus delineates the posterior boundary of the postcentral gyrus. Within the inferior frontal lobule, the two gyri forming Broca's area are shown. Within the parietal lobe, the supramarginal gyrus is shown capping the upper end of the lateral fissure. Within the temporal lobe, the superior and middle temporal gyri are shown separated by the superior temporal sulcus. Inferior to the middle temporal sulcus is the inferior temporal gyrus. The middle temporal sulcus separates the middle and inferior temporal gyri. Several muscles are shown in this section including the masseter, lateral pterygoid, and temporalis muscles. Bony structures shown include the articular tubercle of the temporal bone, condylar process of the mandible, mastoid process of the temporal bone, ramus of the mandible, and zygomatic bone.

# Figure 1-153

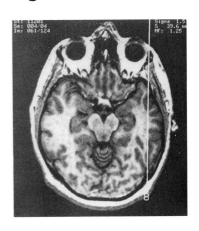

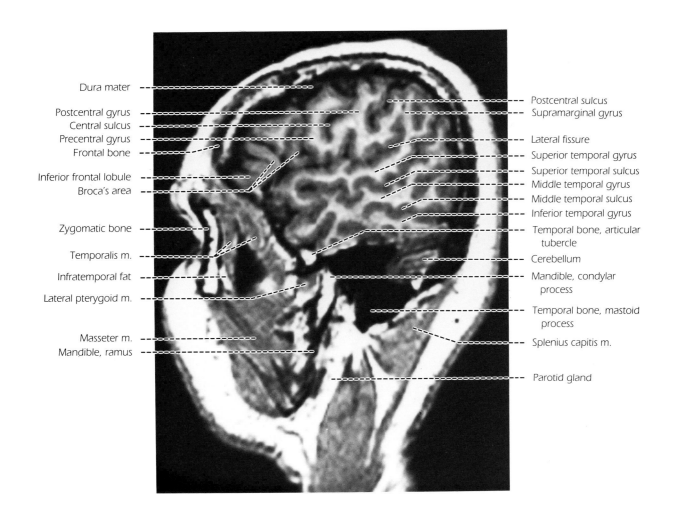

## Figure 1-154

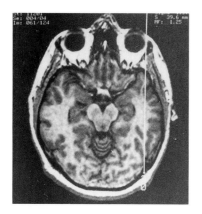

Parasagittal T1-weighted image through the frontal, parietal, and temporal lobes. The lateral fissure separates the frontal and parietal lobes from the temporal lobes. It is capped at its posterior end by the supramarginal gyrus of the parietal lobe. The central sulcus is shown separating the precentral and postcentral gyri. The postcentral sulcus delineates the posterior boundary of the postcentral gyrus. Anterior to the precentral sulcus is Broca's area of motor speech. The tentorium cerebelli is shown separating the cerebral hemisphere from the cerebellum. Bony landmarks shown in this section include the articular tubercle of the temporal bone, condylar process of the mandible, mastoid process, ramus of the mandible, zygomatic bone, and frontal bone. Muscles found in this section include the splenius capitis, masseter, lateral pterygoid, and temporalis muscles.

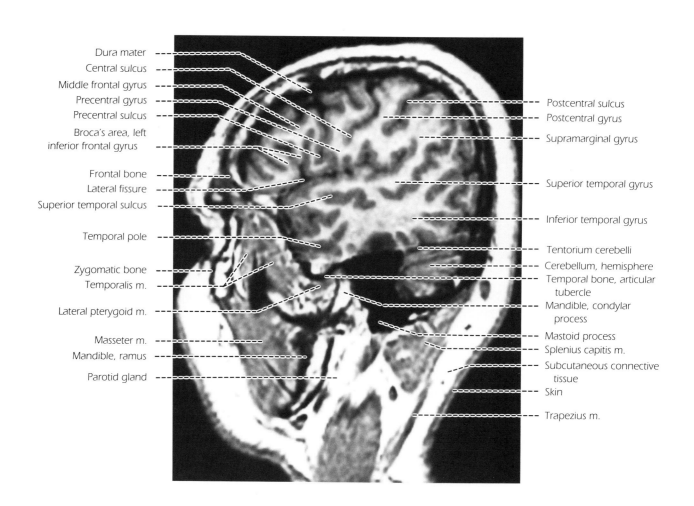

Parasagittal T1-weighted image through the frontal, parietal, and temporal lobes of the left cerebral hemisphere. The lateral (sylvian) fissure separates the frontal and parietal lobes from the temporal lobe. The supramarginal gyrus of the parietal lobe is shown capping the upper end of the lateral fissure. Beneath the supramarginal gyrus is the angular gyrus of the parietal lobe. The central (rolandic) sulcus separates the pre- and postcentral gyri. The postcentral sulcus delineates the posterior boundary of the postcentral gyrus. Within the inferior frontal lobule are shown the opercular part of the inferior frontal lobule and the ascending anterior ramus of the lateral fissure. The inferior longitudinal fasciculus, one of the long association fiber bundles, is shown within the temporal lobe. The tentorium cerebelli separates the cerebral hemisphere from the cerebellum. Caudal to the tentorium cerebelli is the transverse venous sinus. Bony landmarks in this section include the articular tubercle of the temporal bone, mastoid process, ramus of the mandible, condylar process of the mandible, coronoid process of the mandible, maxilla, greater wing of the sphenoid bone, zygomatic bone, and frontal bone. The lacrimal gland is seen within the orbit. Muscles in this section include the masseter, lateral pterygoid, and temporalis muscles.

## Figure 1-155

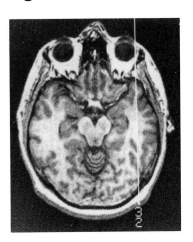

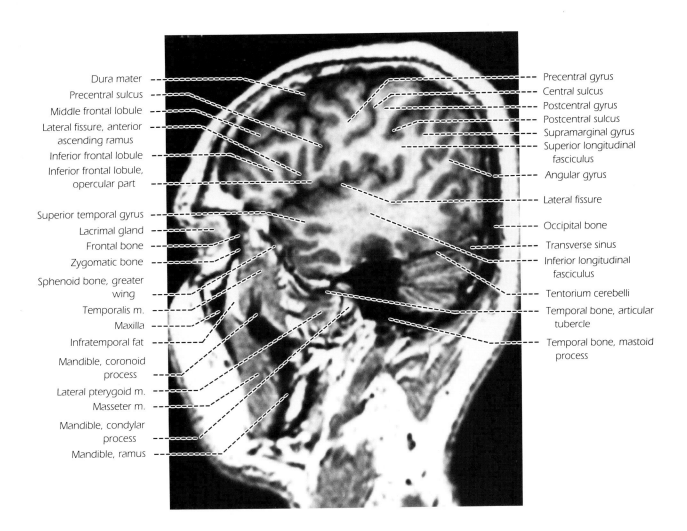

Dura mater
Precentral sulcus
Middle frontal lobule
Lateral fissure, anterior ascending ramus
Inferior frontal lobule
Inferior frontal lobule, opercular part

Superior temporal gyrus
Lacrimal gland
Frontal bone
Zygomatic bone
Sphenoid bone, greater wing
Temporalis m.
Maxilla
Infratemporal fat
Mandible, coronoid process
Lateral pterygoid m.
Masseter m.
Mandible, condylar process
Mandible, ramus

Precentral gyrus
Central sulcus
Postcentral gyrus
Postcentral sulcus
Supramarginal gyrus
Superior longitudinal fasciculus
Angular gyrus
Lateral fissure
Occipital bone
Transverse sinus
Inferior longitudinal fasciculus
Tentorium cerebelli
Temporal bone, articular tubercle
Temporal bone, mastoid process

# Figure 1-156

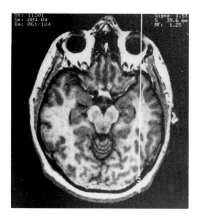

Parasagittal T1-weighted image through the frontal, parietal, and temporal lobes. The lateral fissure is shown separating the frontal and parietal lobes above from the temporal lobe below. The supramarginal gyrus of the parietal lobe caps the upper end of the lateral fissure. The central sulcus separates the frontal and parietal lobes. Rostral to the central sulcus is the precentral gyrus, and caudal to it is the postcentral gyrus. The postcentral sulcus delineates the posterior boundary of the postcentral gyrus. The opercular part of the inferior frontal lobule is seen anterior to the precentral gyrus. Within the temporal lobe, the inferior longitudinal fasciculus, one of the long association fiber bundles, is seen. Within the parietal lobe, another long association fiber bundle, the superior longitudinal fasciculus, is shown. The tentorium cerebelli separates the cerebral hemisphere from the cerebellum. Caudal to the tentorium cerebelli is the transverse sinus. Bony landmarks shown in this section include the petrous part of the temporal bone, coronoid process of the mandible, zygomatic bone, and frontal bone.

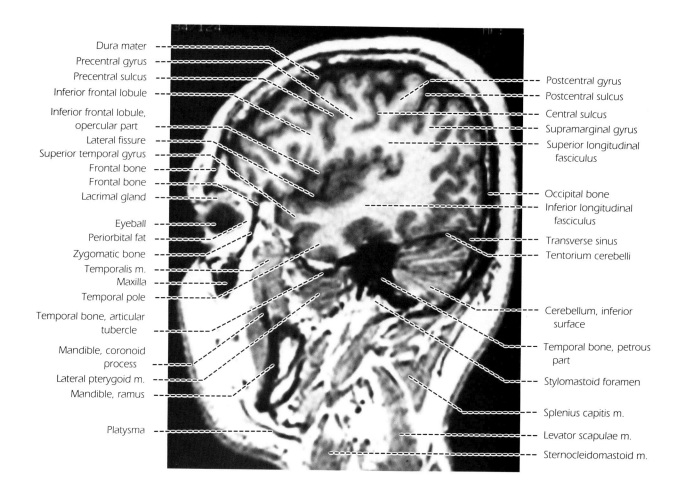

Parasagittal T1-weighted image through the insular cortex (island of Reil). In the frontal lobe, the precentral gyrus, orbital cortex, and ascending anterior ramus of the lateral fissure are shown. The postcentral gyrus of the parietal lobe is shown caudal to the central sulcus. The superior longitudinal (occipitofrontal) fasciculus, one of the long association fiber bundles, is seen in the white matter of the frontal and parietal lobes. The temporal or inferior optic radiation is shown within the temporal lobe. The tentorium cerebelli separates the cerebral hemisphere from the cerebellum. Within the eyeball, the cornea, anterior chamber, and lens are shown. Extraocular muscles shown in this section include the superior rectus, superior palpebrae, and inferior rectus muscles. The transverse venous sinus is shown caudal to the tentorium cerebelli. Bony landmarks include the petrous part of the temporal bone, mandible, greater wing of the sphenoid bone, and frontal bone. Several skeletal muscles are shown including the buccinator, medial pterygoid, temporalis, and lateral pterygoid muscles.

## Figure 1-157

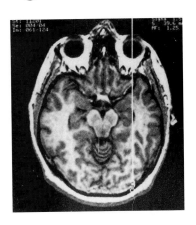

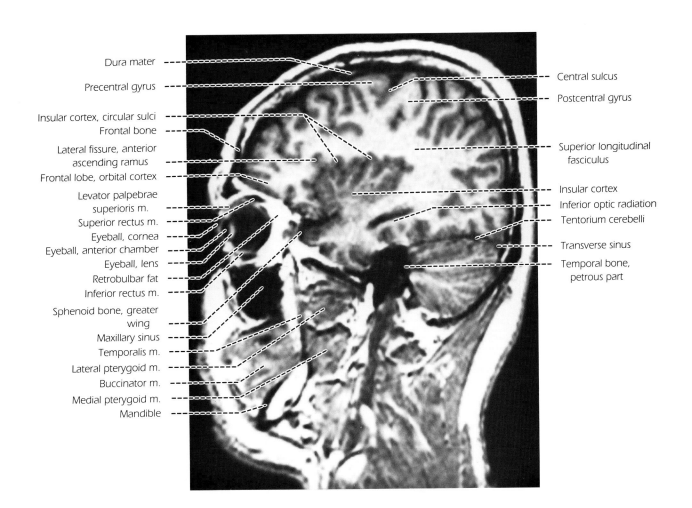

## Figure 1-158

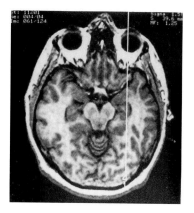

Parasagittal T1-weighted image through the left insular cortex (island of Reil). The insular cortex is surrounded by the circular sulcus. The central sulcus separates the frontal lobe from the parietal lobe. Rostral to the central sulcus is the precentral gyrus, and caudal to it is the postcentral gyrus. In the deep white matter of the frontal and parietal lobes is the superior longitudinal (occipitofrontal) fasciculus, one of the long association fiber bundles. The inferior or temporal optic radiation is shown inferior to the temporal horn of the lateral ventricle. The tentorium cerebelli separates the cerebral hemisphere from the cerebellum. Caudal to the tentorium cerebelli is the transverse venous sinus. Within the eyeball, the cornea, anterior chamber, and lens are shown. Several extraocular muscles are also shown in this section including the inferior rectus, superior rectus, and levator palpebrae superioris muscles. Above the orbit is the orbital cortex of the frontal lobe. Bony landmarks in this section include the petrous part of the temporal bone and the mandible. Several muscles are identified including the buccinator, medial and lateral pterygoid, and extraocular muscles. The maxillary sinus is seen.

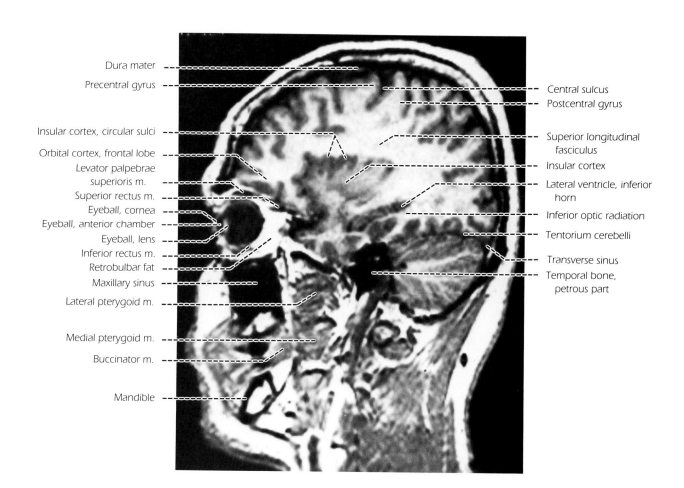

Parasagittal T1-weighted image through the left hemisphere at the level of the lentiform nucleus. The central sulcus separates the pre- and postcentral gyri. The corona radiata containing corticofugal as well as corticopetal fibers is shown in the deep white matter of the frontal and parietal lobes. The medial extension of the insular cortex is shown close to the lentiform nucleus. Caudal to the lentiform nucleus is the posterior limb of the internal capsule. The tentorium cerebelli separates the cerebral hemisphere from the cerebellum. The optic nerve is shown within the optic canal. Bony landmarks include the petrosal part of the temporal bone, mandible, and the first and second molar teeth. Several muscles are shown including the medial and lateral pterygoid, inferior oblique, inferior rectus, superior rectus, and levator palpebrae superioris muscles.

## Figure 1-159

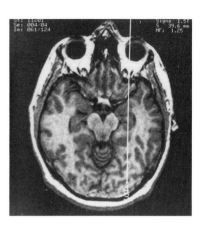

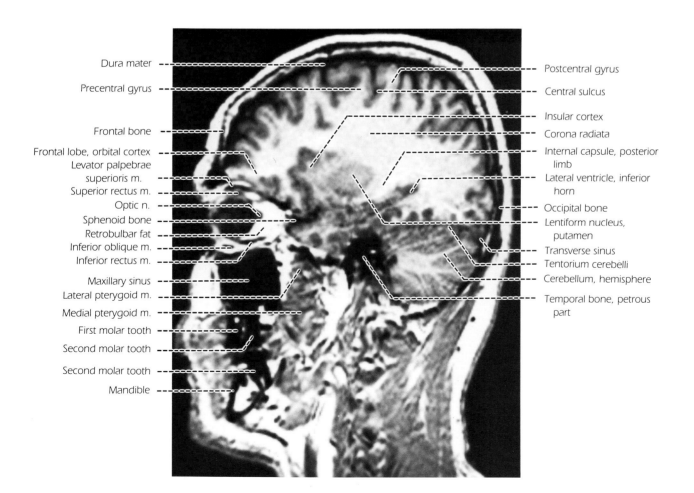

Dura mater
Precentral gyrus

Frontal bone
Frontal lobe, orbital cortex
Levator palpebrae superioris m.
Superior rectus m.
Optic n.
Sphenoid bone
Retrobulbar fat
Inferior oblique m.
Inferior rectus m.
Maxillary sinus
Lateral pterygoid m.
Medial pterygoid m.
First molar tooth
Second molar tooth
Second molar tooth
Mandible

Postcentral gyrus
Central sulcus
Insular cortex
Corona radiata
Internal capsule, posterior limb
Lateral ventricle, inferior horn
Occipital bone
Lentiform nucleus, putamen
Transverse sinus
Tentorium cerebelli
Cerebellum, hemisphere
Temporal bone, petrous part

## Figure 1-160

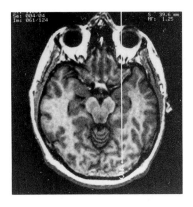

Parasagittal T1-weighted image through the left hemisphere at the level of the lentiform nucleus. The component of the lentiform nucleus shown in this section is the putamen. Caudal to the putamen is the posterior limb of the internal capsule. The corona radiata dominates the deep white matter of the frontal and parietal lobes. The central sulcus separates the frontal lobe from the parietal lobe. The pre- and postcentral gyri delineate the boundaries of the central sulcus. Anterior to the lentiform nucleus is the uncinate fasciculus, one of the long association fiber bundles connecting the frontal and temporal lobes. The optic radiation within the temporal lobe is shown inferior to the trigone of the lateral ventricle. The tentorium cerebelli separates the cerebral hemisphere from the cerebellum. The transverse sinus is caudal to the tentorium. The optic nerve is seen within the optic canal. Several bony landmarks are shown including the petrous part of the temporal bone, sphenoid bone, and frontal bone. The muscles located in this section include the splenius capitis, medial and lateral pterygoid, inferior rectus, inferior oblique, and superior oblique muscles. The maxillary sinus is also shown.

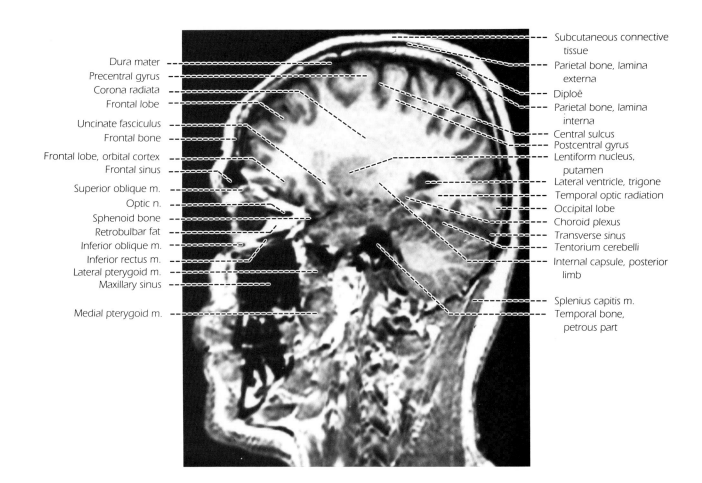

Parasagittal T1-weighted image of the left hemisphere through the putamen nucleus and thalamus. Rostral to the putamen is the uncinate fasciculus, one of the long association fiber bundles connecting the frontal and temporal lobes. The corona radiata dominates the deep white matter of the frontal and parietal lobes. The parietal component of the optic radiation is shown dorsal to the trigone of the lateral ventricle. The central sulcus separates the pre- and postcentral gyri of the frontal and parietal lobes, respectively. Within the temporal lobe, the hippocampus is shown. The fimbria of the fornix is shown arising from the hippocampus. Rostral to the fimbria is the thalamus. The tentorium cerebelli separates the occipital lobe from the cerebellum. Bony landmarks include the petrous part of the temporal bone, molar teeth, and maxilla. The maxillary and sphenoid sinuses are also shown.

## Figure 1-161

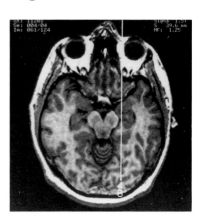

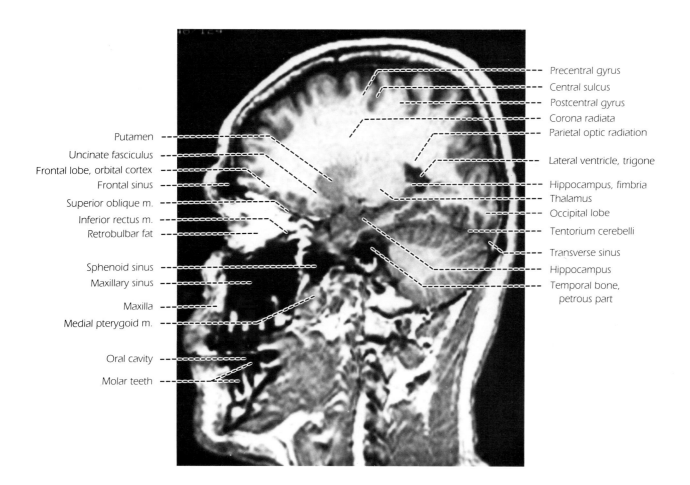

## Figure 1-162

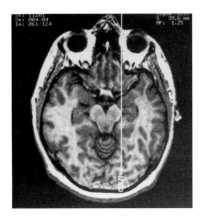

Parasagittal T1-weighted image through the left cerebral hemisphere at the level of the lentiform nucleus and thalamus. Between the lentiform nucleus and thalamus is the posterior limb of the internal capsule. Dorsal to the lentiform nucleus is the anterior limb of the internal capsule. The fimbria is shown arising from the hippocampus. The parietal part of the visual radiation is seen dorsal and posterior to the trigone of the lateral ventricle. The corona radiata dominates the deep white matter of the cerebral hemisphere. The uncinate fasciculus is shown anterior to the lentiform nucleus connecting the frontal and temporal lobes. The tentorium cerebelli separates the occipital lobe from the cerebellum. Bony landmarks shown in this section include the jugular tubercle, hypoglossal canal, occipital condyle, lateral mass of the atlas, mandible, and frontal bone. The trigeminal nerve is shown anterior to the cerebellum. The amygdaloid nucleus is anterior to the hippocampus within the temporal lobe. The orbital cortex of the frontal lobe is anterior to the uncinate fasciculus.

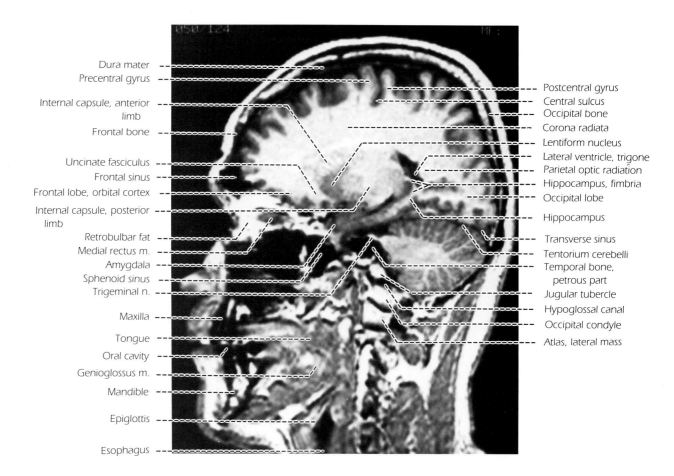

Parasagittal T1-weighted image of the left cerebral hemisphere through the thalamus and basal ganglia. Of the basal ganglia, the caudate nucleus, putamen, and globus pallidus are shown. The anterior limb of the internal capsule separates the head of the caudate nucleus from the putamen, whereas the posterior limb of the internal capsule separates the lentiform nucleus from the thalamus. The genu of the internal capsule is between the anterior and posterior limbs. The corpus callosum overlies the lateral ventricle. The parieto-occipital fissure separates the parietal and occipital lobes. The pulvinar nucleus of the thalamus is shown in the caudal part of the thalamus. The tentorium cerebelli separates the occipital lobe from the cerebellum. In the deep white matter of the cerebellum is the dentate nucleus. The middle cerebellar peduncle (brachium pontis) is shown entering the cerebellum. The uncus of the temporal lobe, optic tract, and orbital cortex of the frontal lobe are shown. The ethmoid and sphenoid sinuses are also shown. Nasal structures in this section include the nares and inferior concha.

## Figure 1-163

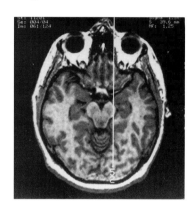

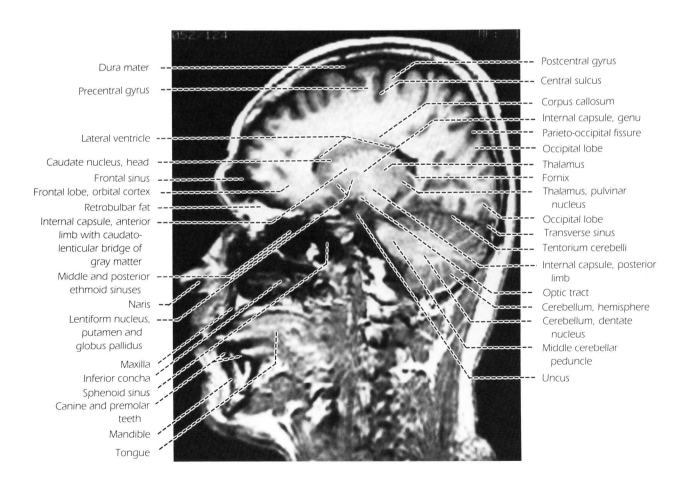

Dura mater

Precentral gyrus

Lateral ventricle

Caudate nucleus, head

Frontal sinus

Frontal lobe, orbital cortex

Retrobulbar fat

Internal capsule, anterior limb with caudato-lenticular bridge of gray matter

Middle and posterior ethmoid sinuses

Naris

Lentiform nucleus, putamen and globus pallidus

Maxilla

Inferior concha

Sphenoid sinus

Canine and premolar teeth

Mandible

Tongue

Postcentral gyrus

Central sulcus

Corpus callosum

Internal capsule, genu

Parieto-occipital fissure

Occipital lobe

Thalamus

Fornix

Thalamus, pulvinar nucleus

Occipital lobe

Transverse sinus

Tentorium cerebelli

Internal capsule, posterior limb

Optic tract

Cerebellum, hemisphere

Cerebellum, dentate nucleus

Middle cerebellar peduncle

Uncus

## Figure 1-164

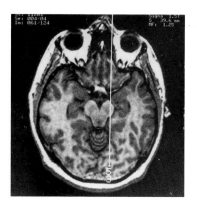

Parasagittal T1-weighted image through the basal ganglia and thalamus. Of the basal ganglia, the caudate nucleus, putamen, and globus pallidus are shown. The anterior limb of the internal capsule separates the head of the caudate nucleus from the putamen, whereas the posterior limb of the internal capsule separates the lentiform nucleus from the thalamus. The genu of the internal capsule is shown between the anterior and posterior limbs. The pulvinar of the thalamus is shown in the caudal part of the thalamus. Close to the pulvinar is the fornix. The central sulcus is shown separating the pre- and postcentral gyri. The parieto-occipital fissure separates the parietal and occipital lobes. The dentate nucleus of the cerebellum is found in the deep white matter. The tentorium cerebelli separates the occipital lobe from the cerebellum. The optic tract is located beneath the basal ganglia and internal capsule. Sphenoid and ethmoid sinuses are also shown. Bony landmarks in this section include the mandible, maxilla, and basiocciput.

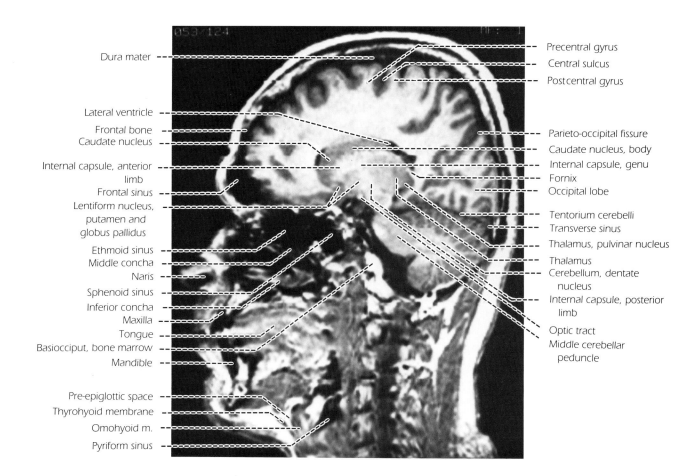

Parasagittal T1-weighted image through the basal ganglia and thalamus. Of the basal ganglia, the caudate and lentiform nuclei are shown. The anterior limb of the internal capsule separates the head of the caudate from the lentiform nucleus, whereas the posterior limb of the internal capsule separates the lentiform nucleus from the thalamus. The genu of the internal capsule is located between the anterior and posterior limbs. The pulvinar nucleus occupies a position in the caudal part of the thalamus. The fornix is shown dorsal to the thalamus. The parieto-occipital fissure is superior to the occipital lobe. The tentorium cerebelli separates the occipital lobe from the cerebellum. The dentate nucleus is in the cerebellar white matter. The basilar pons is shown in the ventral part of the pons. Bony landmarks include the occipital bone, mandible, maxilla, anterior arch of the atlas, and basiocciput. The frontal, ethmoid, and sphenoid sinuses are shown. The epiglottis is also shown.

## Figure 1-165

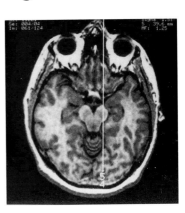

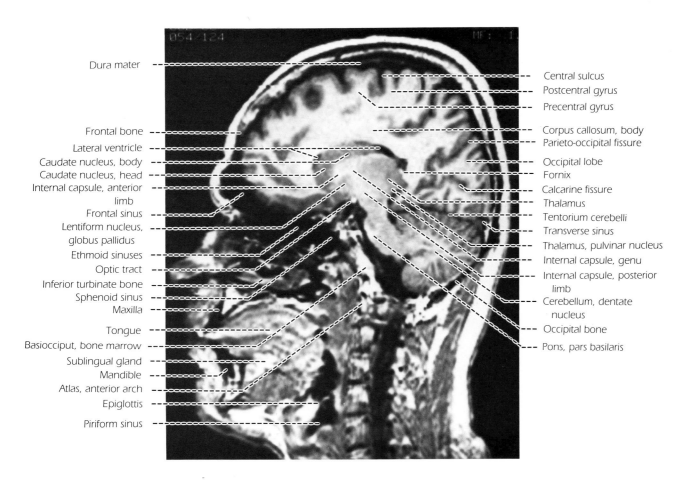

# Figure 1-166

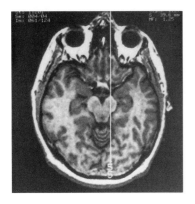

Parasagittal T1-weighted image of the left hemisphere through the thalamus and brain stem. Also shown is the head and body of the caudate nucleus. Dorsal to the body of the lateral ventricle is the body of the corpus callosum. Located within the lateral ventricle is the fornix. The pulvinar nucleus of the thalamus is shown occupying a caudal position in the thalamus. The parieto-occipital fissure separates the parietal and occipital lobes. The tentorium cerebelli separates the occipital lobe from the cerebellum. The middle cerebellar peduncle is shown connecting the pons with the cerebellum. Bony landmarks in this section include the cervical vertebral bodies, anterior arch of the atlas, maxilla, basiocciput, and frontal bone. The intervertebral disks separating cervical vertebrae are shown. The optic tract is shown beneath the thalamus, and the oculomotor nerve is shown leaving the midbrain.

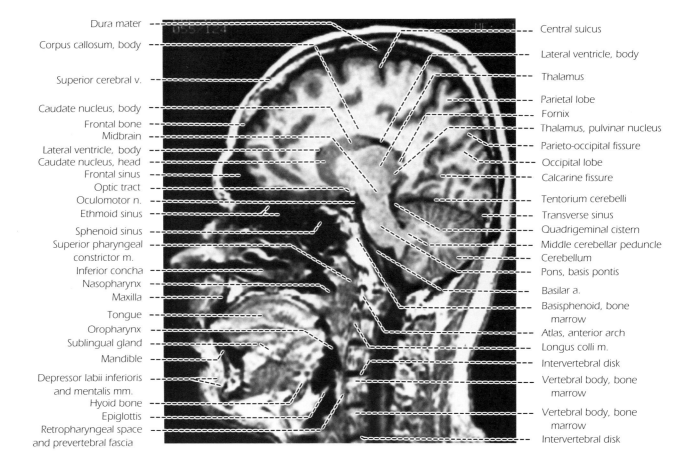

Dura mater

Corpus callosum, body

Superior cerebral v.

Caudate nucleus, body
Frontal bone
Midbrain
Lateral ventricle, body
Caudate nucleus, head
Frontal sinus
Optic tract
Oculomotor n.
Ethmoid sinus

Sphenoid sinus
Superior pharyngeal
constrictor m.
Inferior concha
Nasopharynx
Maxilla
Tongue
Oropharynx
Sublingual gland
Mandible

Depressor labii inferioris
and mentalis mm.
Hyoid bone
Epiglottis
Retropharyngeal space
and prevertebral fascia

Central sulcus

Lateral ventricle, body

Thalamus

Parietal lobe
Fornix
Thalamus, pulvinar nucleus
Parieto-occipital fissure
Occipital lobe
Calcarine fissure

Tentorium cerebelli

Transverse sinus
Quadrigeminal cistern
Middle cerebellar peduncle
Cerebellum
Pons, basis pontis

Basilar a.

Basisphenoid, bone
marrow
Atlas, anterior arch
Longus colli m.
Intervertebral disk

Vertebral body, bone
marrow

Vertebral body, bone
marrow
Intervertebral disk

Parasagittal T1-weighted image through the brain stem and cerebellum. The head of the caudate nucleus is shown bulging into the lateral ventricle. Above the lateral ventricle is the corpus callosum. The pulvinar nucleus of the thalamus is shown occupying a caudal position in the thalamus. The fornix is shown within the lateral ventricle. Caudal to the thalamus is the inferior colliculus. Ventral to the colliculus is the substantia nigra. The tentorium cerebelli separates the occipital lobe from the cerebellum. Caudal to the tentorium is the transverse sinus. The middle cerebellar peduncle is shown connecting the pons with the cerebellum. Caudal to the pons is the medulla oblongata. Beneath the pons is the prepontine cistern. The bright signal intensity of the optic tract is shown inferior to the thalamus. Bony landmarks in this section include the odontoid process (dens), posterior arch of the atlas, vertebral bodies of the cervical spine, hyoid bone, mandible, anterior arch of the atlas, maxilla, basisphenoid, and frontal bone. The frontal, ethmoid, and sphenoid sinuses are also shown. Other structures in this section include the soft palate, uvula, tongue, oropharynx, epiglottis, pharynx, larynx, and trachea.

# Figure 1-167

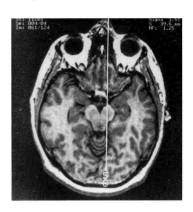

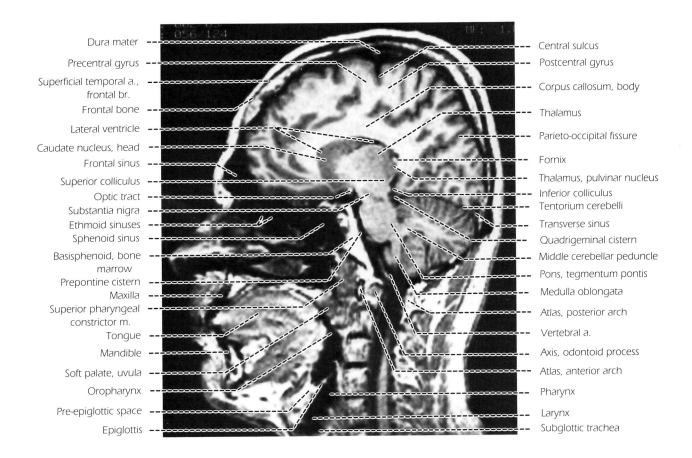

Dura mater
Precentral gyrus
Superficial temporal a., frontal br.
Frontal bone
Lateral ventricle
Caudate nucleus, head
Frontal sinus
Superior colliculus
Optic tract
Substantia nigra
Ethmoid sinuses
Sphenoid sinus
Basisphenoid, bone marrow
Prepontine cistern
Maxilla
Superior pharyngeal constrictor m.
Tongue
Mandible
Soft palate, uvula
Oropharynx
Pre-epiglottic space
Epiglottis

Central sulcus
Postcentral gyrus
Corpus callosum, body
Thalamus
Parieto-occipital fissure
Fornix
Thalamus, pulvinar nucleus
Inferior colliculus
Tentorium cerebelli
Transverse sinus
Quadrigeminal cistern
Middle cerebellar peduncle
Pons, tegmentum pontis
Medulla oblongata
Atlas, posterior arch
Vertebral a.
Axis, odontoid process
Atlas, anterior arch
Pharynx
Larynx
Subglottic trachea

# Figure 1-168

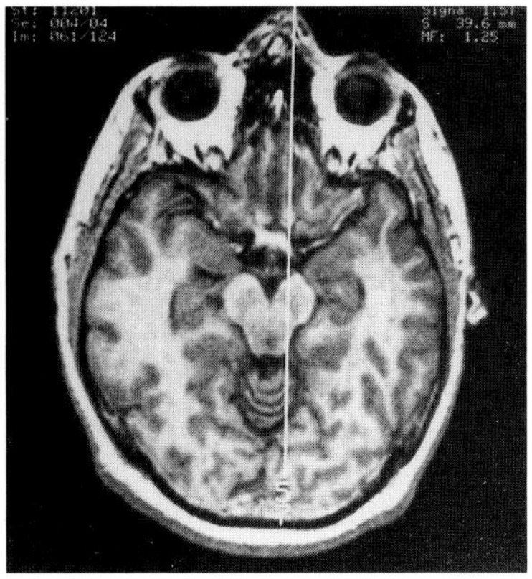

Midsagittal T1-weighted image of the brain. In the cerebral hemispheres, the pre- and postcentral gyri are separated by the central sulcus. The corpus callosum is dorsal to the lateral ventricle. Dorsal to the corpus callosum is the callosal sulcus and cistern. The head of the caudate nucleus is seen bulging into the lateral ventricle. The thalamus is fully developed here. Caudal to the thalamus is the splenium of the corpus callosum and the fornix. The parieto-occipital fissure separates the parietal and occipital lobes. Within the occipital lobe is seen the calcarine fissure. Dorsal to the midbrain is the quadrigeminal cistern. Within the midbrain are the substantia nigra and red nucleus. The tentorium cerebelli is seen dorsal to the cerebellum. The cerebellar tonsils are found above the cisterna magna. Inferior to the cerebellum is the pons and medulla oblongata. The cervical spinal cord is shown. The bright signal intensity of the optic chiasma is shown beneath the thalamus. Bony landmarks in this section include cervical vertebral bodies, mandible, hyoid bone, anterior arch of the atlas, maxilla, basiocciput, and frontal bone. The frontal, ethmoid, and sphenoid air sinuses are also shown. Other important structures in this section include the nasopharynx, choana, pharyngeal constrictor muscles, uvula, and tongue, oropharynx, and epiglottis.

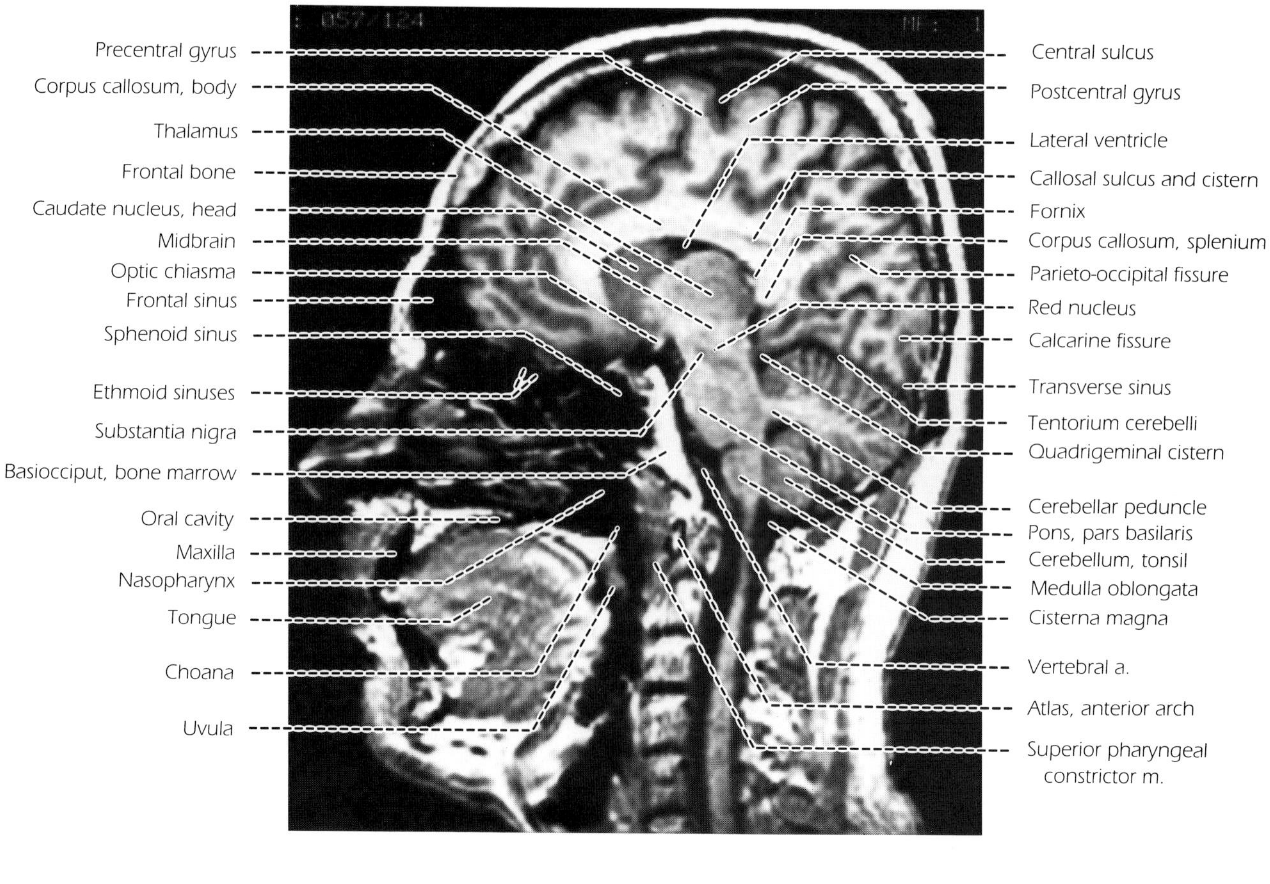
Precentral gyrus
Corpus callosum, body
Thalamus
Frontal bone
Caudate nucleus, head
Midbrain
Optic chiasma
Frontal sinus
Sphenoid sinus
Ethmoid sinuses
Substantia nigra
Basiocciput, bone marrow
Oral cavity
Maxilla
Nasopharynx
Tongue
Choana
Uvula
Central sulcus
Postcentral gyrus
Lateral ventricle
Callosal sulcus and cistern
Fornix
Corpus callosum, splenium
Parieto-occipital fissure
Red nucleus
Calcarine fissure
Transverse sinus
Tentorium cerebelli
Quadrigeminal cistern
Cerebellar peduncle
Pons, pars basilaris
Cerebellum, tonsil
Medulla oblongata
Cisterna magna
Vertebral a.
Atlas, anterior arch
Superior pharyngeal constrictor m.

Midsagittal T1-weighted image of the brain showing the whole extent of the corpus callosum with its different parts: the rostrum, genu, body, and splenium. Beneath the corpus callosum caudally is the fornix. The corpus callosum is separated from the cingulum by the callosal sulcus and cistern. The cingulum is the white matter tract within the cingulate gyrus. In the cerebral hemisphere, the central sulcus separates the pre- and postcentral gyri. Caudally, the parieto-occipital fissure separates the parietal and occipital lobes. Beneath the occipital lobe, and separating it from the cerebellum, is the tentorium cerebelli. Caudal to the tentorium cerebelli is the transverse sinus. The superior cerebellar peduncle (brachium conjunctivum) connects the cerebellum to the midbrain. Seen within the midbrain are the superior colliculus, inferior colliculus, and substantia nigra. Rostral to the midbrain is the thalamus, and caudal to it is the pons. The basilar part of the pons is shown bulging in the inferior aspect of the pons. The fourth ventricle occupies the space between the medulla oblongata and cerebellum. The cervical region of the spinal cord is shown. The caudate nucleus is shown bulging into the cavity of the lateral ventricle. The tonsil of the cerebellum is found above the cisterna magna. Bony landmarks include the posterior arch of the atlas, mandible, anterior arch of the atlas, and basiocciput. Other structures in this section include the orbicularis oris muscle, genioglossus muscle, tongue, oral cavity, nasopharynx, and sphenoid and frontal sinuses. The basilar artery is seen ventral to the pons.

## Figure 1-169

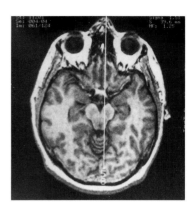

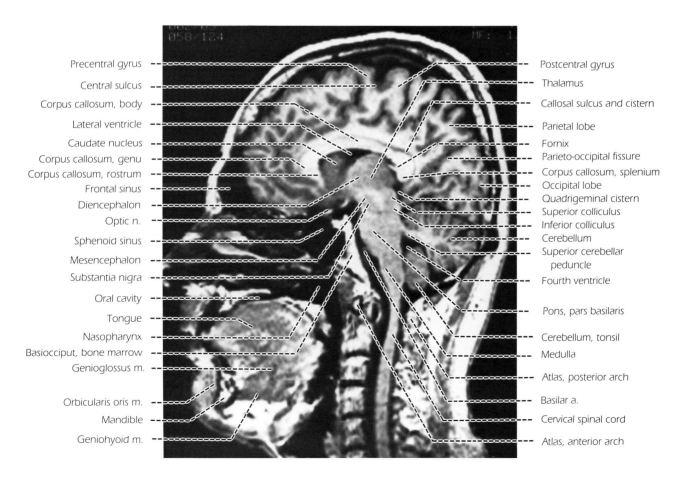

Precentral gyrus

Central sulcus

Corpus callosum, body

Lateral ventricle

Caudate nucleus

Corpus callosum, genu

Corpus callosum, rostrum

Frontal sinus

Diencephalon

Optic n.

Sphenoid sinus

Mesencephalon

Substantia nigra

Oral cavity

Tongue

Nasopharynx

Basiocciput, bone marrow

Genioglossus m.

Orbicularis oris m.

Mandible

Geniohyoid m.

Postcentral gyrus

Thalamus

Callosal sulcus and cistern

Parietal lobe

Fornix

Parieto-occipital fissure

Corpus callosum, splenium

Occipital lobe

Quadrigeminal cistern

Superior colliculus

Inferior colliculus

Cerebellum

Superior cerebellar peduncle

Fourth ventricle

Pons, pars basilaris

Cerebellum, tonsil

Medulla

Atlas, posterior arch

Basilar a.

Cervical spinal cord

Atlas, anterior arch

## Figure 1-170

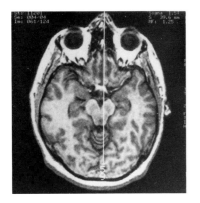

Midsagittal T1-weighted image of the brain showing the full extent of the corpus callosum with its different parts: the rostrum, genu, body, and splenium. Ventral to the corpus callosum is the fornix. The optic chiasma is seen as a bright signal intensity beneath the hypothalamus. Dorsal to the hypothalamus is the thalamus. Dorsal to the corpus callosum is the cingulum, the white matter core of the cingulate gyrus. In the cerebral hemisphere, the paracentral lobule is shown caudal to the paracentral sulcus. The central sulcus separates the pre- and postcentral gyri. The parieto-occipital fissure separates the parietal and occipital lobes. The tentorium cerebelli separates the occipital lobe from the cerebellum. The superior cerebellar peduncle (brachium conjunctivum) connects the cerebellum to the midbrain. Within the midbrain, the superior and inferior colliculi are shown. Dorsal to the colliculi is the quadrigeminal cistern. The tonsil of the cerebellum is dorsal to the cisterna magna. The fourth ventricle is between the pons, medulla, and cerebellum. The basilar artery is inferior to the pons. The cervical spinal cord is caudal to the vertebral bodies of the cervical spine. Bony landmarks seen in this section include the vertebral bodies of the cervical spine, hyoid bone, mandible, maxilla, anterior arch of the atlas, basiocciput, and frontal bone. Other structures found in this section include the epiglottis, orbicularis oris muscle, genioglossus muscle, tongue, oral cavity, nasopharynx, and middle concha. The prepontine cistern is inferior to the pons and contains the basilar artery.

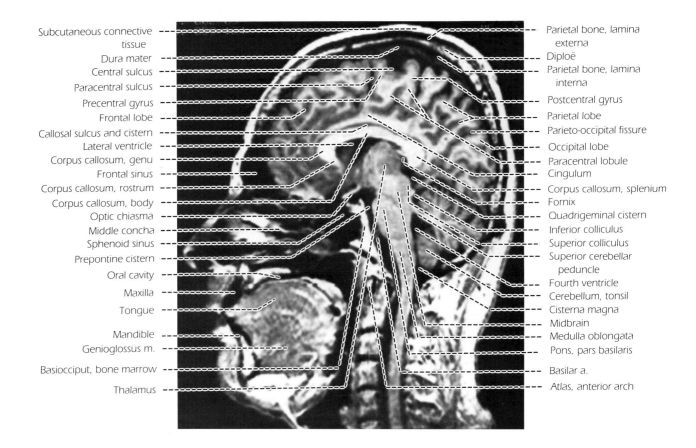

Subcutaneous connective tissue — Parietal bone, lamina externa
Dura mater — Diploë
Central sulcus — Parietal bone, lamina interna
Paracentral sulcus —
Precentral gyrus — Postcentral gyrus
Frontal lobe — Parietal lobe
Callosal sulcus and cistern — Parieto-occipital fissure
Lateral ventricle — Occipital lobe
Corpus callosum, genu — Paracentral lobule
Frontal sinus — Cingulum
Corpus callosum, rostrum — Corpus callosum, splenium
Corpus callosum, body — Fornix
Optic chiasma — Quadrigeminal cistern
Middle concha — Inferior colliculus
Sphenoid sinus — Superior colliculus
Prepontine cistern — Superior cerebellar peduncle
Oral cavity — Fourth ventricle
Maxilla — Cerebellum, tonsil
Tongue — Cisterna magna
— Midbrain
Mandible — Medulla oblongata
Genioglossus m. — Pons, pars basilaris
Basiocciput, bone marrow — Basilar a.
Thalamus — Atlas, anterior arch

Midsagittal T1-weighted image of the brain showing the corpus callosum with its different components: the genu, body, and splenium. Dorsal to the corpus callosum is the callosal sulcus and cistern separating the corpus callosum from the cingulate gyrus. In the cerebral hemisphere, the frontal, parietal, and occipital lobes are seen on their medial surfaces. The paracentral lobule occupies parts of the frontal and parietal lobes. The parieto-occipital fissure separates the parietal and occipital lobes. The straight sinus is shown inferior to the occipital lobe. Also inferior to the occipital lobe is the cerebellum. The superior cerebellar peduncle connects the cerebellum to the midbrain. In the midbrain, the superior and inferior colliculi and the cerebral aqueduct (aqueduct of Sylvius) are shown. Caudal to the midbrain is the pons. The fourth ventricle is located between the cerebellum, pons, and medulla oblongata. The tonsil of the cerebellum is located above the cisterna magna. Rostral to the midbrain is the thalamus and hypothalamus. Coursing within the hypothalamus is the fornix. The optic chiasma is located ventral to the hypothalamus. Bony landmarks in this section include the posterior arch of the atlas, vertebral bodies of the cervical spine, hyoid bone, mandible, odontoid process of the axis, anterior arch of the atlas, and basiocciput. Other important structures include the epiglottis, oropharynx, orbicularis oris muscle, genioglossus muscle, uvula, tongue, oral cavity, nasopharynx, basilar artery, and sphenoid and frontal sinuses.

## Figure 1-171

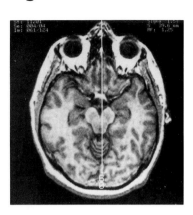

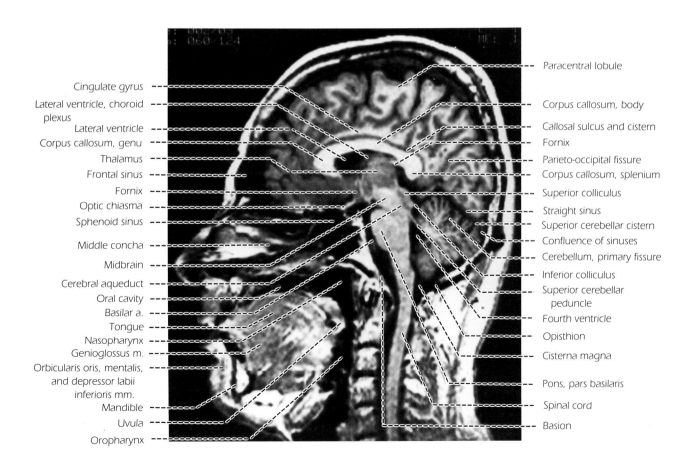

Cingulate gyrus

Lateral ventricle, choroid plexus

Lateral ventricle

Corpus callosum, genu

Thalamus

Frontal sinus

Fornix

Optic chiasma

Sphenoid sinus

Middle concha

Midbrain

Cerebral aqueduct

Oral cavity

Basilar a.

Tongue

Nasopharynx

Genioglossus m.

Orbicularis oris, mentalis, and depressor labii inferioris mm.

Mandible

Uvula

Oropharynx

Paracentral lobule

Corpus callosum, body

Callosal sulcus and cistern

Fornix

Parieto-occipital fissure

Corpus callosum, splenium

Superior colliculus

Straight sinus

Superior cerebellar cistern

Confluence of sinuses

Cerebellum, primary fissure

Inferior colliculus

Superior cerebellar peduncle

Fourth ventricle

Opisthion

Cisterna magna

Pons, pars basilaris

Spinal cord

Basion

## Figure 1-172

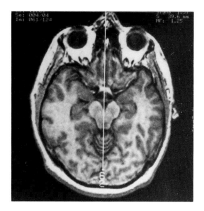

Midsagittal T1-weighted image showing the cerebral hemispheres, corpus callosum, fornix, thalamus, hypothalamus, and brain stem. Within the cerebral hemisphere, the frontal, parietal, and occipital lobes are seen on their medial surfaces. The paracentral lobule occupies part of the frontal and parietal lobes. The parieto-occipital fissure separates the parietal and occipital lobes. The calcarine fissure is seen within the occipital lobe. The straight sinus and confluence of sinuses are shown beneath the occipital lobe. The primary cerebellar fissure is shown within the cerebellum. This fissure separates the cerebellum into anterior and posterior lobes. The anterior medullary velum forms the roof of the fourth ventricle anteriorly or superiorly. The fourth ventricle is located between the cerebellum, pons, and medulla. The tonsil of the cerebellum is located above the cisterna magna. Within the corpus callosum, the genu, body, and splenium are shown. Dorsal to the corpus callosum are the callosal sulcus and cistern separating the corpus callosum from the cingulate gyrus. The cingulate sulcus separates the cingulate gyrus from the rest of the frontal and parietal lobes. The fornix is ventral to the corpus callosum. Ventral to the fornix is the thalamus and hypothalamus. The lamina terminalis delineates the anterior boundary of the hypothalamus. Ventral to the hypothalamus are the optic chiasma and infundibulum. The anterior lobe of the hypophysis is also seen at the inferior border of the infundibulum. Rostral to the cerebellum is the tectum of the mesencephalon, and beneath it is the cerebral aqueduct. The bony landmarks in this section include the posterior arch of the atlas, hyoid bone, mandible, odontoid process of the axis, anterior arch of the atlas, and basisphenoid. Other important structures include the epiglottis, anterior longitudinal ligament, larynx, mentalis muscle, genioglossus muscle, tongue, nasopharynx, inferior and middle conchae of the nose, cruciate ligament, and the basilar artery.

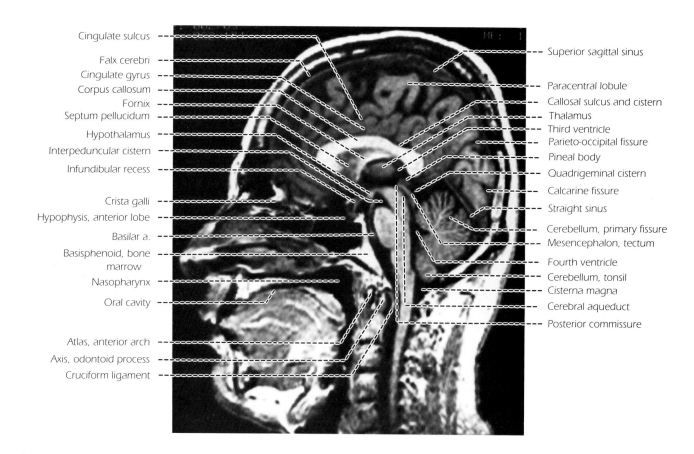

Midsagittal T1-weighted image of the brain and brain stem showing the cerebral hemispheres, corpus callosum, thalamus, hypothalamus, cerebellum, midbrain, pons, and medulla oblongata. Some vascular landmarks are shown in this section including the anterior cerebral artery, pericallosal artery, and frontal branches of the anterior cerebral artery. The superior sagittal venous sinus with arachnoid granulations is shown in the dura mater. Within the corpus callosum are found the genu, body, and splenium. Beneath the corpus callosum is the fornix. Beneath the fornix is the thalamus. The great cerebral vein is ventral to the splenium of the corpus callosum. Caudal to the hypothalamus are the pineal body and habenular and posterior commissures. Dorsal to the tectum of the mesencephalon is the quadrigeminal cistern. Connecting the cerebellum with the tectum is the superior (anterior) medullary velum. The fourth ventricle occupies a position between the medulla oblongata, pons, and cerebellum. The obex is seen in the caudal part of the fourth ventricle. The cervical spinal cord is visible. Ventral to the thalamus is the hypothalamus, which contains the mamillary body in its posterior aspect. The optic chiasma is a bright signal intensity ventral to the hypothalamus. Other important structures include the posterior arch of the atlas, anterior longitudinal ligament, posterior longitudinal ligament, epiglottis, vallecula, hyoid bone, orbicularis oris muscle, mandible, odontoid process of the axis, tongue, soft palate, nasopharynx, basilar artery, and cingulate sulcus and gyrus.

## Figure 1-173

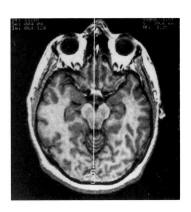

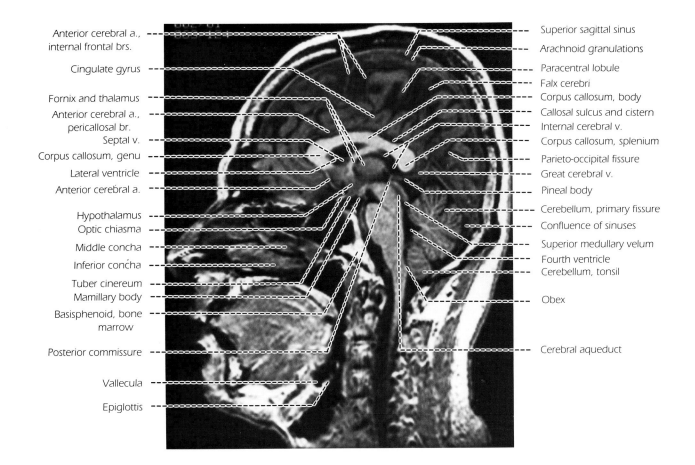

# Figure 1-174

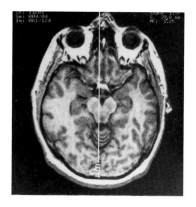

Parasagittal T1-weighted image of the right hemisphere close to the midline. The superior sagittal sinus is seen within the dura mater overlying the hemisphere. The genu, body, and splenium of the corpus callosum are shown. Ventral to the corpus callosum is the fornix. The callosal sulcus and cistern separates the corpus callosum from the cingulate gyrus. Surrounding the cingulate gyrus is the cingulate sulcus. Ventral to the corpus callosum is the thalamus. Anterior to the thalamus is the fornix extending toward the mamillary body. Arising from the mamillary body is the mamillothalamic tract. The optic chiasma is seen as a bright signal intensity anterior to the mamillary body and underneath the hypothalamus. The cerebral aqueduct (aqueduct of Sylvius) is seen beneath the tectum of the midbrain. The primary cerebellar fissure is identified within the cerebellum. The anterior medullary velum is shown connecting the cerebellum with the midbrain. The fourth ventricle occupies a position between the cerebellum, pons, and medulla oblongata. The tonsil of the cerebellum is located dorsal to the cisterna magna. Ventral to the optic chiasma is the posterior lobe of the hypophysis. The basilar artery is shown ventral (anterior) to the pons. Bony landmarks include vertebral bodies of the cervical spine, hyoid bone, mandible, anterior arch of the atlas, and basiocciput. Other important structures include the epiglottis, genu, oropharynx, genioglossus muscle, uvula, tongue, oral cavity, and nasopharynx.

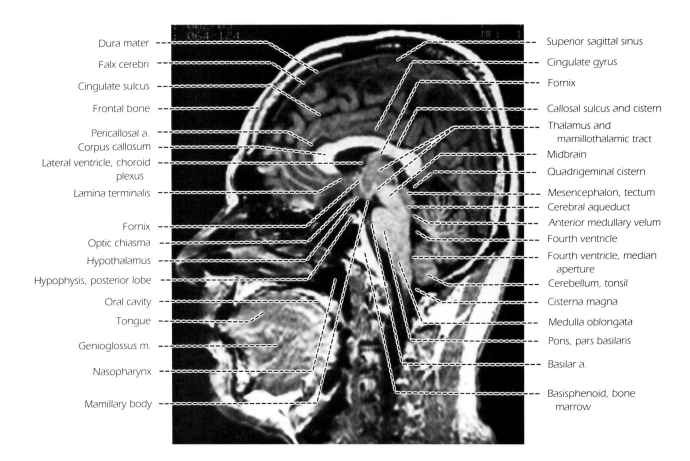

Parasagittal T1-weighted image of the right hemisphere showing the cerebral hemisphere, corpus callosum, thalamus, midbrain, pons, medulla oblongata, and cerebellum. The genu, body, and splenium of the corpus callosum are identified. Ventral to the corpus callosum is the fornix. The callosal sulcus and cistern separate the corpus callosum from the cingulum of the cingulate gyrus. The cingulate sulcus separates the cingulate gyrus from the rest of the cerebral hemisphere. The paracentral lobule is located dorsal to the cingulate sulcus. The sagittal sinus is seen within the dura mater overlying the cerebral hemisphere. The quadrigeminal cistern occupies a position dorsal to the superior and inferior colliculi. The primary cerebellar fissure is found within the cerebellum separating the anterior and posterior lobes of the cerebellum. The fourth ventricle is shown occupying a position between the cerebellum, pons, and medulla oblongata. Anterior to the midbrain is the thalamus capped by the stria medullaris thalami. Bony landmarks include the hyoid bone, mandible, maxilla, basiocciput, and frontal bone. Other important structures seen in this section include the epiglottis, genioglossus muscle, constrictor pharyngeal muscle, tongue, nasopharynx, inferior and middle conchae of the nose, basilar pons, and sphenoid and frontal sinuses.

## Figure 1-175

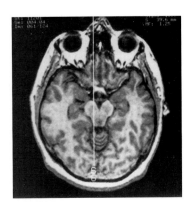

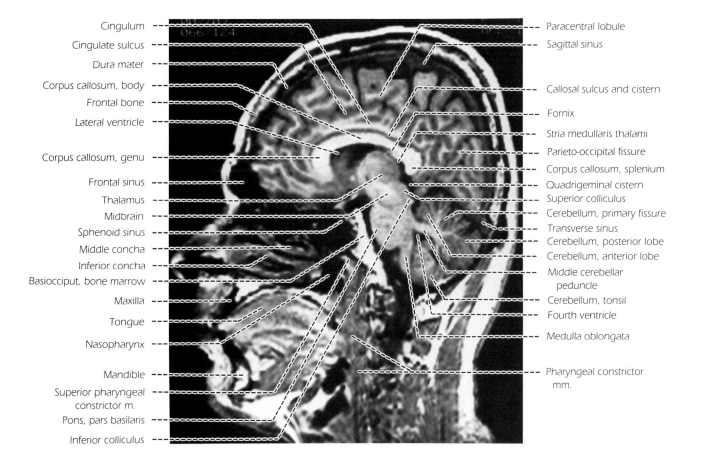

## Figure 1-176

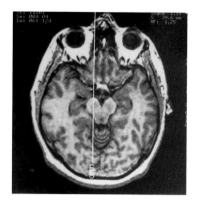

Parasagittal T1-weighted image of the right hemisphere just lateral to the midline. It shows the cerebral hemisphere, corpus callosum, thalamus, midbrain, pons, and cerebellum. The genu, body, and splenium of the corpus callosum are shown. The callosal sulcus and cistern separate the corpus callosum from the cingulum of the cingulate gyrus. The cingulate sulcus separates the cingulate gyrus from the rest of the frontal and parietal lobes. The paracentral lobule is located dorsal to the cingulate sulcus. The parieto-occipital fissure separates the parietal and occipital lobes. The tentorium cerebelli separates the occipital lobe from the cerebellum. The horizontal fissure of the cerebellum separates the cerebellum into superior and inferior surfaces. The middle cerebellar peduncle is shown entering the cerebellum from the pons. The inferior and superior colliculi lie ventral to the quadrigeminal cistern. Rostral to the midbrain is the thalamus. The optic tract is seen inferior to the thalamus. The head of the caudate nucleus is seen bulging into the lateral ventricle. Bony landmarks include the hyoid bone, mandible, maxilla, basiocciput, and frontal bone. Other important structures seen in this section include the transverse sinus, epiglottis, tongue, constrictor muscles of the pharynx, genioglossus muscle, middle and inferior conchae, prepontine cistern, and sphenoid and frontal sinuses.

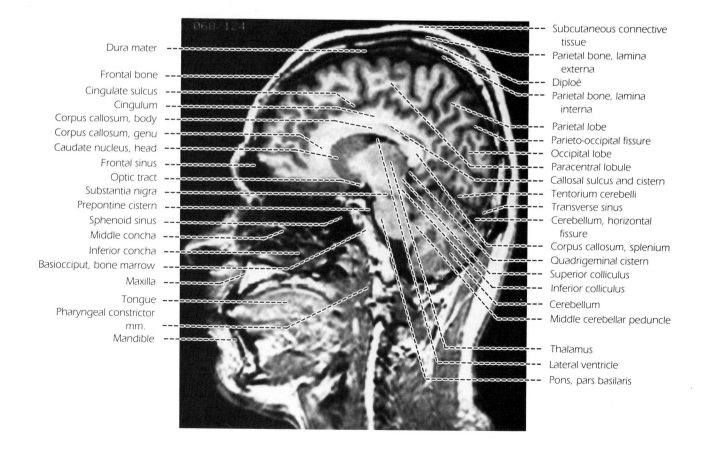

Parasagittal T1-weighted image of the right hemisphere showing the cerebral hemisphere, thalamus, corpus callosum, midbrain, pons, and cerebellum. The body of the corpus callosum is shown beneath the cingulum of the cingulate gyrus and is separated from it by the callosal sulcus and cistern. The cingulate sulcus separates the cingulum from the paracentral lobule. The parieto-occipital fissure separates the parietal and occipital lobes. The splenium of the corpus callosum is located in the caudal part of the corpus callosum. Beneath the corpus callosum is the fornix. The quadrigeminal cistern is located dorsal to the midbrain. The middle cerebellar peduncle is shown extending from the basis pontis or basilar pons to the cerebellum. Rostral to the midbrain is the thalamus. The internal capsule separates the thalamus from the head of the caudate nucleus. The tentorium cerebelli separates the occipital lobe from the cerebellum. Caudal to the tentorium is the transverse sinus. Bony landmarks include the occipital bone, hyoid bone, mandible, maxilla, basiocciput, and frontal bone. Other important structures seen in this section include the tongue; pharyngeal constrictor muscles; prepontine cistern; frontal, ethmoid, and sphenoid sinuses; optic tract; and dura mater.

## Figure 1-177

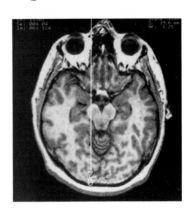

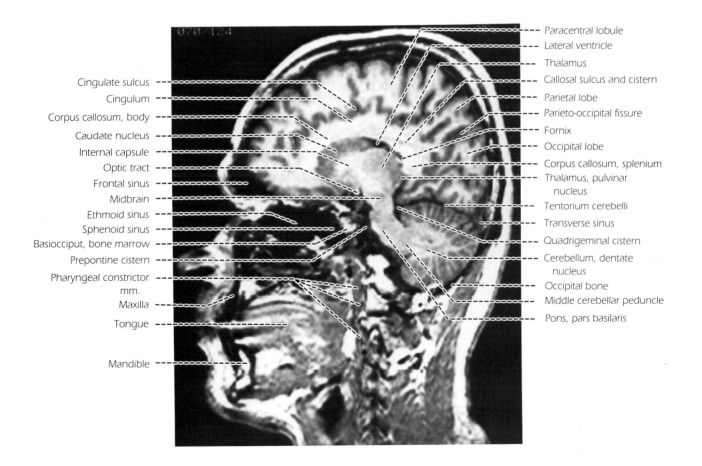

## Figure 1-178

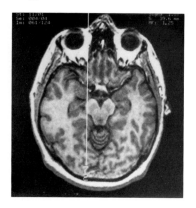

Parasagittal T1-weighted image through the right cerebral hemisphere showing the basal ganglia, internal capsule, thalamus, and cerebellum. The corpus callosum is seen dorsal to the lateral ventricle. The caudate nucleus is seen bulging into the lateral ventricle. The lentiform nucleus is separated from the caudate nucleus by the anterior limb of the internal capsule. The posterior limb of the internal capsule separates the lentiform nucleus from the thalamus. The pulvinar nucleus of the thalamus occupies a caudal position within the thalamus. Ventral to the corpus callosum is the fornix. The middle cerebellar peduncle is shown entering the cerebellum. The dentate nucleus of the cerebellum is seen within the white matter core of the cerebellum. The tentorium cerebelli separates the occipital lobe from the cerebellum. Caudal to the tentorium is the transverse sinus. The trigeminal nerve is seen as a bright signal intensity rostral to the cerebellum. Other important structures seen in this section include the mandible, tongue, maxilla, ethmoid and sphenoid sinuses, optic tract, and dura mater.

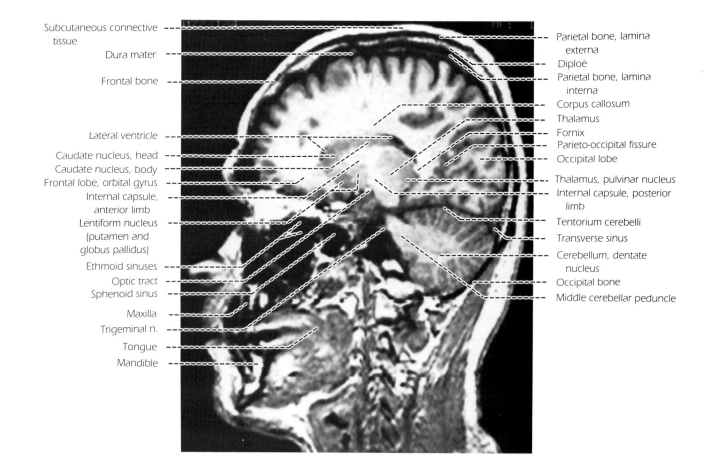

Parasagittal T1-weighted image through the right hemisphere showing the basal ganglia, thalamus, and cerebellum. The corona radiata is shown within the deep white matter of the cerebral hemisphere. The lentiform nucleus is separated from the thalamus by the posterior limb of the internal capsule. Ventral to the trigone of the lateral ventricle is the fornix. The parietal optic radiation is seen dorsal and caudal to the trigone. The tentorium cerebelli separates the occipital lobe from the cerebellum. The uncinate fasciculus, one of the long association fiber bundles, is seen connecting the frontal and temporal lobes. Other important structures seen in this section include the tongue, oral cavity, pharyngeal constrictor muscles, maxilla, trigeminal nerve, maxillary and sphenoid sinuses, medial rectus muscle, and orbital cortex of the frontal lobe.

## Figure 1-179

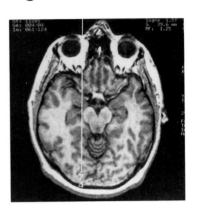

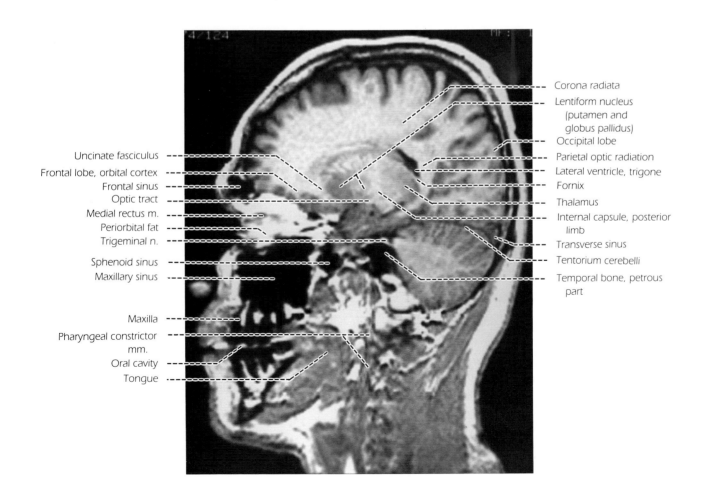

Corona radiata

Lentiform nucleus (putamen and globus pallidus)

Occipital lobe

Uncinate fasciculus

Frontal lobe, orbital cortex

Frontal sinus

Optic tract

Medial rectus m.

Periorbital fat

Trigeminal n.

Sphenoid sinus

Maxillary sinus

Maxilla

Pharyngeal constrictor mm.

Oral cavity

Tongue

Parietal optic radiation

Lateral ventricle, trigone

Fornix

Thalamus

Internal capsule, posterior limb

Transverse sinus

Tentorium cerebelli

Temporal bone, petrous part

## Figure 1-180

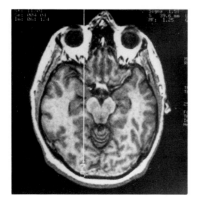

Parasagittal T1-weighted image through the right hemisphere showing the lentiform nucleus and cerebellum. The corona radiata occupies the deep white matter core of the cerebral hemisphere. The putamen nucleus is shown beneath the corona radiata. The parietal optic radiation is seen caudal and dorsal to the trigone of the lateral ventricle. The uncinate fasciculus, connecting the frontal and temporal lobes, is seen rostral to the putamen. Within the temporal lobe is seen the hippocampus. Other important structures seen in this section include the petrous part of the temporal bone, transverse sinus, tentorium cerebelli, maxillary sinus, maxilla, sphenoid sinus, inferior oblique, inferior rectus and medial rectus muscles, frontal sinus, optic tract, and superior frontal gyrus.

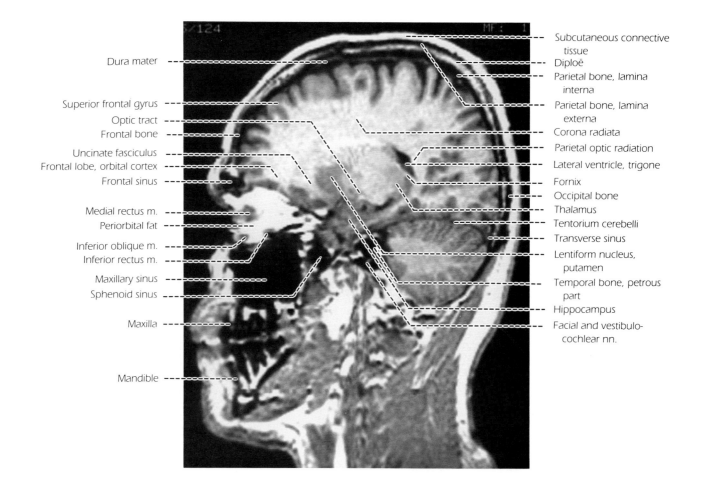

Dura mater

Superior frontal gyrus
Optic tract
Frontal bone

Uncinate fasciculus
Frontal lobe, orbital cortex
Frontal sinus

Medial rectus m.
Periorbital fat

Inferior oblique m.
Inferior rectus m.

Maxillary sinus
Sphenoid sinus

Maxilla

Mandible

Subcutaneous connective tissue
Diploë
Parietal bone, lamina interna
Parietal bone, lamina externa
Corona radiata
Parietal optic radiation
Lateral ventricle, trigone
Fornix
Occipital bone
Thalamus
Tentorium cerebelli
Transverse sinus
Lentiform nucleus, putamen
Temporal bone, petrous part
Hippocampus
Facial and vestibulo-cochlear nn.

Parasagittal T1-weighted image through the right cerebral hemisphere showing the lentiform nucleus and cerebellum. Within the right hemisphere, the central sulcus separates the pre- and postcentral gyri. The corona radiata occupies the deep white matter of the cerebral hemisphere. The uncinate fasciculus is seen rostral to the lentiform nucleus. This fasciculus is one of the long association fiber bundles connecting the frontal and temporal lobes. The optic parietal radiation is shown caudal to the trigone of the lateral ventricle. The fimbria of the fornix is seen arising from the hippocampus. The transverse sinus is seen caudal to the tentorium cerebelli, which separates the occipital lobe from the cerebellum. Other important structures seen in this section include the petrous part of the temporal bone, mandible, oral cavity, maxilla, medial pterygoid muscle, maxillary sinus, inferior rectus and oblique muscles, superior oblique muscle, and orbital cortex of the frontal lobe.

## Figure 1-181

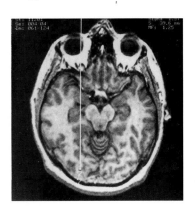

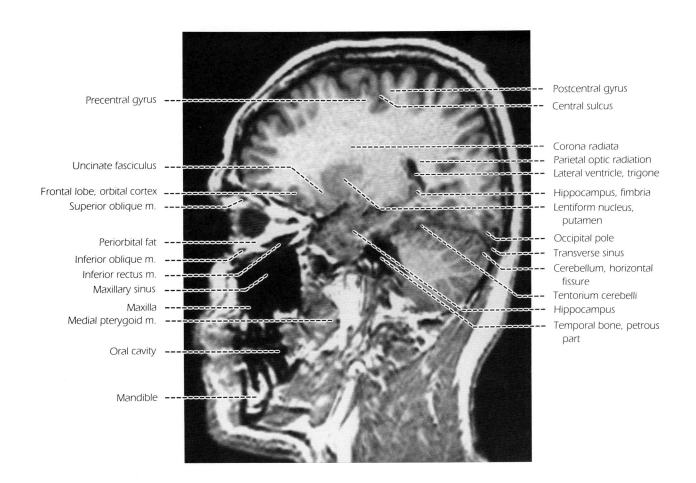

## Figure 1-182

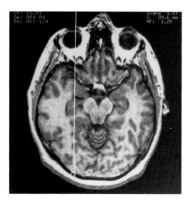

Parasagittal T1-weighted image through the right hemisphere showing the lentiform nucleus and cerebellum. In the cerebral hemisphere, the central sulcus separates the pre- and postcentral gyri. The corona radiata occupies the deep white matter core of the cerebral hemisphere. The parietal optic radiation occupies the dorsal and caudal parts of the trigone of the lateral ventricle. The fimbria is seen arising from the hippocampus. The transverse sinus is seen caudal to the tentorium cerebelli. Other important structures seen in this section include the petrous part of the temporal bone, mandible, medial and lateral pterygoid muscles, maxillary sinus, inferior oblique and rectus muscles, superior rectus muscle, anterior chamber of the eyeball, and frontal bone.

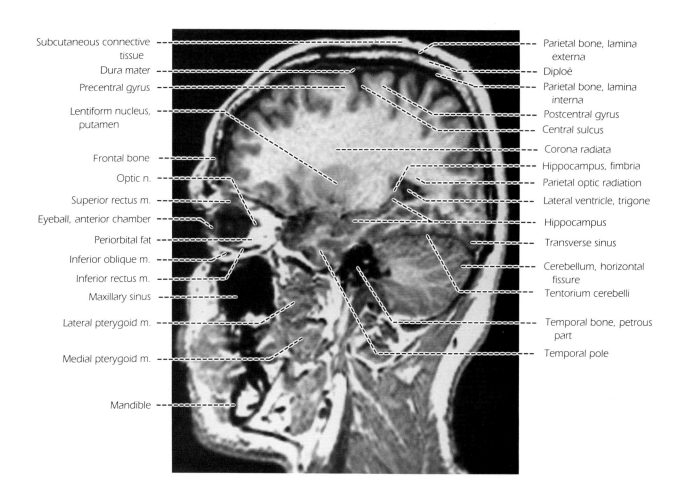

Parasagittal T1-weighted image through the right cerebral hemisphere. The central sulcus is seen separating the pre- and postcentral gyri. The dura mater caps the cerebral hemisphere. The corona radiata forms the deep white matter core of the cerebral hemisphere. The tentorium cerebelli is located between the occipital lobe and cerebellum. The insular cortex (island of Reil) is seen. The cornea, lens, and anterior chamber of the eyeball are seen. Muscles of extraocular movement seen in this section include superior rectus, inferior oblique, and medial rectus. Other structures seen in this section include the levator palpebrae superioris muscle, petrous part of the temporal bone, mandible, medial and lateral pterygoid muscles, maxillary sinus, frontal bone, and orbital cortex of the frontal lobe.

## Figure 1-183

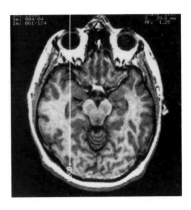

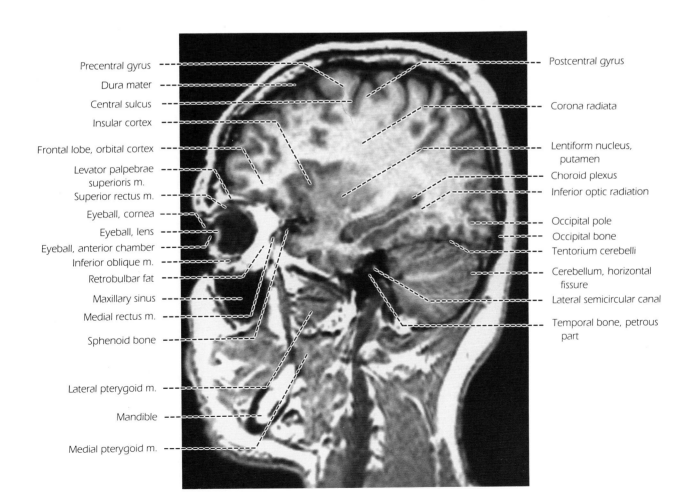

Precentral gyrus

Dura mater

Central sulcus

Insular cortex

Frontal lobe, orbital cortex

Levator palpebrae superioris m.

Superior rectus m.

Eyeball, cornea

Eyeball, lens

Eyeball, anterior chamber

Inferior oblique m.

Retrobulbar fat

Maxillary sinus

Medial rectus m.

Sphenoid bone

Lateral pterygoid m.

Mandible

Medial pterygoid m.

Postcentral gyrus

Corona radiata

Lentiform nucleus, putamen

Choroid plexus

Inferior optic radiation

Occipital pole

Occipital bone

Tentorium cerebelli

Cerebellum, horizontal fissure

Lateral semicircular canal

Temporal bone, petrous part

## Figure 1-184

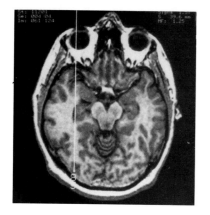

Parasagittal T1-weighted image through the right hemisphere showing the insular cortex (island of Reil). The superior longitudinal (occipitofrontal) fasciculus occupies the white matter of the frontal and parietal lobes. The central sulcus separates the pre- and post-central gyri. The optic radiation is shown on each side of the inferior horn of the lateral ventricle. The tentorium cerebelli overlies the cerebellum. Caudal to it is the transverse sinus. The cornea, lens, and anterior chamber of the eyeball are seen. One muscle of extraocular movement, the inferior oblique, is seen in this section. Other important structures include the lateral semicircular canal, petrous part of the temporal bone, facial cranial nerve, mandible, levator palpebrae superioris muscle, medial and lateral pterygoid muscles, maxillary sinus, sphenoid bone, and orbital cortex of the frontal lobe.

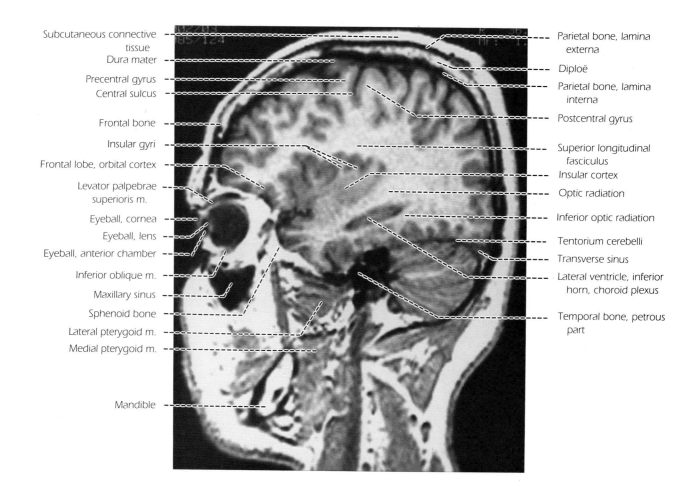

Parasagittal T1-weighted image through the right hemisphere at the level of the insular cortex (island of Reil). The central sulcus separates the pre- and postcentral gyri. The superior longitudinal fasciculus is seen within the white matter of the frontal and parietal lobes. The inferior longitudinal fasciculus, another of the long association fiber bundles, is seen within the temporal lobe. The inferior optic radiation is seen beneath the inferior (temporal) horn of the lateral ventricle. The tentorium cerebelli caps the cerebellum. Caudal to the tentorium is the transverse sinus. Other important structures include the dura mater, orbital cortex of the frontal lobe, superior rectus muscle, greater wing of the sphenoid bone, lateral rectus muscle, maxillary sinus, lateral and medial pterygoid muscles, and temporalis muscle.

## Figure 1-185

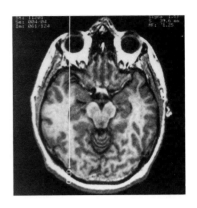

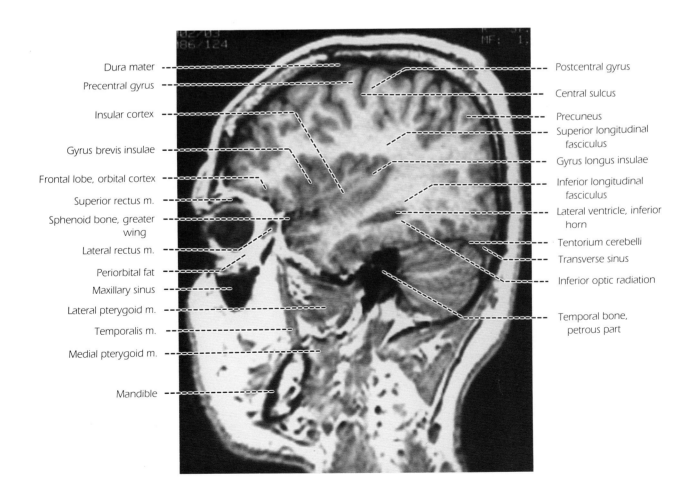

## Figure 1-186

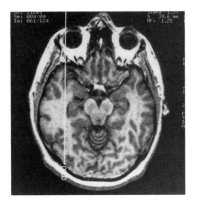

Parasagittal T1-weighted image through the right hemisphere at the level of the insular cortex (island of Reil). The central sulcus separates the pre- and postcentral gyri. Two long association fiber bundles, the superior and inferior longitudinal fasciculi, are seen coursing in the white matter of the frontal, parietal, and temporal lobes. The tentorium cerebelli separates the occipital lobe from the cerebellum. The opercular and triangular parts of the inferior frontal lobule are shown overlying the insular cortex. Other important structures include the petrous part of the temporal bone, ramus of the mandible, masseter muscle, lateral pterygoid muscle, maxilla, temporalis muscle, articular tubercle of temporal bone, zygomatic bone, lateral rectus muscle, and frontal bone.

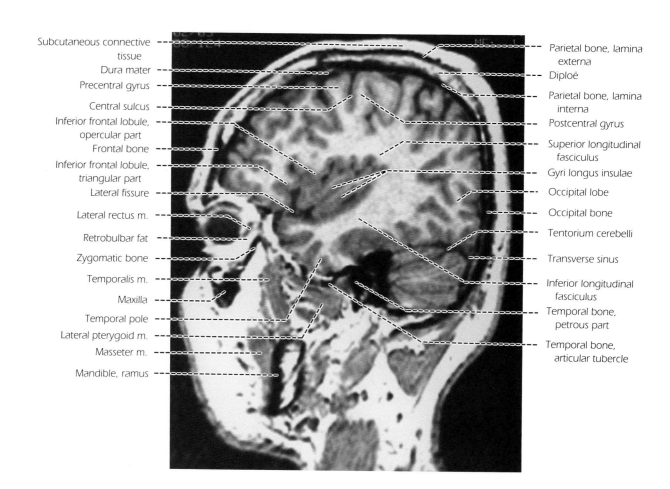

Parasagittal T1-weighted image through the right cerebral hemisphere and the cerebellum. The central sulcus separates the pre- and postcentral gyri. Rostral to the precentral gyrus is the precentral sulcus. The superior and inferior longitudinal fasciculi occupy the white matter of the frontal, parietal, and temporal lobes. The supramarginal gyrus is seen within the parietal lobe. The tentorium cerebelli caps the cerebellum. Caudal to the tentorium is the transverse sinus. The opercular and triangular parts of the inferior frontal lobule are seen. Bony landmarks in this section include the ramus of the mandible, condylar process of the mandible, articular tubercle of the temporal bone, coronoid process of the mandible, zygomatic bone, and frontal bone. Other important structures include the dura mater (overlying, the cerebral hemisphere), middle frontal gyrus, lateral cerebral fissure, superior temporal gyrus, temporal pole, temporalis and masseter muscles, and lateral pterygoid muscle.

## Figure 1-187

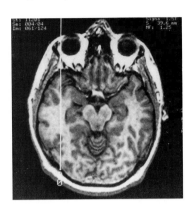

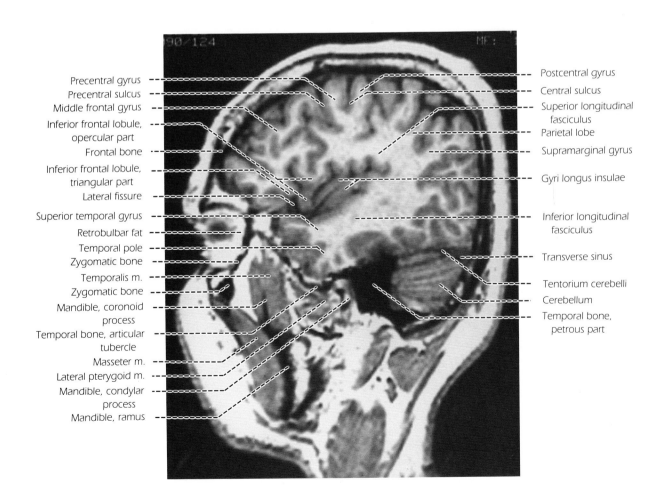

# Figure 1-188

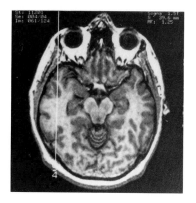

Parasagittal T1-weighted image through the right cerebral hemisphere showing parts of the frontal, parietal, and temporal lobes and section of the cerebellar hemisphere. The supramarginal gyrus is capping the lateral fissure, whereas the angular gyrus is capping the superior temporal sulcus. Within the temporal lobe, the superior and middle temporal gyri are seen separated by the superior temporal sulcus. The central sulcus separates the post- and precentral gyri. Rostral to the lower part of the precentral gyrus is the triangular part of the inferior frontal lobule. Other important structures include the frontal bone; temporalis, masseter, and lateral pterygoid muscles; zygomatic bone; ramus of the mandible; coronoid process of the mandible; condylar process of the mandible; mastoid process of the temporal bone; and internal jugular vein.

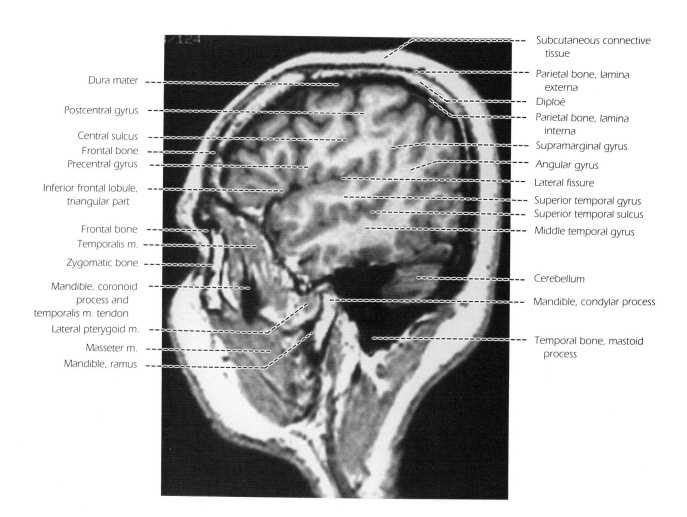

Parasagittal T1-weighted image through the right cerebral hemisphere. It shows parts of the frontal, parietal, and temporal lobes. Within the frontal lobe, the central sulcus separates the pre- and postcentral gyri. The triangular part of the inferior frontal gyrus is located anterior to the ascending ramus of the lateral sulcus. The supramarginal gyrus of the parietal lobe caps the lateral fissure, whereas the superior temporal sulcus separates the superior and middle temporal gyri. Ventral to the middle temporal gyrus is the inferior temporal gyrus. A portion of the lateral hemisphere of the cerebellum is seen. Other important structures include the occipital bone; articular tubercle of the temporal bone; condylar and coronoid processes of the mandible; mastoid process; masseter, lateral pterygoid, and temporalis muscles; temporalis muscle tendon; zygomatic bone; and frontal bone.

## Figure 1-189

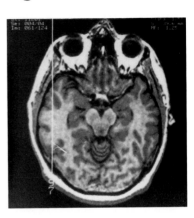

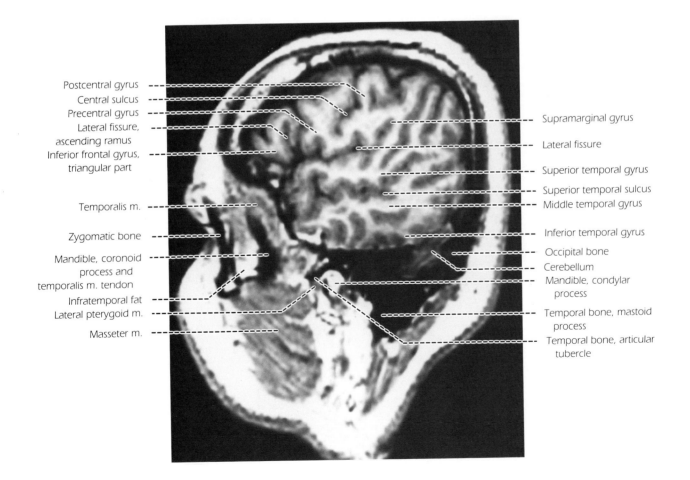

## Figure 1-190

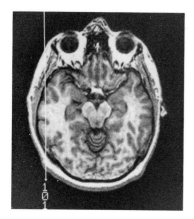

Parasagittal T1-weighted image through the right cerebral hemisphere showing portions of the parietal and temporal lobes. The supramarginal gyrus caps the terminal end of the lateral fissure. Within the temporal lobe, the superior temporal sulcus separates the superior and middle temporal gyri. Inferior to the middle temporal gyrus is the inferior temporal gyrus. Other important structures include the mastoid process, masseter muscle, zygomatic arch, and frontal bone.

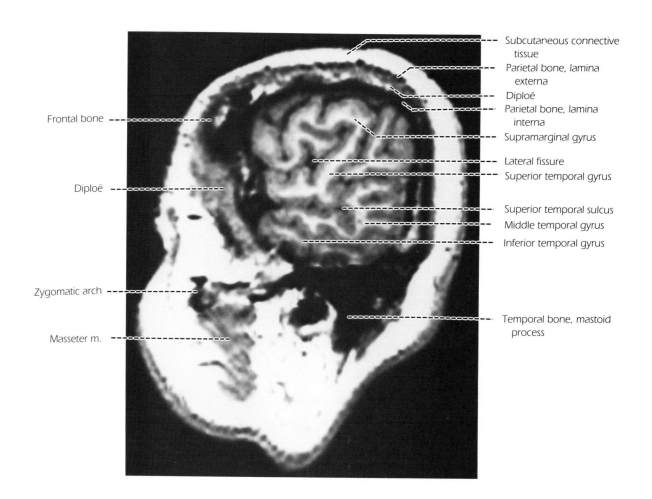

Parasagittal T1-weighted image through the temporal lobe showing the superior and middle temporal gyri separated by the superior temporal sulcus. Other important structures include the temporal bone, frontal bone, and zygomatic process of the temporal bone.

## Figure 1-191

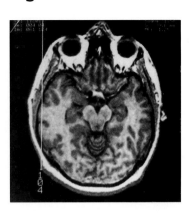

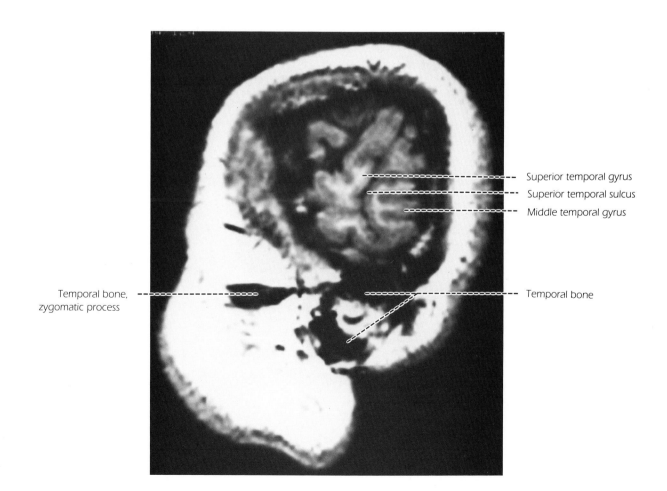

# Figure 1-192

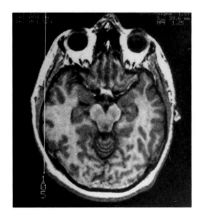

Parasagittal T1-weighted image through the temporal lobe of the right hemisphere showing the superior and middle temporal gyri separated by the superior temporal sulcus. Other important structures include the temporal bone, zygomatic process of the temporal bone, and frontal bone.

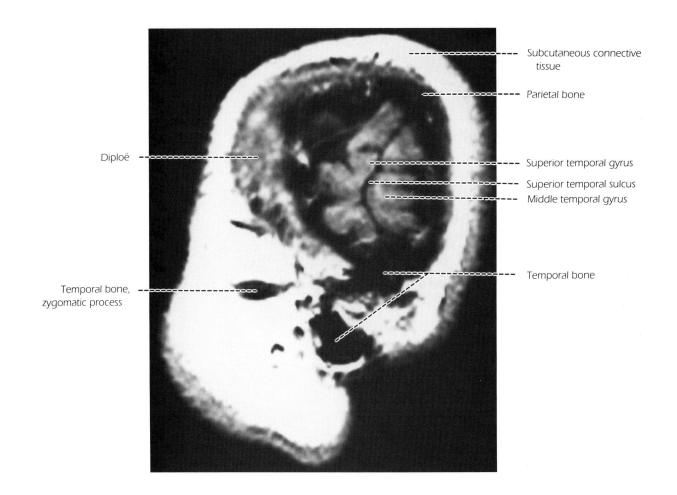

Subcutaneous connective tissue

Parietal bone

Diploë

Superior temporal gyrus

Superior temporal sulcus

Middle temporal gyrus

Temporal bone

Temporal bone, zygomatic process

Parasagittal T2-weighted image showing the most lateral part of the left cerebral hemisphere. The middle meningeal artery is seen coursing superficial to the dura mater.

Figure 1-193

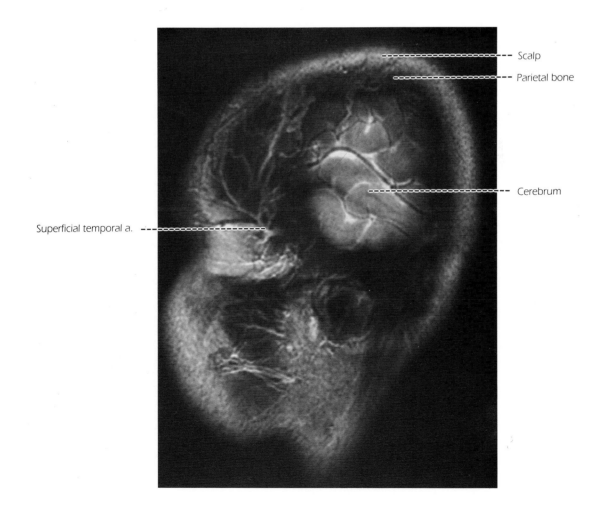

## Figure 1-194

Parasagittal T2-weighted image of the left hemisphere showing the frontal, parietal, and temporal lobes. Branches of the middle cerebral artery are seen in the lateral fissure. Bony landmarks in this section include the frontal bone, zygomatic bone, articular tubercle of the temporal bone, condylar process of the mandible, and mastoid bone.

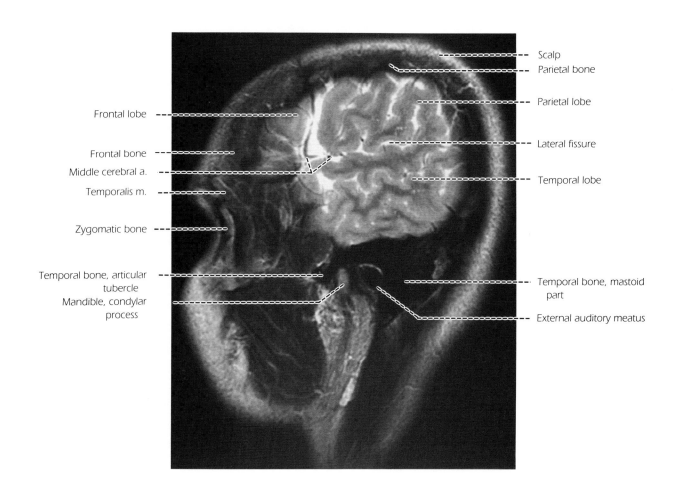

Frontal lobe

Frontal bone
Middle cerebral a.
Temporalis m.

Zygomatic bone

Temporal bone, articular tubercle
Mandible, condylar process

Scalp
Parietal bone

Parietal lobe

Lateral fissure

Temporal lobe

Temporal bone, mastoid part

External auditory meatus

Parasagittal T2-weighted image of the left hemisphere showing the lateral fissure separating the frontal and parietal lobes from the temporal lobe. The central sulcus separates the pre- and postcentral gyri. The precentral sulcus delineates the anterior boundary of the precentral gyrus. The postcentral sulcus delineates the posterior boundary of the postcentral gyrus. The sulci are seen as bright signal intensities in the T2-weighted image because they contain cerebrospinal fluid. Capping the lateral fissure is the supramarginal gyrus. Within the temporal lobe, the superior and middle temporal gyri are separated by the superior temporal sulcus. The cerebellum is found beneath the temporal lobe. Arising from the lateral fissure is the anterior ascending ramus of the lateral fissure. Caudal to this sulcus is the opercular part (pars opercularis), and rostral to it is the triangular part (pars triangularis) of the inferior frontal lobule. These two gyri in the left hemisphere constitute Broca's area of speech. Bony landmarks include the petrous part of the temporal bone, condylar process of the mandible, zygomatic bone, coronoid process of the mandible, and zygomatic bone.

Figure 1-195

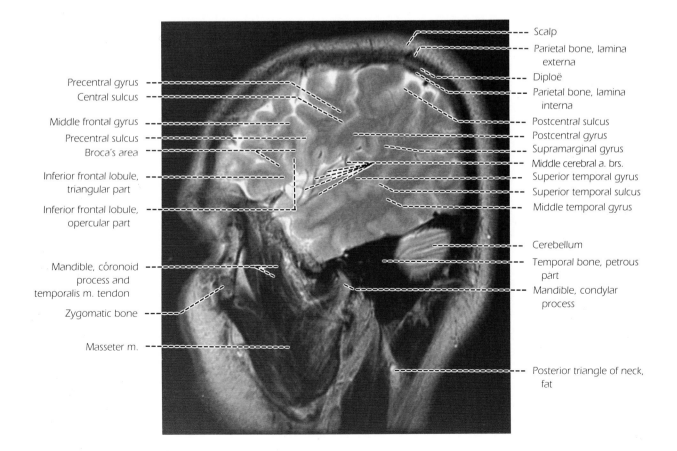

# Figure 1-196

Parasagittal T2-weighted image through the left hemisphere. The central sulcus separates the pre- and postcentral gyri. The precentral sulcus delineates the anterior boundary of the precentral gyrus, whereas the postcentral sulcus delineates the posterior boundary of the postcentral gyrus. The ascending ramus of the lateral fissure separates the opercular and triangular parts of the inferior frontal lobule. The horizontal ramus of the lateral fissure separates the triangular and orbital parts of the inferior frontal lobule. The triangular and opercular parts of the inferior frontal lobule in the left hemisphere constitute Broca's area of speech. The middle cerebral artery is found deep within the lateral fissure. The superior and inferior longitudinal fasciculi, two of the long association fiber bundles, are seen in the frontal, parietal, and temporal lobes. The cerebellum and its horizontal fissure are seen. The eyeball is surrounded by periorbital fat. Bony landmarks include the occipital bone, petrous part of the temporal bone, and mandible. The maxillary air sinus is seen beneath the orbit. Skeletal muscles seen in this section include the lateral pterygoid, temporalis, and superior palpebrae muscles. The transverse venous sinus is seen dorsal and caudal to the cerebellum. The semicircular canals are seen ventral to the temporal lobe.

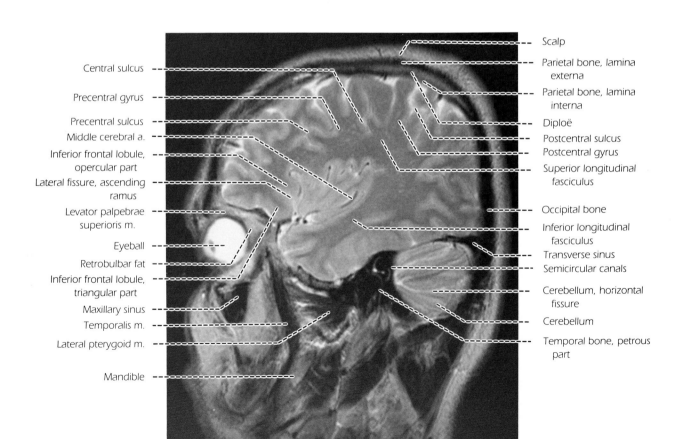

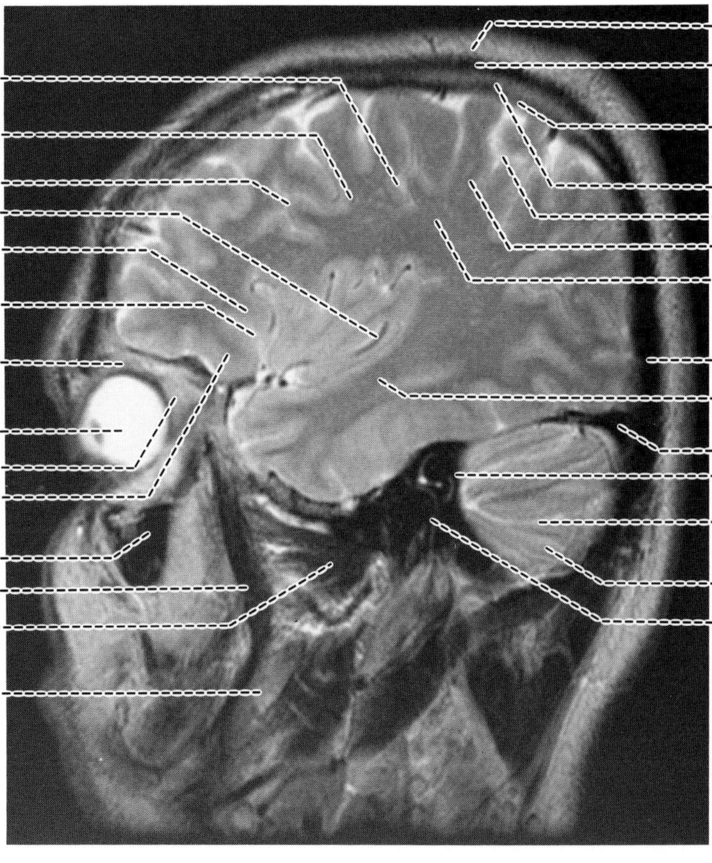
Central sulcus
Precentral gyrus
Precentral sulcus
Middle cerebral a.
Inferior frontal lobule, opercular part
Lateral fissure, ascending ramus
Levator palpebrae superioris m.
Eyeball
Retrobulbar fat
Inferior frontal lobule, triangular part
Maxillary sinus
Temporalis m.
Lateral pterygoid m.
Mandible
Scalp
Parietal bone, lamina externa
Parietal bone, lamina interna
Diploë
Postcentral sulcus
Postcentral gyrus
Superior longitudinal fasciculus
Occipital bone
Inferior longitudinal fasciculus
Transverse sinus
Semicircular canals
Cerebellum, horizontal fissure
Cerebellum
Temporal bone, petrous part

Parasagittal T2-weighted image through the left cerebral hemisphere. The insular cortex (island of Reil) is seen in the middle of this section. In the frontal lobe, the precentral gyrus is found anterior to the central sulcus. The postcentral gyrus is seen caudal to the central sulcus within the parietal lobe. The superior longitudinal fasciculus is found in the deep white matter of the frontal and parietal lobes. The circular sulcus of the insular cortex surrounds the insular cortex. The inferior or temporal horn of the lateral ventricle is found in the temporal lobe. The tentorium cerebelli separates the cerebellum from the cerebral hemisphere. Caudal to the tentorium cerebelli is the transverse venous sinus. The inferior (temporal) optic radiation is seen inferior to the inferior horn of the lateral ventricle. The inner ear is seen as a bright signal intensity beneath the temporal lobe. The lens is a low signal intensity within the eyeball. The optic nerve is seen within the periorbital fat. The superior and inferior rectus and superior palpebrae muscles surround the eyeball. The frontal and maxillary sinuses are identified. The middle cerebral artery is located rostral to the insular cortex.

Figure 1-197

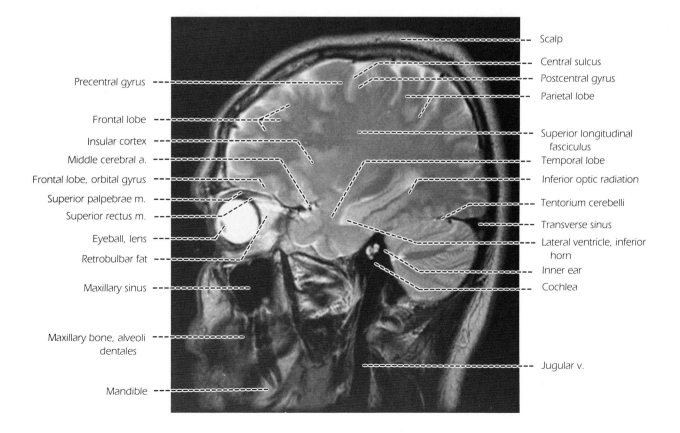

## Figure 1-198

Parasagittal T2-weighted image through the left hemisphere and cerebellum. The central sulcus separates the pre- and postcentral gyri. The corona radiata forms the core of the white matter of the hemisphere. The trigone of the lateral ventricle is a bright signal intensity. The putamen is seen ventral to the corona radiata. The tentorium cerebelli separates the cerebral hemisphere from the cerebellum. Caudal to the tentorium is the transverse venous sinus. The eyeball has a bright signal intensity. The superior and inferior oblique muscles are seen dorsal and ventral to the eyeball. The uncinate fasciculus connecting the frontal and temporal lobes is located rostral to the lentiform nucleus. The frontal and maxillary sinuses are identified.

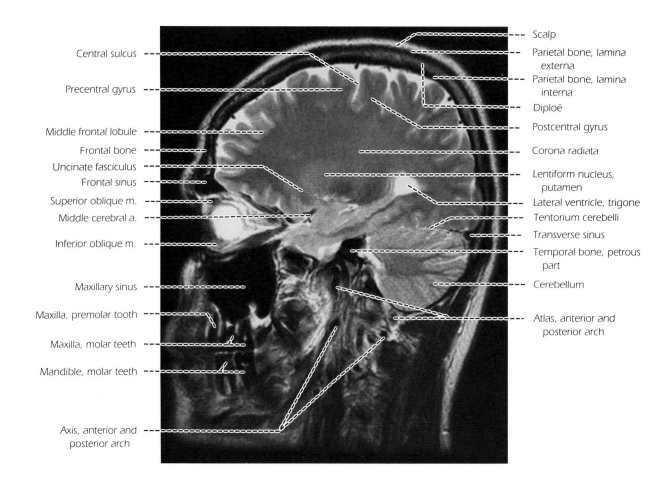

Parasagittal T2-weighted image through the cerebral hemisphere and cerebellum. The central sulcus separates the pre- and postcentral gyri. The centrum semiovale forms the deep white matter core of the hemisphere. Bright signal intensities of the lateral ventricles are seen. Dorsal to the lateral ventricle is the corpus callosum. Ventral to the lateral ventricle is the head and body of the caudate nucleus. Ventral to the caudate nucleus is the genu of the internal capsule. The posterior limb of the internal capsule is found ventral and almost at right angles to the genu of the internal capsule. The tentorium cerebelli separates the cerebral hemisphere from the cerebellum. The suprasellar cistern is seen as a bright signal intensity in front of the cerebellum. The internal carotid artery is located ventral to the suprasellar cistern. The putamen nucleus is seen ventral to the head of the caudate nucleus. The globus pallidus is seen adjacent to the putamen. Close to the globus pallidus is the anterior commissure shown in cross section. Other important structures include the nasopharynx; inferior concha; eustachian tube; sphenoid, ethmoid, and frontal sinuses; maxilla; premolar teeth; and mandible.

# Figure 1-199

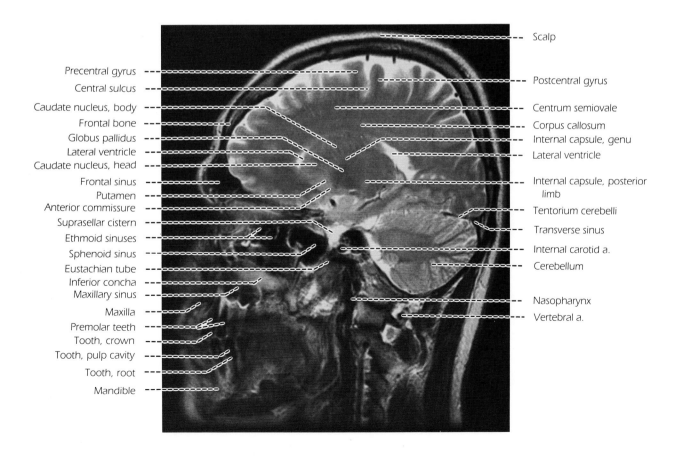

# Figure 1-200

Parasagittal T2-weighted image of the left hemisphere through the thalamus. In the hemisphere, the central sulcus separates the pre- and postcentral gyri. Coursing on the surface of the hemisphere are superior cerebral veins. The tentorium cerebelli separates the cerebral hemisphere from the cerebellum. Caudal to the tentorium cerebelli is the transverse sinus. Rostral to the cerebellum is the quadrigeminal cistern, overlying the brain stem. Caudal within the thalamus is the pulvinar nucleus. Capping the thalamus is the lateral ventricle. The head of the caudate is located rostral to the thalamus. Ventral to the head of the caudate is the putamen. The body of the corpus callosum is seen dorsal to the lateral ventricle. The middle cerebellar peduncle (brachium pontis) connects the pons with the cerebellum. The basis pontis is the ventral bulge in the pons. The vertebral artery is seen in the subarachnoid space beneath and caudal to the pons. The frontal, ethmoid, and sphenoid sinuses are seen. The uvula, tongue, salpingopharyngeal fold, incisive canal, pharyngeal recess, and torus tubarius are visible. Besides the vertebral artery, several other arteries are found in this section including the sphenopalatine artery, greater palatine artery, anterior ethmoidal branch of the sphenopalatine artery, and branches of the anterior cerebral artery.

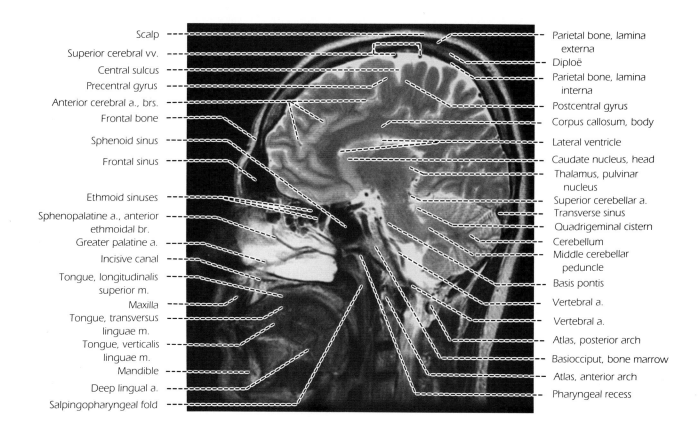

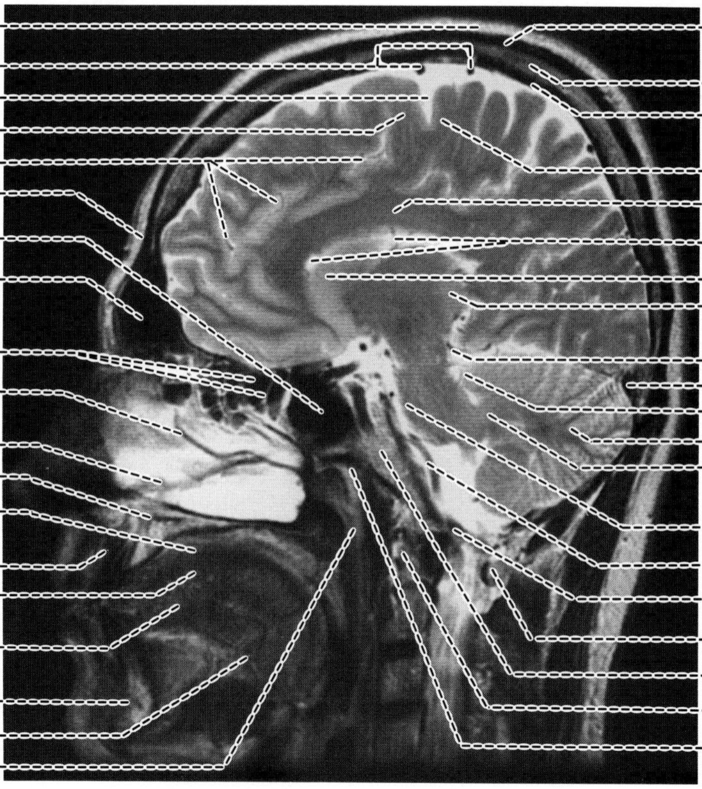
Scalp
Superior cerebral vv.
Central sulcus
Precentral gyrus
Anterior cerebral a., brs.
Frontal bone
Sphenoid sinus
Frontal sinus
Ethmoid sinuses
Sphenopalatine a., anterior ethmoidal br.
Greater palatine a.
Incisive canal
Tongue, longitudinalis superior m.
Maxilla
Tongue, transversus linguae m.
Tongue, verticalis linguae m.
Mandible
Deep lingual a.
Salpingopharyngeal fold
Parietal bone, lamina externa
Diploë
Parietal bone, lamina interna
Postcentral gyrus
Corpus callosum, body
Lateral ventricle
Caudate nucleus, head
Thalamus, pulvinar nucleus
Superior cerebellar a.
Transverse sinus
Quadrigeminal cistern
Cerebellum
Middle cerebellar peduncle
Basis pontis
Vertebral a.
Vertebral a.
Atlas, posterior arch
Basiocciput, bone marrow
Atlas, anterior arch
Pharyngeal recess

Parasagittal T2-weighted image showing the corpus callosum and lateral ventricle. Ventral to the lateral ventricle is the thalamus. Dorsal and caudal within the thalamus is the pulvinar nucleus of the thalamus. The tentorium cerebelli separates the cerebellum from the cerebral hemispheres. Flow voids of the superior cerebellar, posterior inferior cerebellar, and vertebral arteries are seen. Other structures seen in this section include the transverse sinus, posterior arch of the atlas, torus tubarius, uvula, tongue, and frontal sinus.

Figure 1-201

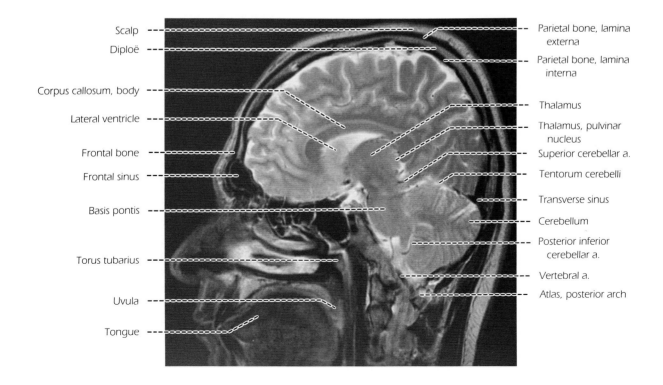

Scalp

Diploë

Corpus callosum, body

Lateral ventricle

Frontal bone

Frontal sinus

Basis pontis

Torus tubarius

Uvula

Tongue

Parietal bone, lamina externa

Parietal bone, lamina interna

Thalamus

Thalamus, pulvinar nucleus

Superior cerebellar a.

Tentorum cerebelli

Transverse sinus

Cerebellum

Posterior inferior cerebellar a.

Vertebral a.

Atlas, posterior arch

## Figure 1-202

Midsagittal T2-weighted image at the level of the thalamus and brain stem. The low signal intensity of the corpus callosum is seen along its extent. The body and splenium of the corpus callosum are identified. Surrounding the corpus callosum is the callosal sulcus and cistern. Dorsal to the callosal sulcus is the cingulate gyrus. Dorsal to the cingulate gyrus is the cingulate sulcus, which separates it from the paracentral lobule. Close to the paracentral lobule are paracentral branches of the anterior cerebral artery. Ventral to the body of the corpus callosum and just rostral to the splenium is the fornix. The thalamus is seen ventral to the corpus callosum, between it and the lateral ventricle. Ventral to the splenium of the corpus callosum is the great cerebral vein (Galen's vein), and adjacent to it is the basal vein (Rosenthal's vein). The anterior medullary velum connects the cerebellum with the tectum of the midbrain. Ventral to the cerebellum is the fourth ventricle, and caudal to it is the cisterna magna. The basilar artery is found ventral to the basis pontis. The parieto-occipital fissure separates the parietal and occipital lobes. The sella turcica, containing the hypophysis, is dorsal to the sphenoid sinus. Dorsal to the sella is the suprasellar cistern. The internal cerebral vein courses dorsal to the thalamus. The quadrigeminal cistern is dorsal to the tectum of the mesencephalon. The anterior cerebral artery is ventral to the rostrum of the corpus callosum. Several branches of the anterior cerebral artery are seen including the frontopolar, pericallosal, paracentral, callosomarginal, and internal frontal. The medulla oblongata is seen caudal to the pons and inferior to the cerebellum. In continuity with the medulla oblongata is the spinal cord. Cervical vertebral bodies, intervertebral disks, and laminae are visible. Other important structures seen in this section include the epiglottis, uvula, tongue, soft palate, nasopharynx, odontoid process of the axis, posterior arch of the atlas vertebrae, mandible, maxilla, anterior arch of the atlas, hard palate, and bone marrow of the basiocciput.

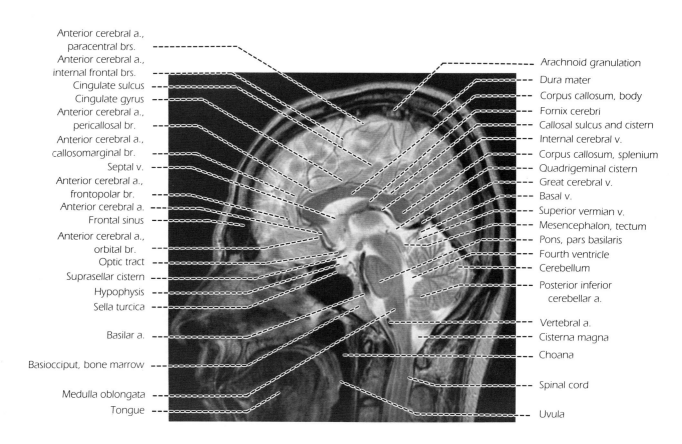

Figure 1-203

Sagittal T2-weighted image through the thalamus and brain stem. The genu, body, and splenium of the corpus callosum are visualized in the midline. Dorsal to the corpus callosum is the callosal sulcus and cistern. The cingulate gyrus is located beneath the callosal sulcus and the cingulate sulcus. Dorsal to the cingulate sulcus is the paracentral lobule. The paracentral sulcus delineates the anterior boundary of the paracentral lobule. Arachnoid granulations are seen dorsal to the hemisphere. The parieto-occipital fissure separates the parietal and occipital lobes. Ventral to the corpus callosum and rostral to the splenium is the fornix. The great cerebral vein (Galen's vein) is seen inferior and caudal to the splenium of the corpus callosum. The thalamus is located ventral to the lateral ventricle. The superior and inferior colliculi form the tectum of the midbrain. The fourth ventricle is between the pons, medulla oblongata, and cerebellum. The vertebral artery is seen inferior to the medulla oblongata, and the basilar artery is inferior to the pons. The hypophysis is seen ventral to the suprasellar cistern. The quadrigeminal cistern is dorsal to the superior and inferior colliculi. The optic tract is dorsal to the suprasellar cistern. The callosomarginal branch of the anterior cerebral artery is dorsal to the cingulate gyrus. The frontal, ethmoid, and sphenoid sinuses are identified. Other important structures include the epiglottis, hyoid bone, mandible, tongue, uvula, soft palate, hard palate, basiocciput, and anterior and posterior arches of the atlas vertebrae.

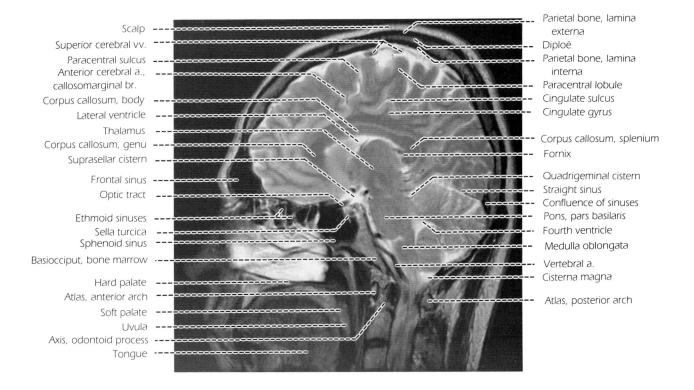

Scalp

Superior cerebral vv.

Paracentral sulcus

Anterior cerebral a., callosomarginal br.

Corpus callosum, body

Lateral ventricle

Thalamus

Corpus callosum, genu

Suprasellar cistern

Frontal sinus

Optic tract

Ethmoid sinuses

Sella turcica

Sphenoid sinus

Basiocciput, bone marrow

Hard palate

Atlas, anterior arch

Soft palate

Uvula

Axis, odontoid process

Tongue

Parietal bone, lamina externa

Diploë

Parietal bone, lamina interna

Paracentral lobule

Cingulate sulcus

Cingulate gyrus

Corpus callosum, splenium

Fornix

Quadrigeminal cistern

Straight sinus

Confluence of sinuses

Pons, pars basilaris

Fourth ventricle

Medulla oblongata

Vertebral a.

Cisterna magna

Atlas, posterior arch

## Figure 1-204

Parasagittal T2-weighted image of the right hemisphere through the thalamus. On the medial surface of the hemisphere, the central sulcus separates the pre- and postcentral gyri. The corpus callosum, a massive white matter bundle connecting the two hemispheres, is seen above the lateral ventricle. The caudate nucleus is found inferior to the lateral ventricle. The fornix is inferior to the caudal part of the corpus callosum. The pulvinar nucleus of the thalamus occupies a caudal position within the thalamus. The parieto-occipital fissure separates the parietal and occipital lobes. The superior cerebral vein and arachnoid granulations are located dorsal to the cerebral hemisphere. Other important structures seen in this section include the transverse venous sinus, vertebral artery, mandible, tongue, maxilla, sphenoid and ethmoid sinuses, internal carotid artery, and frontal bone.

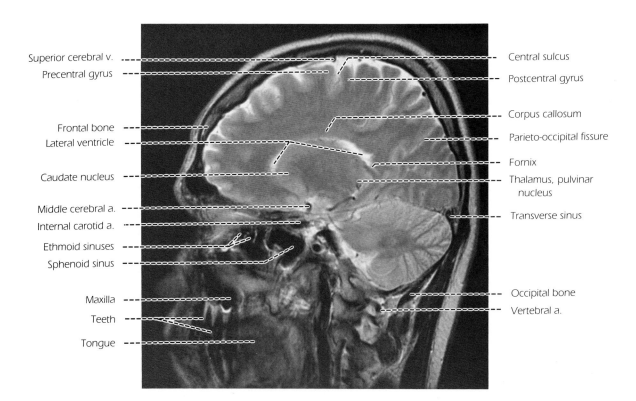

Superior cerebral v.
Precentral gyrus
Frontal bone
Lateral ventricle
Caudate nucleus
Middle cerebral a.
Internal carotid a.
Ethmoid sinuses
Sphenoid sinus
Maxilla
Teeth
Tongue

Central sulcus
Postcentral gyrus
Corpus callosum
Parieto-occipital fissure
Fornix
Thalamus, pulvinar nucleus
Transverse sinus
Occipital bone
Vertebral a.

Sagittal T2-weighted image through the thalamus and basal ganglia. The superior cerebral veins and arachnoid granulations are located dorsal to the cerebral hemisphere. The corona radiata is the deep white matter core of the cerebral hemisphere. The trigone of the lateral ventricle is seen. Dorsal and caudal to the trigone is the parietal portion of the visual radiation. Ventral to the trigone is the fornix. Frontal and anterior to the fornix is the thalamus. The lentiform nucleus is composed of the putamen and the darker globus pallidus. The tentorium cerebelli separates the occipital lobe from the cerebellum. Caudal to the tentorium cerebelli is the transverse sinus. The optic nerve is caudal to the eyeball, and the inferior rectus muscle is ventral to the eyeball. The uncinate fasciculus, one of the long association fiber bundles, is rostral to the putamen. The orbital cortex of the frontal lobe is located in the ventral part of the frontal lobe. The central sulcus separates the pre- and postcentral gyri. Other important structures include the petrous part of the temporal bone, molar and premolar teeth, maxilla, maxillary and sphenoid sinuses, and frontal bone.

Figure 1-205

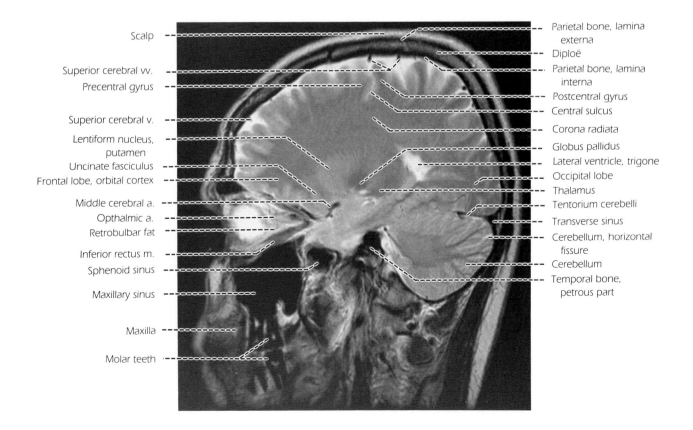

Scalp
Superior cerebral vv.
Precentral gyrus
Superior cerebral v.
Lentiform nucleus, putamen
Uncinate fasciculus
Frontal lobe, orbital cortex
Middle cerebral a.
Opthalmic a.
Retrobulbar fat
Inferior rectus m.
Sphenoid sinus
Maxillary sinus
Maxilla
Molar teeth

Parietal bone, lamina externa
Diploë
Parietal bone, lamina interna
Postcentral gyrus
Central sulcus
Corona radiata
Globus pallidus
Lateral ventricle, trigone
Occipital lobe
Thalamus
Tentorium cerebelli
Transverse sinus
Cerebellum, horizontal fissure
Cerebellum
Temporal bone, petrous part

## Figure 1-206

Parasagittal T2-weighted image through the right hemisphere. The superior cerebral veins are dorsal to the cerebral hemisphere. The central sulcus separates the pre- and postcentral gyri. The corona radiata is the white matter core of the cerebral hemisphere. The optic radiation is seen dorsal and caudal to the trigone of the lateral ventricle. The hippocampus is located within the temporal lobe. The tentorium cerebelli separates the occipital lobes from the cerebellum. Caudal to the tentorium is the transverse venous sinus. The anterior chamber and the lens of the eyeball are identified. The temporal pole is anterior to the hippocampus. Other structures seen in this section include the petrous part of the temporal bone, the bright signal intensity of the vestibule, mandible, lateral pterygoid muscle, maxillary sinus, and frontal bone.

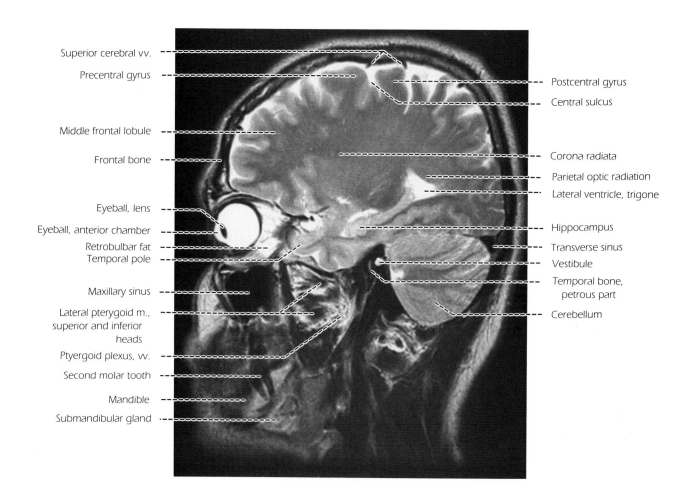

Superior cerebral vv.
Precentral gyrus
Middle frontal lobule
Frontal bone
Eyeball, lens
Eyeball, anterior chamber
Retrobulbar fat
Temporal pole
Maxillary sinus
Lateral pterygoid m., superior and inferior heads
Ptyergoid plexus, vv.
Second molar tooth
Mandible
Submandibular gland

Postcentral gyrus
Central sulcus
Corona radiata
Parietal optic radiation
Lateral ventricle, trigone
Hippocampus
Transverse sinus
Vestibule
Temporal bone, petrous part
Cerebellum

Parasagittal T2-weighted image through the right cerebral hemisphere showing the insular cortex (island of Reil) within the lateral fissure. The circular sulcus of the insular cortex surrounds the insular cortex. Dorsal to the insular cortex is the superior longitudinal fasciculus, one of the long association fiber bundles. The central sulcus separates the pre- and postcentral gyri. The inferior horn of the lateral ventricle is seen in the temporal lobe. Ventral to the ventricle is the inferior optic radiation. The tentorium cerebelli is dorsal to the cerebellum. Caudal to the tentorium is the transverse sinus. The external auditory meatus, cochlea, and semicircular canals are identified. The cornea is located in the front of the eyeball. The orbital cortex of the frontal lobe is in the inferior part of the frontal lobe. Branches of the middle cerebral artery are found rostral to the insular cortex. The lateral pterygoid and temporalis muscles are seen.

Figure 1-207

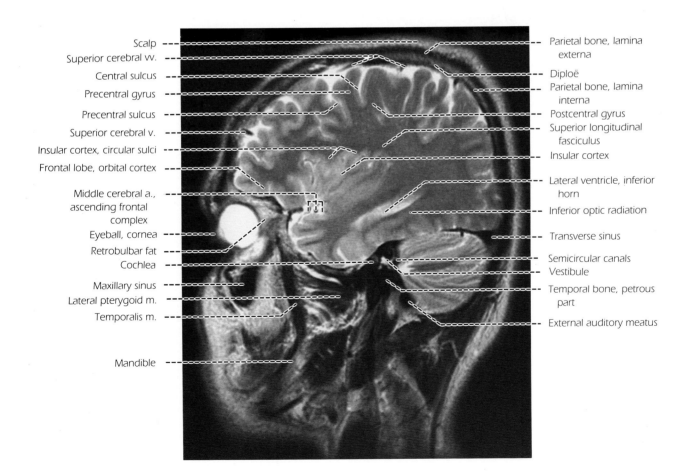

## Figure 1-208

Parasagittal T2-weighted image through the right hemisphere. The central sulcus separates the pre- and postcentral gyri. Branches of the middle cerebral artery are seen in the lateral fissure. The opercular and triangular parts of the inferior frontal lobule are separated by the anterior ascending ramus of the lateral fissure. The inferior longitudinal fasciculus is located in the white matter core of the temporal lobe. Other structures seen in this section include the petrous part of the temporal bone, cerebellar hemisphere, zygomatic bone, temporalis muscle, and infratemporal fat.

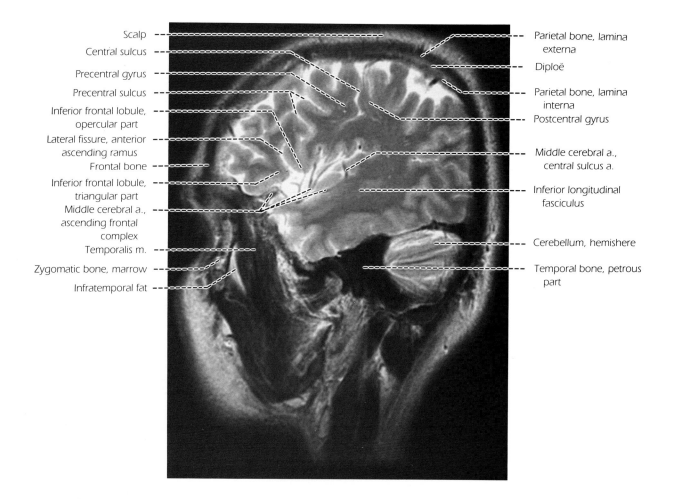

Parasagittal T2-weighted image through the frontal, parietal, and temporal lobes. The lateral fissure separates the frontal and parietal lobes from the temporal lobe. The supramarginal gyrus caps the posterior end of the lateral fissure. Within the temporal lobe, the superior and middle temporal gyri are separated by the superior temporal sulcus. The angular gyrus of the temporal lobe caps the upper end of the superior temporal sulcus. A portion of the lateral hemisphere is seen in the cerebellum. Orbital frontal branches of the middle cerebral artery are located in the orbital part of the frontal lobe. Other important structures include the zygomatic bone, temporalis muscle, masseter muscle, mastoid process, and condylar process of the mandible.

# Figure 1-209

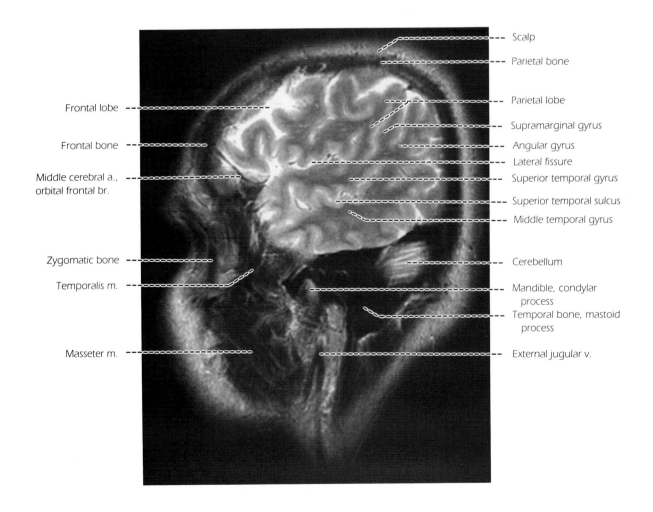

Frontal lobe

Frontal bone

Middle cerebral a., orbital frontal br.

Zygomatic bone

Temporalis m.

Masseter m.

Scalp

Parietal bone

Parietal lobe

Supramarginal gyrus

Angular gyrus

Lateral fissure

Superior temporal gyrus

Superior temporal sulcus

Middle temporal gyrus

Cerebellum

Mandible, condylar process

Temporal bone, mastoid process

External jugular v.

# 2

# NECK

# AXIAL VIEWS

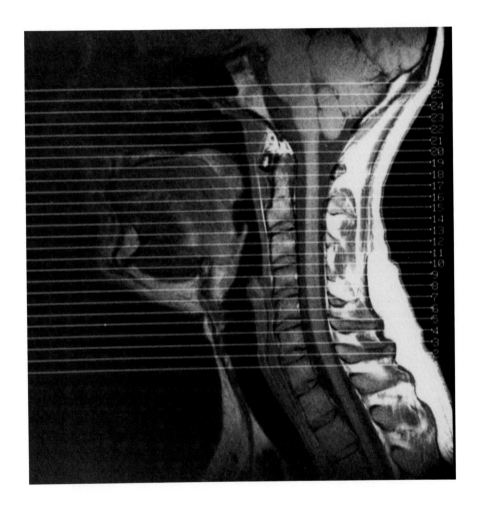

Key to the axial planes of inspection for T1-weighted images.

## Figure 2-1

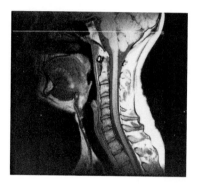

Axial T1-weighted image of several cuts above the neck, showing the facial and vestibulocochlear nerves (cranial nerves VII and VIII). Elements of the facial nerve include the geniculate ganglion (vertical and horizontal parts) and the greater petrosal nerve. Meckel's cavity, containing the semilunar ganglion of the trigeminal nerve (cranial nerve V), is identified. The orbicularis oculi, temporalis, and semispinalis capitis muscles are shown. Bony elements include the nasal septum, basisphenoid, occipital bone, mastoid air cells, greater wing of the sphenoid, zygomatic arch, mandible, zygomatic bone, and maxillary sinus. The arteries include the basilar, superficial temporal, and internal carotid. The retromandibular vein is shown.

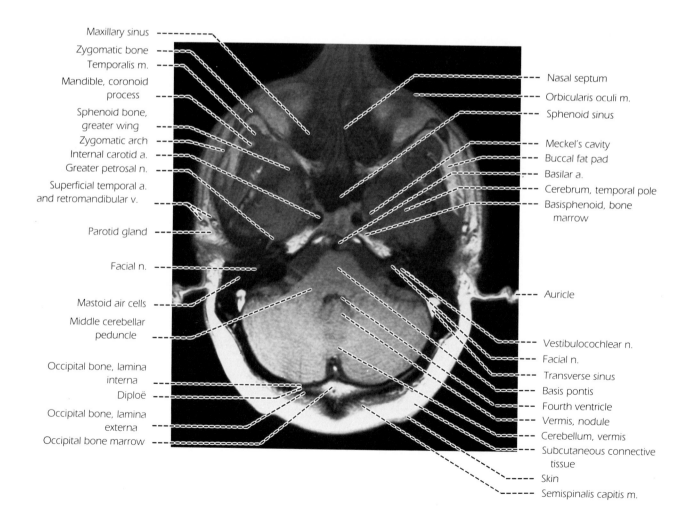

Axial T1-weighted image showing elements of the glossopharyngeal and vagus nerves (cranial nerves IX and X). Important blood vessels include the basilar and superficial temporal arteries, retromandibular vein, and transverse sinus. The muscles of the region include the orbicularis oculi, splenius capitis, semispinalis capitis, masseter, and temporalis. Bony structures include the middle nasal concha, pterygoid plate, temporal bone, mastoid air cells, occipital bone and bone marrow, basiocciput, mandible and its coronoid and condylar processes, nasal septum, and zygomatic bone/arch. Note the cerebellopontine cistern, auricle, and external auditory meatus.

## Figure 2-2

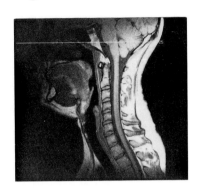

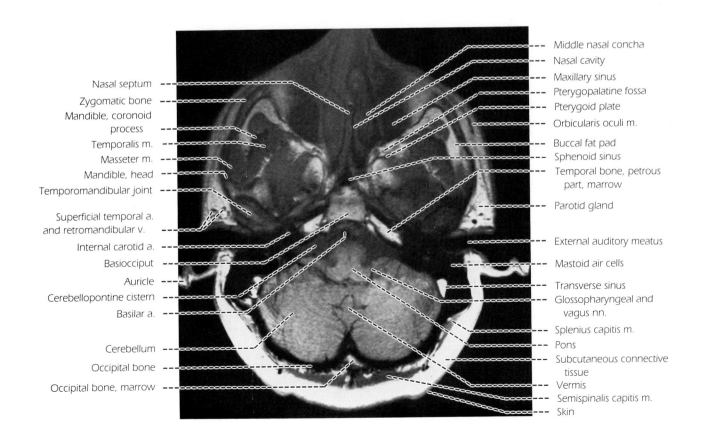

Middle nasal concha
Nasal cavity
Maxillary sinus
Nasal septum
Pterygopalatine fossa
Zygomatic bone
Pterygoid plate
Mandible, coronoid
process
Orbicularis oculi m.
Temporalis m.
Buccal fat pad
Masseter m.
Sphenoid sinus
Mandible, head
Temporal bone, petrous
part, marrow
Temporomandibular joint
Parotid gland
Superficial temporal a.
and retromandibular v.
External auditory meatus
Internal carotid a.
Mastoid air cells
Basiocciput
Transverse sinus
Auricle
Glossopharyngeal and
Cerebellopontine cistern
vagus nn.
Basilar a.
Splenius capitis m.
Pons
Cerebellum
Subcutaneous connective
tissue
Occipital bone
Vermis
Occipital bone, marrow
Semispinalis capitis m.
Skin

# Figure 2-3

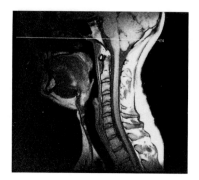

Important muscles visible in this axial T1-weighted image include the orbicularis oculi, splenius capitis, sternocleidomastoid, semispinalis capitis, tensor veli palatini, lateral pterygoid, masseter, and temporalis. The superficial temporal and internal carotid arteries and the retromandibular and internal jugular veins are identified. Bony structures include the inferior concha, coronoid and condylar processes of the mandible, vomer, mastoid air cells of the temporal bone, basiocciput, eustachian tube, and nasal septum. The ligamentum nuchae is seen arising from the external occipital protuberance. Note that the external auditory meatus leads to elements of the vestibular apparatus and cochlea.

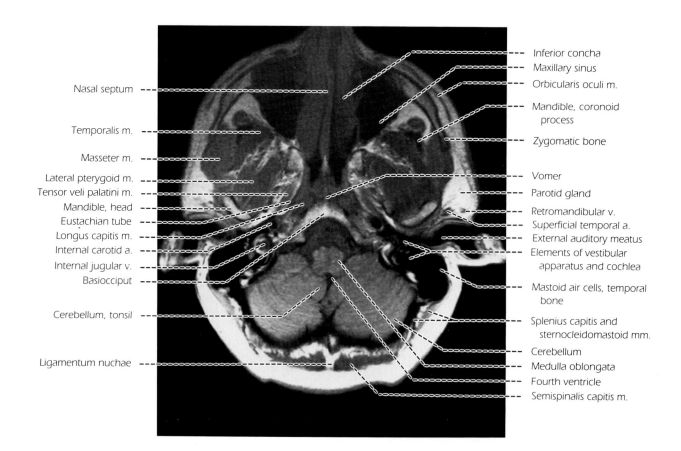

Nasal septum

Temporalis m.

Masseter m.

Lateral pterygoid m.
Tensor veli palatini m.
Mandible, head
Eustachian tube
Longus capitis m.
Internal carotid a.
Internal jugular v.
Basiocciput

Cerebellum, tonsil

Ligamentum nuchae

Inferior concha
Maxillary sinus
Orbicularis oculi m.

Mandible, coronoid
  process
Zygomatic bone

Vomer
Parotid gland
Retromandibular v.
Superficial temporal a.
External auditory meatus
Elements of vestibular
  apparatus and cochlea

Mastoid air cells, temporal
  bone

Splenius capitis and
  sternocleidomastoid mm.
Cerebellum
Medulla oblongata
Fourth ventricle
Semispinalis capitis m.

The blood vessels shown in this axial T1-weighted image include the angular, maxillary, sphenopalatine, superficial temporal, occipital, internal carotid, and deep temporal arteries, and the angular, retromandibular, occipital, and internal jugular veins. The glossopharyngeal, vagus, and spinal accessory nerves (cranial nerves IX, X, and XI) are identified. The pterygopalatine parasympathetic ganglion (cranial nerve) is seen. The condylar and coronoid processes of the mandible, inferior nasal concha, eustachian tube, and mastoid process of the temporal bone are shown. Note the deviated nasal septum and the nasopharynx and its lateral recess. Muscles include the levator labii superioris, orbicularis oculi, zygomaticus major, tensor veli palatini, longus capitis, rectus capitis anterior, splenius capitis, rectus capitis posterior major and minor, semi-spinalis capitis, lateral and medial pterygoids, masseter, and temporalis.

## Figure 2-4

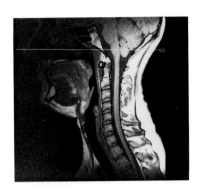

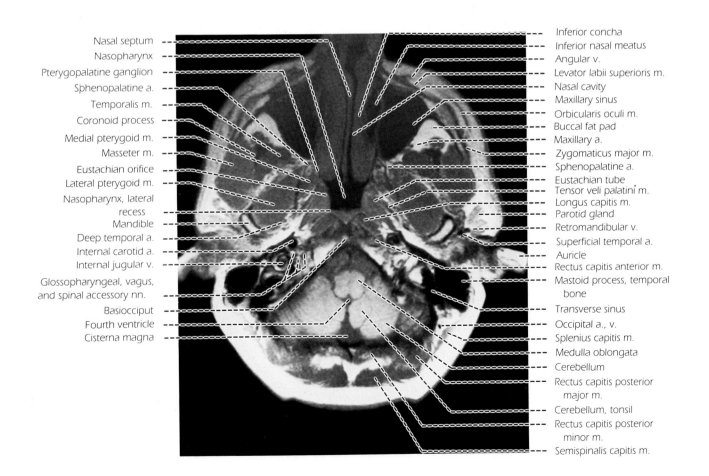

# Figure 2-5

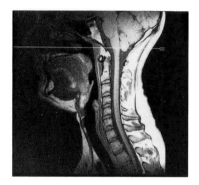

The blood vessels seen in this axial T1-weighted image include the descending palatine, superficial temporal, vertebral, internal carotid, and middle meningeal arteries, and the retromandibular and posterior facial veins. The glossopharyngeal, vagus, and spinal accessory nerves (cranial nerves IX, X, and XI) are identified. Muscles of the head and neck include the levator labii superioris, orbicularis oculi, zygomaticus major, longus capitis, rectus capitis anterior, rectus capitis lateralis, digastric (posterior belly), obliquus capitis superioris, longissimus capitis, splenius capitis, rectus capitis posterior major and minor, semispinalis capitis, trapezius, sternocleidomastoid, lateral and medial pterygoids, and temporalis. Note the pharyngobasilar fascia, parapharyngeal fat, lymph node belonging to the internal jugular group, pharyngeal tubercle, and nasopharynx.

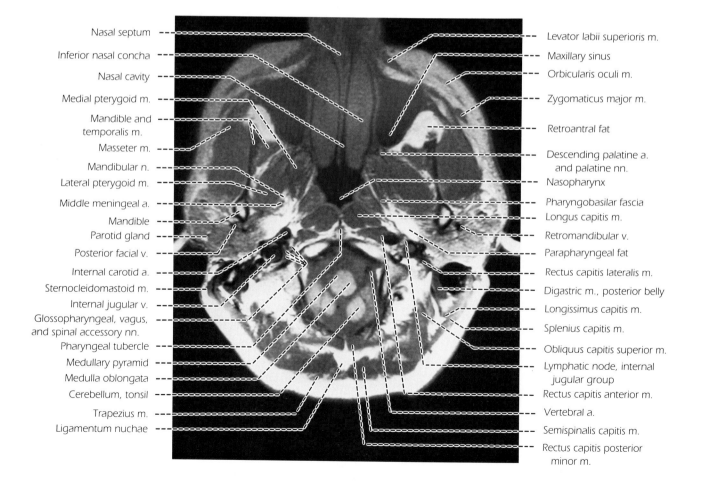

Nasal septum

Inferior nasal concha

Nasal cavity

Medial pterygoid m.

Mandible and temporalis m.

Masseter m.

Mandibular n.

Lateral pterygoid m.

Middle meningeal a.

Mandible

Parotid gland

Posterior facial v.

Internal carotid a.

Sternocleidomastoid m.

Internal jugular v.

Glossopharyngeal, vagus, and spinal accessory nn.

Pharyngeal tubercle

Medullary pyramid

Medulla oblongata

Cerebellum, tonsil

Trapezius m.

Ligamentum nuchae

Levator labii superioris m.

Maxillary sinus

Orbicularis oculi m.

Zygomaticus major m.

Retroantral fat

Descending palatine a. and palatine nn.

Nasopharynx

Pharyngobasilar fascia

Longus capitis m.

Retromandibular v.

Parapharyngeal fat

Rectus capitis lateralis m.

Digastric m., posterior belly

Longissimus capitis m.

Splenius capitis m.

Obliquus capitis superior m.

Lymphatic node, internal jugular group

Rectus capitis anterior m.

Vertebral a.

Semispinalis capitis m.

Rectus capitis posterior minor m.

In this axial T1-weighted image, the parotid gland has reached its maximum size. Note the retromandibular vein within the gland. The muscles located at the back of the head include the digastric (posterior belly), obliquus capitis superioris, splenius capitis, longissimus capitis, rectus capitis posterior major and minor, semispinalis capitis, and trapezius. Note the ligamentum nuchae and anterior and posterior longitudinal ligaments. In relation to the nasopharynx, note the medial pterygoid, tensor veli palatini, palatopharyngeus, and longus capitis and colli muscles. The occipital condyles are seen. The glossopharyngeal, vagus, and spinal accessory nerves, (cranial nerves IX, X, and XI) are clustered with the internal jugular vein and internal carotid artery.

## Figure 2-6

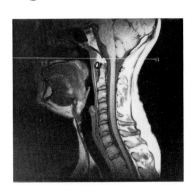

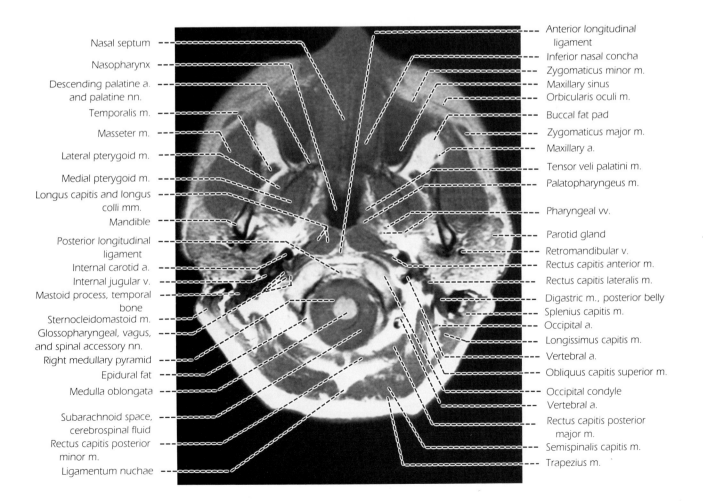

Nasal septum

Nasopharynx

Descending palatine a.
and palatine nn.

Temporalis m.

Masseter m.

Lateral pterygoid m.

Medial pterygoid m.

Longus capitis and longus
colli mm.

Mandible

Posterior longitudinal
ligament

Internal carotid a.

Internal jugular v.

Mastoid process, temporal
bone

Sternocleidomastoid m.

Glossopharyngeal, vagus,
and spinal accessory nn.

Right medullary pyramid

Epidural fat

Medulla oblongata

Subarachnoid space,
cerebrospinal fluid

Rectus capitis posterior
minor m.

Ligamentum nuchae

Anterior longitudinal
ligament

Inferior nasal concha

Zygomaticus minor m.

Maxillary sinus

Orbicularis oculi m.

Buccal fat pad

Zygomaticus major m.

Maxillary a.

Tensor veli palatini m.

Palatopharyngeus m.

Pharyngeal vv.

Parotid gland

Retromandibular v.

Rectus capitis anterior m.

Rectus capitis lateralis m.

Digastric m., posterior belly

Splenius capitis m.

Occipital a.

Longissimus capitis m.

Vertebral a.

Obliquus capitis superior m.

Occipital condyle

Vertebral a.

Rectus capitis posterior
major m.

Semispinalis capitis m.

Trapezius m.

# Figure 2-7

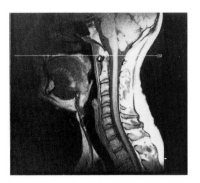

In this axial T1-weighted image the following muscles are identified: zygomaticus minor (infraorbital head), zygomaticus major, buccinator, palatopharyngeus, digastric (posterior belly), obliquus capitis superior, longissimus capitis, sternocleidomastoid, splenius capitis, rectus capitis posterior major, semispinalis capitis, trapezius, longus capitis and colli, stylohyoid, styloglossus, stylopharyngeus, tensor veli palatini, medial and lateral pterygoid, masseter, and tensor and levator palatini. Also shown are the anterior arch of the atlas and its superior articular facet, the bifid spinous process of the axis and its odontoid process, and the alar ligament. The parotid duct (Stensen's duct) and the parotid gland are identified.

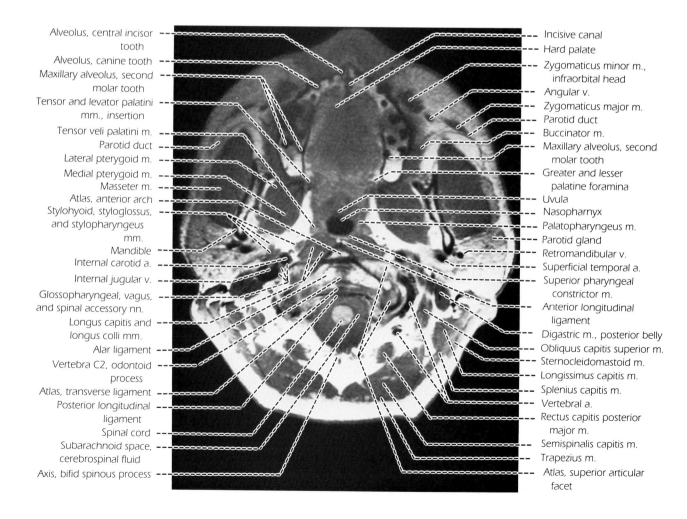

Alveolus, central incisor tooth
Alveolus, canine tooth
Maxillary alveolus, second molar tooth
Tensor and levator palatini mm., insertion
Tensor veli palatini m.
Parotid duct
Lateral pterygoid m.
Medial pterygoid m.
Masseter m.
Atlas, anterior arch
Stylohyoid, styloglossus, and stylopharyngeus mm.
Mandible
Internal carotid a.
Internal jugular v.
Glossopharyngeal, vagus, and spinal accessory nn.
Longus capitis and longus colli mm.
Alar ligament
Vertebra C2, odontoid process
Atlas, transverse ligament
Posterior longitudinal ligament
Spinal cord
Subarachnoid space, cerebrospinal fluid
Axis, bifid spinous process

Incisive canal
Hard palate
Zygomaticus minor m., infraorbital head
Angular v.
Zygomaticus major m.
Parotid duct
Buccinator m.
Maxillary alveolus, second molar tooth
Greater and lesser palatine foramina
Uvula
Nasopharynx
Palatopharyngeus m.
Parotid gland
Retromandibular v.
Superficial temporal a.
Superior pharyngeal constrictor m.
Anterior longitudinal ligament
Digastric m., posterior belly
Obliquus capitis superior m.
Sternocleidomastoid m.
Longissimus capitis m.
Splenius capitis m.
Vertebral a.
Rectus capitis posterior major m.
Semispinalis capitis m.
Trapezius m.
Atlas, superior articular facet

Important blood vessels shown in this axial T1-weighted image include the vertebral, deep cervical, internal and external carotid, ascending pharyngeal, lingual, and facial arteries, and the external and internal jugular and facial veins. Muscles in this part of the neck include the genioglossus, mylohyoideus, hyoglossus, stylopharyngeus, palatopharyngeus, pharyngeal constrictor, sternocleidomastoid, anterior scalene, middle scalene, and posterior scalene, longus colli and capitis, trapezius, splenius cervicis and capitis, semispinalis cervicis and capitis, multifidus, longissimus cervicis and capitis, levator scapulae, digastric (posterior belly), stylohyoideus, platysma, and tongue. The anterior and posterior longitudinal ligaments and the ligamentum flavum and nuchae are seen. The arch and articular process of the third cervical vertebra are seen. Note the fourth cervical nerve.

## Figure 2-8

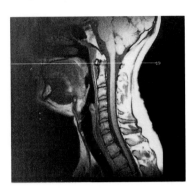

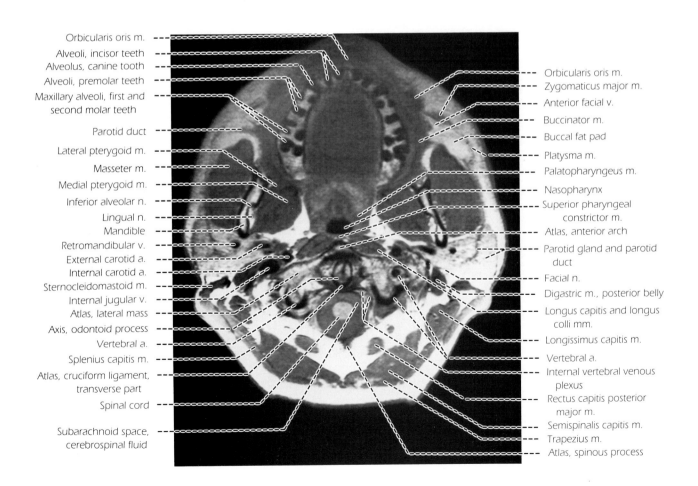

Orbicularis oris m.
Alveoli, incisor teeth
Alveolus, canine tooth
Alveoli, premolar teeth
Maxillary alveoli, first and second molar teeth
Parotid duct
Lateral pterygoid m.
Masseter m.
Medial pterygoid m.
Inferior alveolar n.
Lingual n.
Mandible
Retromandibular v.
External carotid a.
Internal carotid a.
Sternocleidomastoid m.
Internal jugular v.
Atlas, lateral mass
Axis, odontoid process
Vertebral a.
Splenius capitis m.
Atlas, cruciform ligament, transverse part
Spinal cord
Subarachnoid space, cerebrospinal fluid

Orbicularis oris m.
Zygomaticus major m.
Anterior facial v.
Buccinator m.
Buccal fat pad
Platysma m.
Palatopharyngeus m.
Nasopharynx
Superior pharyngeal constrictor m.
Atlas, anterior arch
Parotid gland and parotid duct
Facial n.
Digastric m., posterior belly
Longus capitis and longus colli mm.
Longissimus capitis m.
Vertebral a.
Internal vertebral venous plexus
Rectus capitis posterior major m.
Semispinalis capitis m.
Trapezius m.
Atlas, spinous process

## Figure 2-9

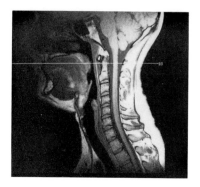

In this axial T1-weighted image the inferior alveolar (cranial nerve V, mandibular division) and second cervical nerve and its sensory ganglion are identified. The bony structures include the lateral mass and posterior arch of the atlas and odontoid process of the axis. Important blood vessels include the inferior alveolar, vertebral, external carotid, and internal carotid arteries, and the facial, inferior alveolar, internal jugular, and retromandibular veins. Parts of the tongue shown are the transversus linguae muscle, root of the tongue and lingual tonsils, foramen cecum, and median lingual sulcus. The muscles of the neck and head include the longissimus capitis, splenius capitis, obliquus capitis inferior, semispinalis capitis, rectus capitis posterior major, trapezius, and sternocleidomastoid.

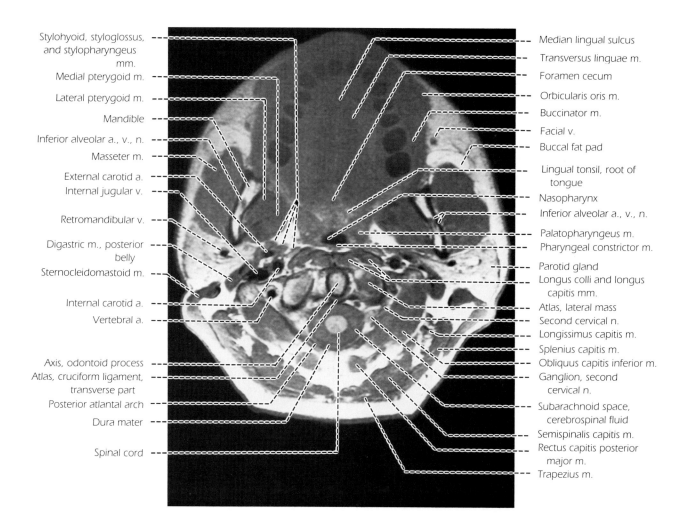

Stylohyoid, styloglossus, and stylopharyngeus mm.

Medial pterygoid m.

Lateral pterygoid m.

Mandible

Inferior alveolar a., v., n.

Masseter m.

External carotid a.

Internal jugular v.

Retromandibular v.

Digastric m., posterior belly

Sternocleidomastoid m.

Internal carotid a.

Vertebral a.

Axis, odontoid process

Atlas, cruciform ligament, transverse part

Posterior atlantal arch

Dura mater

Spinal cord

Median lingual sulcus

Transversus linguae m.

Foramen cecum

Orbicularis oris m.

Buccinator m.

Facial v.

Buccal fat pad

Lingual tonsil, root of tongue

Nasopharynx

Inferior alveolar a., v., n.

Palatopharyngeus m.

Pharyngeal constrictor m.

Parotid gland

Longus colli and longus capitis mm.

Atlas, lateral mass

Second cervical n.

Longissimus capitis m.

Splenius capitis m.

Obliquus capitis inferior m.

Ganglion, second cervical n.

Subarachnoid space, cerebrospinal fluid

Semispinalis capitis m.

Rectus capitis posterior major m.

Trapezius m.

The muscles of the head and neck shown in this axial section include the longus colli and cervicis, splenius cervicis, levator scapulae, obliquus capitis inferior, longissimus capitis, splenius capitis, semispinalis capitis, rectus capitis posterior major, and sternocleidomastoid. The muscles of the pharynx include the palatopharyngeus, stylopharyngeus, and superior pharyngeal constrictor. The muscles of the tongue include the genioglossus, palatoglossus, and hyoglossus. The relationships among the masseter, mandible, and pterygoid muscles are shown. Within the mandibular canal, the inferior alveolar nerve (cranial nerve V, mandibular division) can be identified. Note the spinal cord, subarachnoid space filled with cerebrospinal fluid, and dura mater in the vertebral foramen of the axis. The important internal vertebral arterial and venous plexuses are also identified.

## Figure 2-10

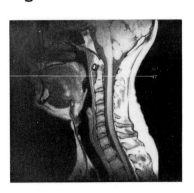

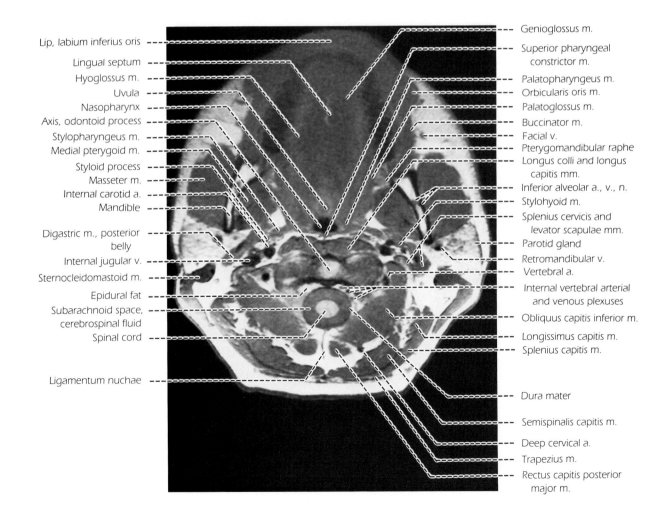

Lip, labium inferius oris

Lingual septum

Hyoglossus m.

Uvula

Nasopharynx

Axis, odontoid process

Stylopharyngeus m.

Medial pterygoid m.

Styloid process

Masseter m.

Internal carotid a.

Mandible

Digastric m., posterior belly

Internal jugular v.

Sternocleidomastoid m.

Epidural fat

Subarachnoid space, cerebrospinal fluid

Spinal cord

Ligamentum nuchae

Genioglossus m.

Superior pharyngeal constrictor m.

Palatopharyngeus m.

Orbicularis oris m.

Palatoglossus m.

Buccinator m.

Facial v.

Pterygomandibular raphe

Longus colli and longus capitis mm.

Inferior alveolar a., v., n.

Stylohyoid m.

Splenius cervicis and levator scapulae mm.

Parotid gland

Retromandibular v.

Vertebral a.

Internal vertebral arterial and venous plexuses

Obliquus capitis inferior m.

Longissimus capitis m.

Splenius capitis m.

Dura mater

Semispinalis capitis m.

Deep cervical a.

Trapezius m.

Rectus capitis posterior major m.

# Figure 2-11

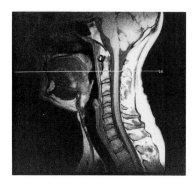

The parts of the second cervical vertebra shown in this axial T1-weighted image include the body, arch, bifid spinous process, transverse foramina containing the vertebral arteries, and vertebral foramen containing the spinal cord. The lingual nerve (cranial nerve V, mandibular division) is adjacent to the medial side of the mandible. The inferior alveolar nerve (cranial nerve V, mandibular division) is seen in the mandibular canal. The muscles include the genioglossus, orbicularis oris, depressor anguli oris, buccinator, palatopharyngeus, stylopharyngeus, pharyngeal constrictor, longus colli and capitis, intertransversarius, scalenus medius, splenius cervicis, levator scapulae, longissimus capitis and cervicis, splenius capitis, obliquus capitis inferior, semispinalis capitis, trapezius, sternocleidomastoid, digastric (posterior belly), stylohyoid, masseter, mylohyoideus, and hyoglossus. The parotid gland is still present, and the palatine tonsils are shown.

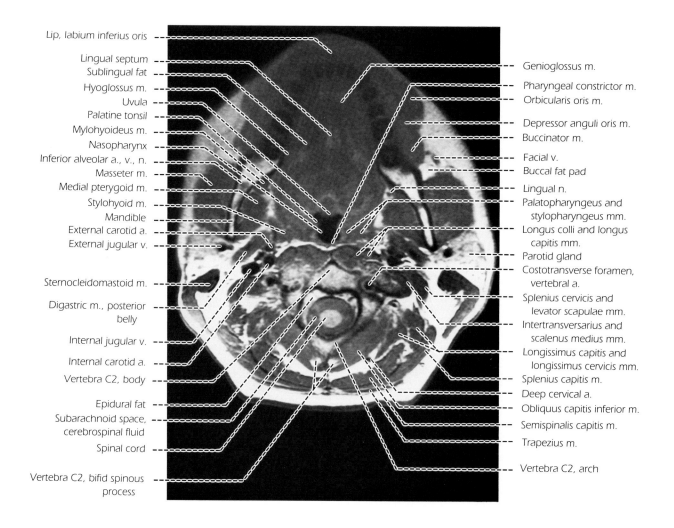

Lip, labium inferius oris
Lingual septum
Sublingual fat
Hyoglossus m.
Uvula
Palatine tonsil
Mylohyoideus m.
Nasopharynx
Inferior alveolar a., v., n.
Masseter m.
Medial pterygoid m.
Stylohyoid m.
Mandible
External carotid a.
External jugular v.

Sternocleidomastoid m.

Digastric m., posterior belly

Internal jugular v.

Internal carotid a.
Vertebra C2, body

Epidural fat
Subarachnoid space, cerebrospinal fluid
Spinal cord

Vertebra C2, bifid spinous process

Genioglossus m.
Pharyngeal constrictor m.
Orbicularis oris m.
Depressor anguli oris m.
Buccinator m.
Facial v.
Buccal fat pad
Lingual n.
Palatopharyngeus and stylopharyngeus mm.
Longus colli and longus capitis mm.
Parotid gland
Costotransverse foramen, vertebral a.
Splenius cervicis and levator scapulae mm.
Intertransversarius and scalenus medius mm.
Longissimus capitis and longissimus cervicis mm.
Splenius capitis m.
Deep cervical a.
Obliquus capitis inferior m.
Semispinalis capitis m.
Trapezius m.

Vertebra C2, arch

Important blood vessels in this axial T1-weighted image include the inferior alveolar, external carotid, internal carotid, vertebral, and deep cervical arteries, and the inferior alveolar, internal jugular, pharyngeal, and retromandibular veins. The nervous system is represented by the inferior alveolar (cranial nerve V, mandibular division), and third cervical nerves, and the spinal cord. Bony structures include the vertebral body of the axis, posterior arch of the axis, bifid spinous process of the axis, and mandible. Muscles of the neck and head include the platysma, sternocleidomastoid, levator scapulae, splenius cervicis and capitis, semispinalis cervicis, trapezius, longus colli and capitis, and scalenus medius and posterior. Note the ligamenta nuchae and flavum. The muscles of the mouth and pharynx include the hyoglossus, masseter, stylohyoideus, genioglossus, orbicularis oris, depressor anguli oris, buccinator, mylohyoideus, styloglossus, medial pterygoid, palatopharyngeus, stylopharyngeus, and pharyngeal constrictor. Note also the palatine tonsil and the diminished size of the parotid gland.

## Figure 2-12

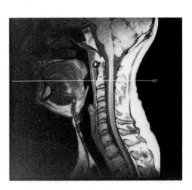

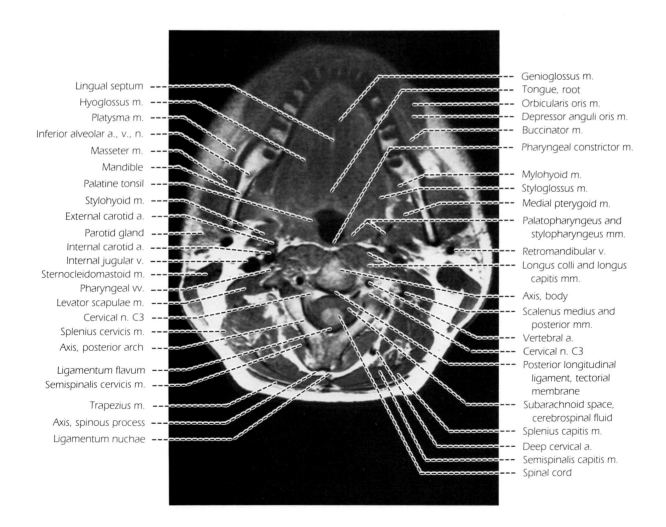

## Figure 2-13

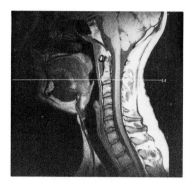

Bony structures visible in this axial T1-weighted image include the body of the axis and an articular facet. The vagus (cranial nerve X), second cervical, and greater occipital nerves are identified. The epiglottis, valleculae, and pharyngoepiglottic fold are present in this section. Other pharyngeal structures include the stylopharyngeus, palatopharyngeus, and pharyngeal constrictor muscles. Three ligaments are shown: posterior longitudinal and tectorial membrane, ligamentum flavum, and ligamentum nuchae. The sublingual, parotid, and submandibular salivary glands are present.

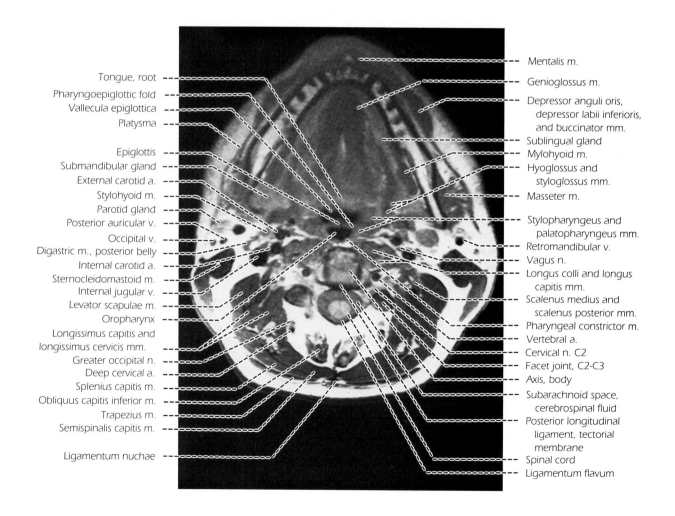

Important blood vessels shown in this axial T1-weighted image include the vertebral, deep cervical, internal carotid, external carotid, facial, and lingual arteries, and the retromandibular, vertebral venous rete, internal jugular, facial, and sublingual veins. The vagus nerve (cranial nerve X) is identified. The body, superior articular process, and transverse foramen of the third vertebra are present. The ligamenta flavum and nuchae and anterior and posterior longitudinal ligaments are identified. The scalenus anterior, medius, and posterior muscles are seen.

# Figure 2-14

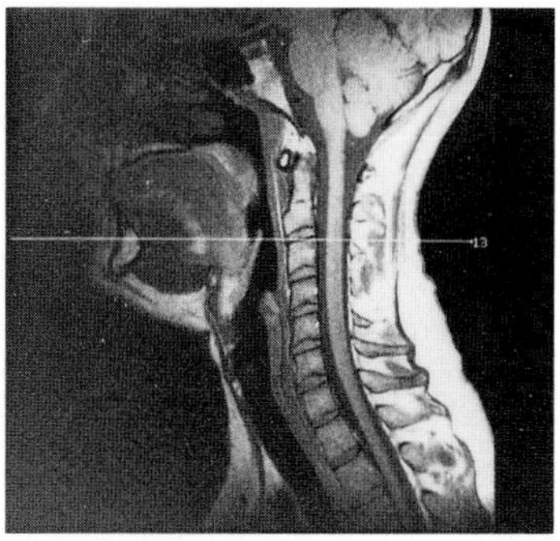

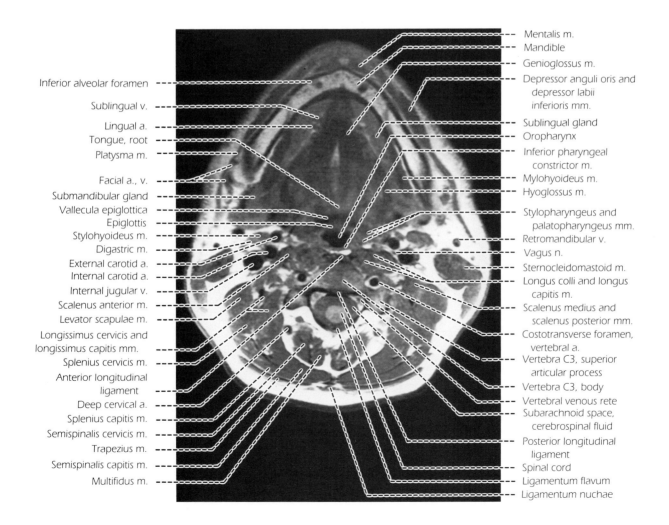

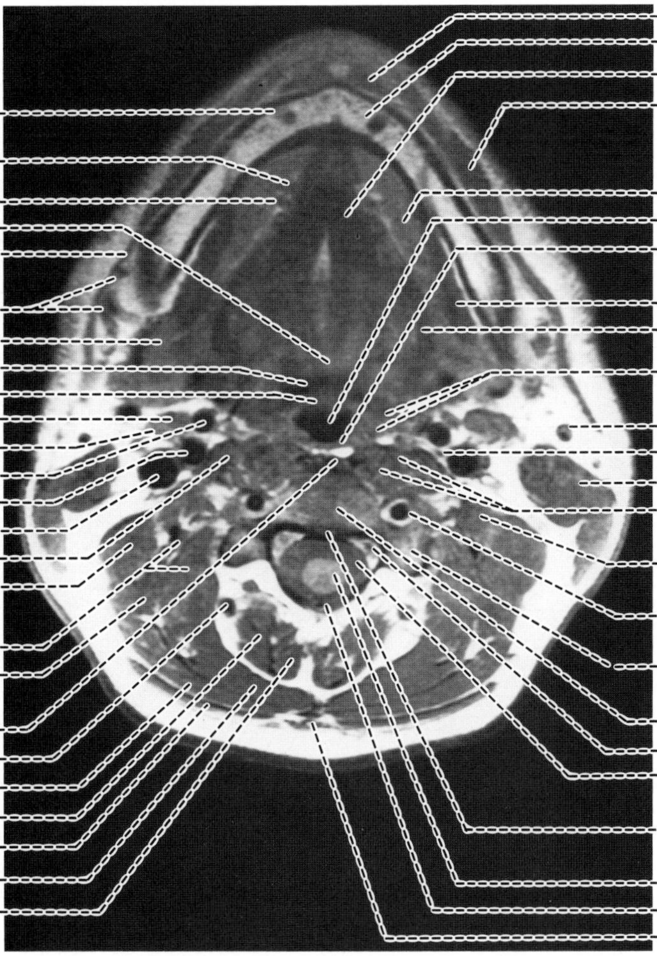
Inferior alveolar foramen
Sublingual v.
Lingual a.
Tongue, root
Platysma m.
Facial a., v.
Submandibular gland
Vallecula epiglottica
Epiglottis
Stylohyoideus m.
Digastric m.
External carotid a.
Internal carotid a.
Internal jugular v.
Scalenus anterior m.
Levator scapulae m.
Longissimus cervicis and longissimus capitis mm.
Splenius cervicis m.
Anterior longitudinal ligament
Deep cervical a.
Splenius capitis m.
Semispinalis cervicis m.
Trapezius m.
Semispinalis capitis m.
Multifidus m.
Mentalis m.
Mandible
Genioglossus m.
Depressor anguli oris and depressor labii inferioris mm.
Sublingual gland
Oropharynx
Inferior pharyngeal constrictor m.
Mylohyoideus m.
Hyoglossus m.
Stylopharyngeus and palatopharyngeus mm.
Retromandibular v.
Vagus n.
Sternocleidomastoid m.
Longus colli and longus capitis m.
Scalenus medius and scalenus posterior mm.
Costotransverse foramen, vertebral a.
Vertebra C3, superior articular process
Vertebra C3, body
Vertebral venous rete
Subarachnoid space, cerebrospinal fluid
Posterior longitudinal ligament
Spinal cord
Ligamentum flavum
Ligamentum nuchae

# Figure 2-15

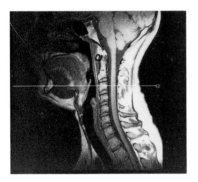

Important blood vessels shown in this axial T1-weighted image include the vertebral, deep cervical, internal and external carotid, ascending pharyngeal, lingual, and facial arteries, and the external and internal jugular and facial veins. Muscles in this part of the neck include the genioglossus, mylohyoideus, hyoglossus, stylopharyngeus, palatopharyngeus, pharyngeal constrictor, sternocleidomastoid, anterior scalene, middle scalene, and posterior scalene, longus colli and capitis, trapezius, splenius cervicis and capitis, semispinalis cervicis and capitis, multifidus, longissimus cervicis and capitis, levator scapulae, digastric (posterior belly), stylohyoideus, platysma, and tongue. The anterior and posterior longitudinal ligaments and the ligamentum flavum and nuchae are seen. The arch and articular process of the third cervical vertebra are seen. Note the fourth cervical nerve.

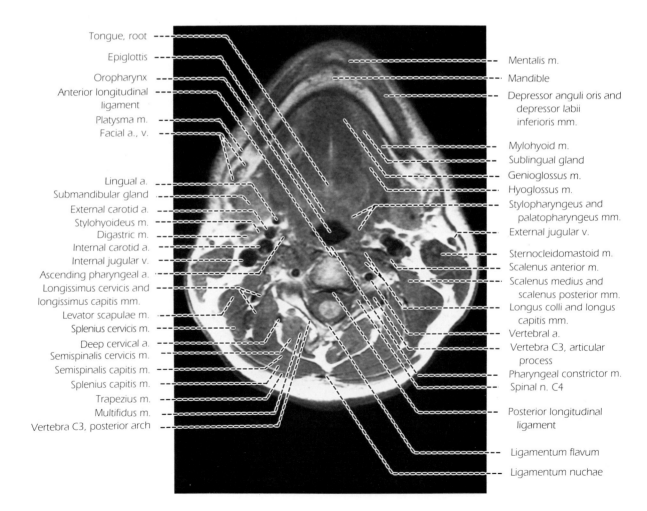

Tongue, root
Epiglottis
Oropharynx
Anterior longitudinal ligament
Platysma m.
Facial a., v.

Lingual a.
Submandibular gland
External carotid a.
Stylohyoideus m.
Digastric m.
Internal carotid a.
Internal jugular v.
Ascending pharyngeal a.
Longissimus cervicis and longissimus capitis mm.
Levator scapulae m.
Splenius cervicis m.
Deep cervical a.
Semispinalis cervicis m.
Semispinalis capitis m.
Splenius capitis m.
Trapezius m.
Multifidus m.
Vertebra C3, posterior arch

Mentalis m.
Mandible
Depressor anguli oris and depressor labii inferioris mm.
Mylohyoid m.
Sublingual gland
Genioglossus m.
Hyoglossus m.
Stylopharyngeus and palatopharyngeus mm.
External jugular v.
Sternocleidomastoid m.
Scalenus anterior m.
Scalenus medius and scalenus posterior mm.
Longus colli and longus capitis mm.
Vertebral a.
Vertebra C3, articular process
Pharyngeal constrictor m.
Spinal n. C4
Posterior longitudinal ligament
Ligamentum flavum
Ligamentum nuchae

The body and inferior articular process of the third cervical vertebra are identified in this axial T1-weighted image. Note the fourth cervical nerve. The vertebral foramen of the third cervical vertebra can be identified by the spinal cord and subarachnoid space; the costotransverse foramen can be identified by the presence of the vertebral artery. The anterior and posterior longitudinal ligaments and ligamentum nuchae can be seen. Important blood vessels include the vertebral, deep cervical, external and internal carotid, superior thyroid, lingual, and facial arteries; and the external and internal jugular, ascending pharyngeal, deep facial, common facial, and facial veins. Muscles associated with the stability of the vertebral column include the multifidus, interspinales, longissimus cervicis, longus colli, semispinalis cervicis, splenius cervicis, and the scalenes (anterior, middle, and posterior).

# Figure 2-16

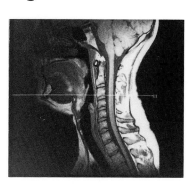

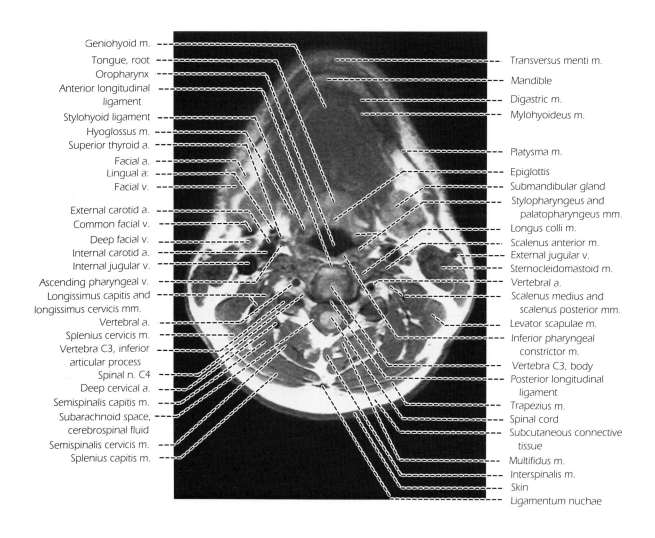

Geniohyoid m.
Tongue, root
Oropharynx
Anterior longitudinal ligament
Stylohyoid ligament
Hyoglossus m.
Superior thyroid a.
Facial a.
Lingual a.
Facial v.
External carotid a.
Common facial v.
Deep facial v.
Internal carotid a.
Internal jugular v.
Ascending pharyngeal v.
Longissimus capitis and longissimus cervicis mm.
Vertebral a.
Splenius cervicis m.
Vertebra C3, inferior articular process
Spinal n. C4
Deep cervical a.
Semispinalis capitis m.
Subarachnoid space, cerebrospinal fluid
Semispinalis cervicis m.
Splenius capitis m.

Transversus menti m.
Mandible
Digastric m.
Mylohyoideus m.
Platysma m.
Epiglottis
Submandibular gland
Stylopharyngeus and palatopharyngeus mm.
Longus colli m.
Scalenus anterior m.
External jugular v.
Sternocleidomastoid m.
Vertebral a.
Scalenus medius and scalenus posterior mm.
Levator scapulae m.
Inferior pharyngeal constrictor m.
Vertebra C3, body
Posterior longitudinal ligament
Trapezius m.
Spinal cord
Subcutaneous connective tissue
Multifidus m.
Interspinalis m.
Skin
Ligamentum nuchae

# Figure 2-17

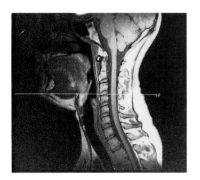

Structures in the pharyngeal region visible in this axial T1-weighted image include the pre-epiglottic space; epiglottis; laryngeal vestibule; stylopharyngeus, palatopharyngeus, and inferior pharyngeal constrictor muscles; piriform sinus; aryepiglottic fold; and hyoid bone. The fourth vertebral body, transverse foramen, and transverse process are identified as is the spinal cord in the vertebral foramen. Note the vertebral artery and vein in the transverse foramen. Several important nerves identified in this section include the phrenic, vagus (cranial nerve X), and internal laryngeal (cranial nerve X). Important blood vessels include the vertebral, deep cervical, external and internal carotid, and superior laryngeal arteries, and the common facial, vertebral, external and internal jugular, and superior laryngeal veins.

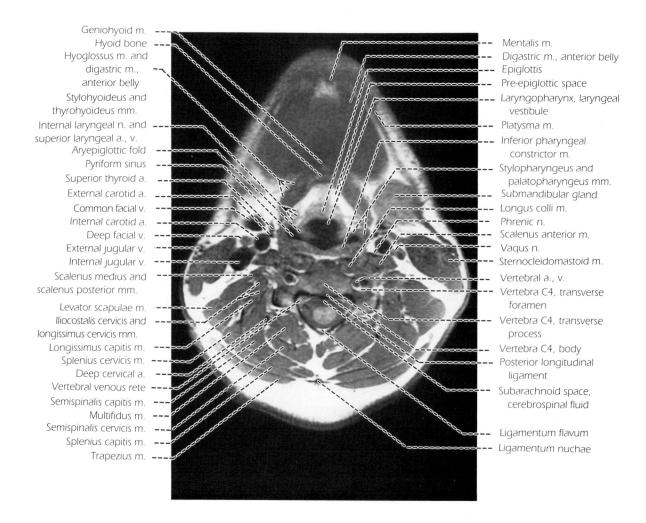

Muscles visible in this axial T1-weighted image include the digastric (anterior belly), geniohyoid, platysma, sternohyoid, thyrohyoid, sternocleidomastoid, scalenes (anterior, medius, and posterior), longus colli, levator scapulae, trapezius, splenius capitis and cervicis, multifidus, semispinalis capitis and cervicis, iliocostalis cervicis, and longissimus cervicis. Note the thyroid cartilage and its superior cornu. The fourth cervical vertebral body, posterior arch, articular process, and bifid spinous process are identified. The cervical spinal nerve is also present. In the laryngeal region are the pre-epiglottic space, aryepiglottic fold, petiolus of the epiglottis, laryngeal vestibule, and the internal laryngeal artery, vein, and nerve. The anterior and posterior longitudinal ligaments and the ligamenta flavum and nuchae are identified.

## Figure 2-18

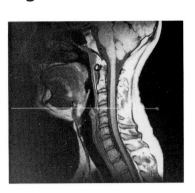

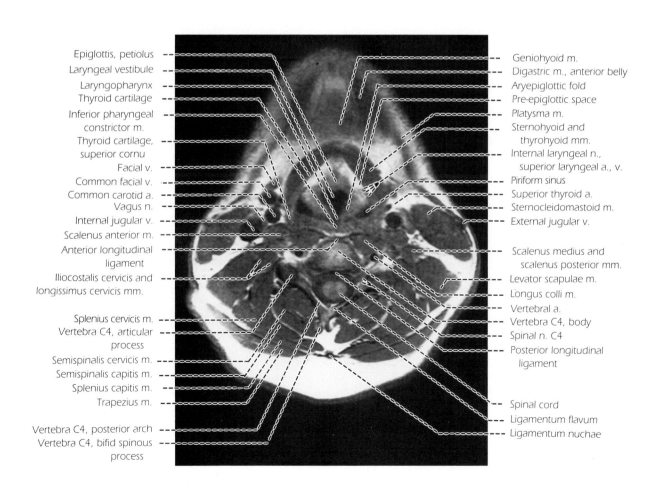

Epiglottis, petiolus
Laryngeal vestibule
Laryngopharynx
Thyroid cartilage
Inferior pharyngeal constrictor m.
Thyroid cartilage, superior cornu
Facial v.
Common facial v.
Common carotid a.
Vagus n.
Internal jugular v.
Scalenus anterior m.
Anterior longitudinal ligament
Iliocostalis cervicis and longissimus cervicis mm.
Splenius cervicis m.
Vertebra C4, articular process
Semispinalis cervicis m.
Semispinalis capitis m.
Splenius capitis m.
Trapezius m.
Vertebra C4, posterior arch
Vertebra C4, bifid spinous process

Geniohyoid m.
Digastric m., anterior belly
Aryepiglottic fold
Pre-epiglottic space
Platysma m.
Sternohyoid and thyrohyoid mm.
Internal laryngeal n., superior laryngeal a., v.
Piriform sinus
Superior thyroid a.
Sternocleidomastoid m.
External jugular v.
Scalenus medius and scalenus posterior mm.
Levator scapulae m.
Longus colli m.
Vertebral a.
Vertebra C4, body
Spinal n. C4
Posterior longitudinal ligament
Spinal cord
Ligamentum flavum
Ligamentum nuchae

# Figure 2-19

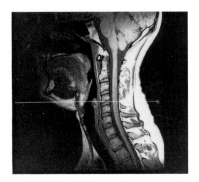

In this axial T1-weighted image, the spinal accessory nerve (cranial nerve XI) is present along with two muscles it supplies, the sternocleidomastoid and trapezius. The fourth cervical vertebra is represented by several parts, including the body and articular process. The spinal cord is in the fourth vertebral foramen and the vertebral arteries are in the fourth transverse foramen. The dorsal and ventral roots of the fifth cervical nerve have been resolved. The thyroid cartilage is still present, but the epiglottis is represented only by its stalk (petiolus).

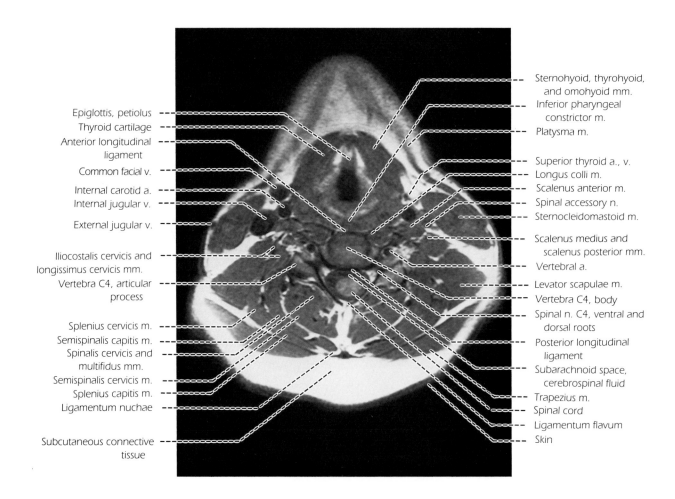

Epiglottis, petiolus
Thyroid cartilage
Anterior longitudinal ligament
Common facial v.
Internal carotid a.
Internal jugular v.
External jugular v.

Iliocostalis cervicis and longissimus cervicis mm.
Vertebra C4, articular process

Splenius cervicis m.
Semispinalis capitis m.
Spinalis cervicis and multifidus mm.
Semispinalis cervicis m.
Splenius capitis m.
Ligamentum nuchae

Subcutaneous connective tissue

Sternohyoid, thyrohyoid, and omohyoid mm.
Inferior pharyngeal constrictor m.
Platysma m.

Superior thyroid a., v.
Longus colli m.
Scalenus anterior m.
Spinal accessory n.
Sternocleidomastoid m.

Scalenus medius and scalenus posterior mm.
Vertebral a.
Levator scapulae m.
Vertebra C4, body
Spinal n. C4, ventral and dorsal roots
Posterior longitudinal ligament
Subarachnoid space, cerebrospinal fluid
Trapezius m.
Spinal cord
Ligamentum flavum
Skin

Axial T1-weighted image through the rima glottidis and vocal cord as well as some of the muscles and associated structures involved in voice and sound production including the thyroid and arytenoid cartilages and the thyroarytenoideus and arytenoideus muscles. Important blood vessels found in this section include the superior thyroid, vertebral, deep cervical, and common carotid arteries, and the anterior jugular, superior thyroid, and external and internal jugular veins. The vertebral arteries are in the transverse foramina. The spinal cord is in the vertebral foramen of the fifth cervical vertebra.

## Figure 2-20

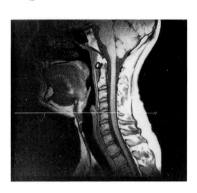

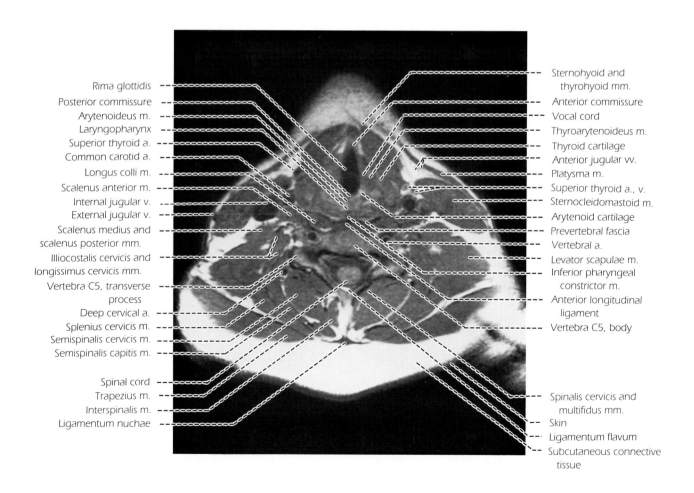

Rima glottidis

Posterior commissure

Arytenoideus m.

Laryngopharynx

Superior thyroid a.

Common carotid a.

Longus colli m.

Scalenus anterior m.

Internal jugular v.

External jugular v.

Scalenus medius and scalenus posterior mm.

Illiocostalis cervicis and longissimus cervicis mm.

Vertebra C5, transverse process

Deep cervical a.

Splenius cervicis m.

Semispinalis cervicis m.

Semispinalis capitis m.

Spinal cord

Trapezius m.

Interspinalis m.

Ligamentum nuchae

Sternohyoid and thyrohyoid mm.

Anterior commissure

Vocal cord

Thyroarytenoideus m.

Thyroid cartilage

Anterior jugular vv.

Platysma m.

Superior thyroid a., v.

Sternocleidomastoid m.

Arytenoid cartilage

Prevertebral fascia

Vertebral a.

Levator scapulae m.

Inferior pharyngeal constrictor m.

Anterior longitudinal ligament

Vertebra C5, body

Spinalis cervicis and multifidus mm.

Skin

Ligamentum flavum

Subcutaneous connective tissue

## Figure 2-21

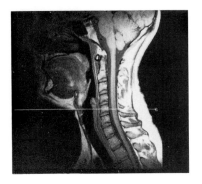

The muscles of the neck region visible in this axial T1-weighted image include the sternohyoid, thyrohyoid, platysma, sternocleidomastoid, levator scapulae, iliocostalis cervicis, longissimus cervicis, trapezius, splenius cervicis, spinalis cervicis, multifidus, semispinalis cervicis, semispinalis capitis, splenius capitis, scalenus anterior, scalenus medius, scalenus posterior, longus colli, and inferior pharyngeal constrictor. The phrenic nerve and fifth cervical spinal nerve are present. The fifth cervical nerve, with some nerve fibers from the fourth cervical nerve, begins its contributions to the brachial plexus of nerves, which innervates the upper limb.

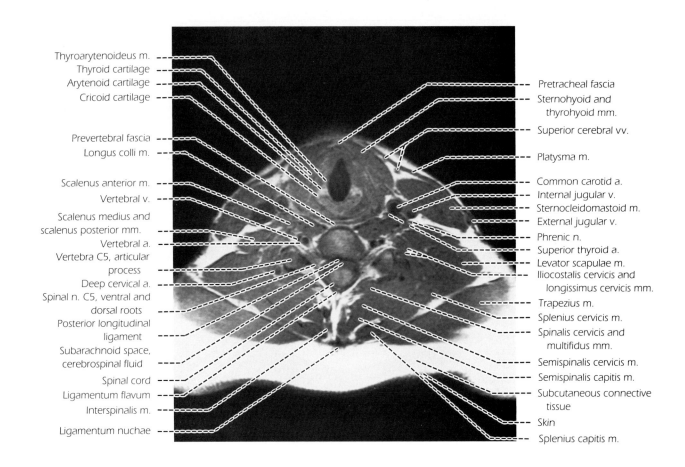

In this axial T1-weighted image, the body, arch, inferior articular process, and spinous process of the fifth cervical vertebra are seen. The vertebral foramen is filled with the spinal cord and its membranes, cerebrospinal fluid, fat, and blood vessels. The vertebral arteries and veins fill the transverse foramina of the fifth cervical vertebra. The blood vessels identified in this section include the common carotid, superior thyroid, ascending cervical, deep cervical, and vertebral arteries, and the anterior jugular, internal jugular, and vertebral veins. The inferior cornu of the thyroid cartilage and cricothyroid muscle are seen for the first time.

## Figure 2-22

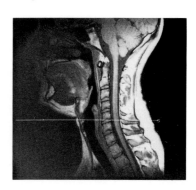

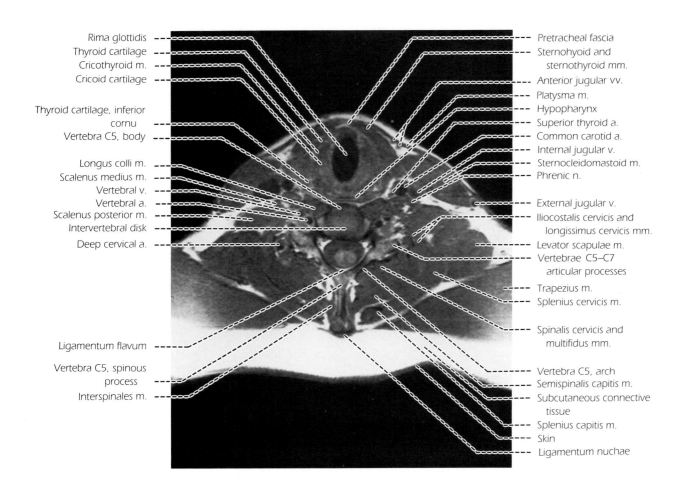

Rima glottidis
Thyroid cartilage
Cricothyroid m.
Cricoid cartilage

Thyroid cartilage, inferior cornu
Vertebra C5, body

Longus colli m.
Scalenus medius m.
Vertebral v.
Vertebral a.
Scalenus posterior m.
Intervertebral disk
Deep cervical a.

Ligamentum flavum

Vertebra C5, spinous process
Interspinales m.

Pretracheal fascia
Sternohyoid and sternothyroid mm.
Anterior jugular vv.
Platysma m.
Hypopharynx
Superior thyroid a.
Common carotid a.
Internal jugular v.
Sternocleidomastoid m.
Phrenic n.

External jugular v.
Iliocostalis cervicis and longissimus cervicis mm.
Levator scapulae m.
Vertebrae C5–C7 articular processes
Trapezius m.
Splenius cervicis m.

Spinalis cervicis and multifidus mm.

Vertebra C5, arch
Semispinalis capitis m.
Subcutaneous connective tissue
Splenius capitis m.
Skin
Ligamentum nuchae

# Figure 2-23

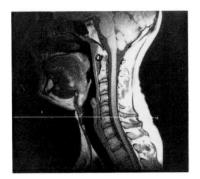

The thyroid gland and esophagus are present in this axial T1-weighted image. Several nerves are identifiable including the supraclavicular, vagus, and spinal accessory (cranial nerves X and XI), fifth and sixth cervical, and phrenic. The sixth cervical vertebral body, articular process, and spinous process are seen. At the level of the sixth cervical vertebra, the transverse foramen is filled in about 90 percent of cases with entering vertebral arteries and veins. Significantly fewer vessels enter either the seventh (about 3 percent) or fifth (about 10 percent) transverse foramen. Important neck muscles include the levator scapulae, iliocostalis cervicis, longissimus cervicis, trapezius, splenius cervicis, semispinalis cervicis, spinalis cervicis, multifidus, longus colli, and the anterior, middle, and posterior scalenes.

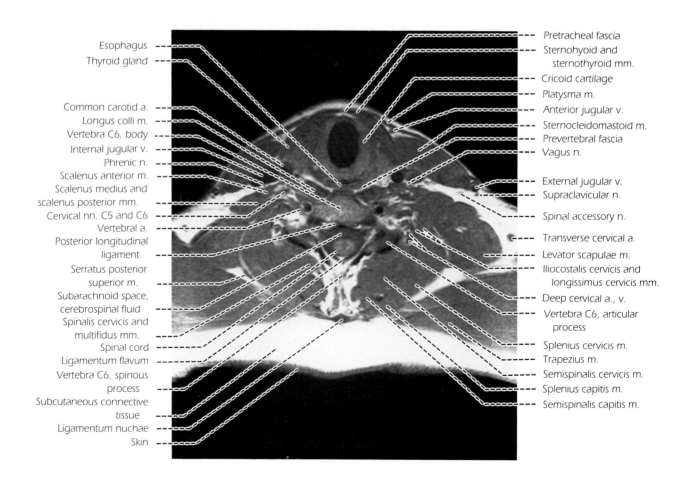

In this axial T1-weighted image, the vagus (cranial nerve X), inferior laryngeal, phrenic, and fifth and sixth cervical nerves are seen. The fifth and sixth cervical nerves both contribute to the formation of the brachial plexus of nerves. The ventral roots of the fifth cervical nerve through the first thoracic nerve usually pass between the anterior and middle scalene muscles. The visceral compartment of the neck contains the trachea, thyroid gland, esophagus, and blood vessels; they are separated from the vertebral column and its associated muscles by the retropharyngeal space and prevertebral fascia. The prevertebral muscles seen in this section include the anterior, middle, and posterior scalene and longus colli muscles.

## Figure 2-24

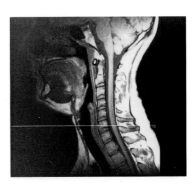

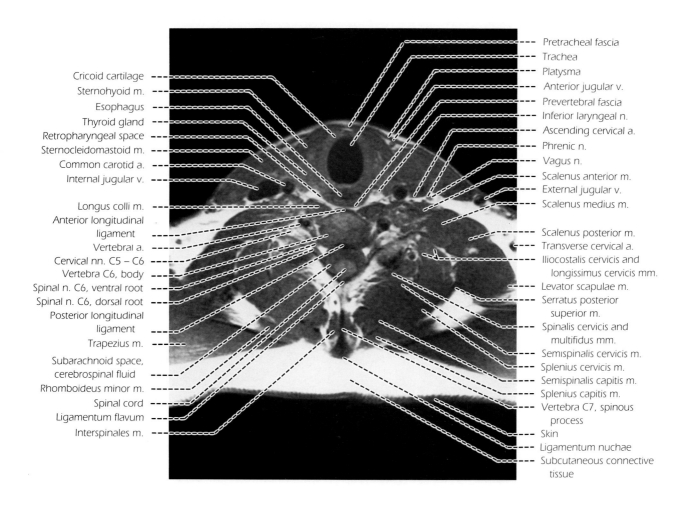

Cricoid cartilage

Sternohyoid m.

Esophagus

Thyroid gland

Retropharyngeal space

Sternocleidomastoid m.

Common carotid a.

Internal jugular v.

Longus colli m.

Anterior longitudinal ligament

Vertebral a.

Cervical nn. C5 – C6

Vertebra C6, body

Spinal n. C6, ventral root

Spinal n. C6, dorsal root

Posterior longitudinal ligament

Trapezius m.

Subarachnoid space, cerebrospinal fluid

Rhomboideus minor m.

Spinal cord

Ligamentum flavum

Interspinales m.

Pretracheal fascia

Trachea

Platysma

Anterior jugular v.

Prevertebral fascia

Inferior laryngeal n.

Ascending cervical a.

Phrenic n.

Vagus n.

Scalenus anterior m.

External jugular v.

Scalenus medius m.

Scalenus posterior m.

Transverse cervical a.

Iliocostalis cervicis and longissimus cervicis mm.

Levator scapulae m.

Serratus posterior superior m.

Spinalis cervicis and multifidus mm.

Semispinalis cervicis m.

Splenius cervicis m.

Semispinalis capitis m.

Splenius capitis m.

Vertebra C7, spinous process

Skin

Ligamentum nuchae

Subcutaneous connective tissue

## Figure 2-25

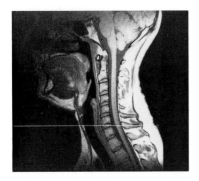

Important nerves found in this axial T1-weighted image include the sympathetic trunk, supraclavicular nerve, phrenic nerve, fifth, sixth, and seventh cervical nerves, and inferior laryngeal nerve (cranial nerve X). The following blood vessels are seen: the inferior thyroid, transverse cervical, deep cervical, vertebral, and common carotid arteries, and the anterior jugular, inferior thyroid, external jugular, superficial cervical, transverse cervical, and vertebral veins. The vertebral arteries are not in the transverse foramen of the seventh cervical vertebra.

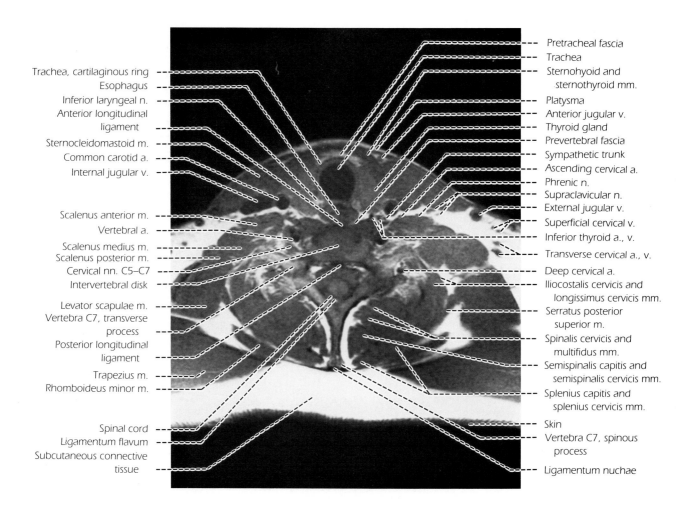

In this axial T1-weighted image, the following nerves are seen: the phrenic, sympathetic trunk, fifth, sixth, and seventh cervical nerves (these cervical nerves participate in the formation of the brachial plexus), and the inferior laryngeal, which is a branch of the vagus (cranial nerve X). Important blood vessels include the inferior thyroid, ascending cervical, deep cervical, vertebral, and common carotid arteries, and the inferior thyroid, external jugular, and vertebral veins. The seventh cervical vertebra is represented by its body and transverse process. Ligaments associated with the spinal column include the ligamentum nuchae, supraspinal ligament, ligamentum flavum, and anterior and posterior longitudinal ligaments. Note the trachea and its cartilage and the thyroid gland. Cervical muscles include the scalenes, longus colli, iliocostalis cervicis, longissimus cervicis, spinalis cervicis, and splenius cervicis.

## Figure 2-26

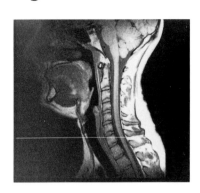

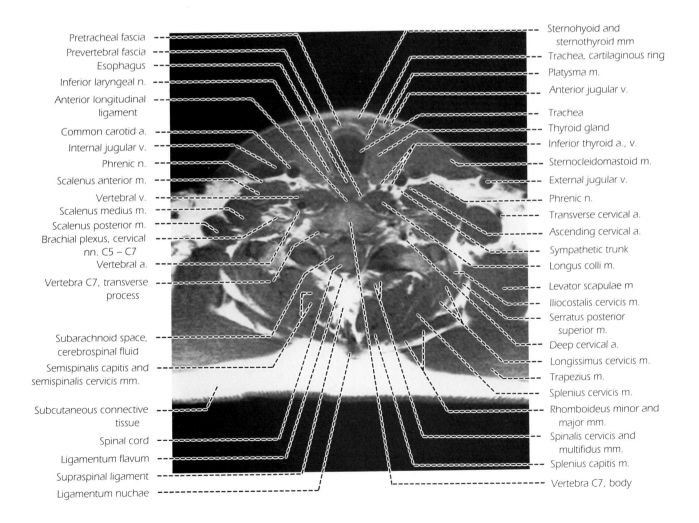

# Figure 2-27

The muscles identified in this axial T2-weighted image include the platysma, sternohyoid, sternothyroid in the visceral compartment; the three scalenes and longus colli in the prevertebral region; and the iliocostalis cervicis, longissimus cervicis, splenius cervicis, and multifidus in the vertebral region. The body, arch and spinous process of the fifth cervical vertebra is seen. The thyroid gland extends above the level of the trachea to the infraglottic region of the larynx and is at the level of the cricoid cartilage in this section.

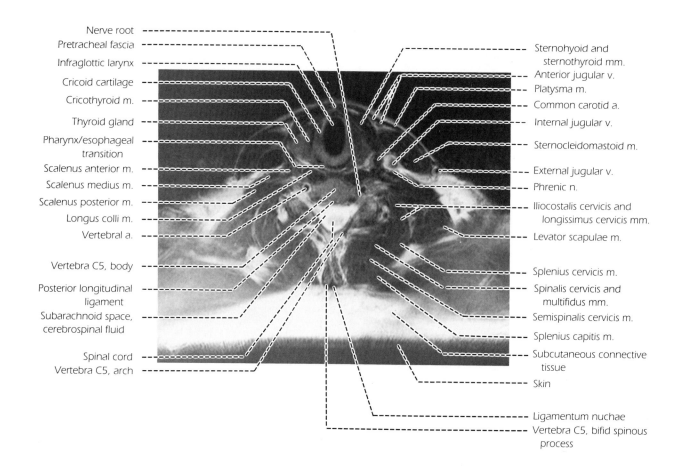

Nerve root
Pretracheal fascia
Infraglottic larynx
Cricoid cartilage
Cricothyroid m.
Thyroid gland
Pharynx/esophageal transition
Scalenus anterior m.
Scalenus medius m.
Scalenus posterior m.
Longus colli m.
Vertebral a.

Vertebra C5, body
Posterior longitudinal ligament
Subarachnoid space, cerebrospinal fluid

Spinal cord
Vertebra C5, arch

Sternohyoid and sternothyroid mm.
Anterior jugular v.
Platysma m.
Common carotid a.
Internal jugular v.
Sternocleidomastoid m.
External jugular v.
Phrenic n.
Iliocostalis cervicis and longissimus cervicis mm.
Levator scapulae m.
Splenius cervicis m.
Spinalis cervicis and multifidus mm.
Semispinalis cervicis m.
Splenius capitis m.
Subcutaneous connective tissue
Skin
Ligamentum nuchae
Vertebra C5, bifid spinous process

# CORONAL VIEWS

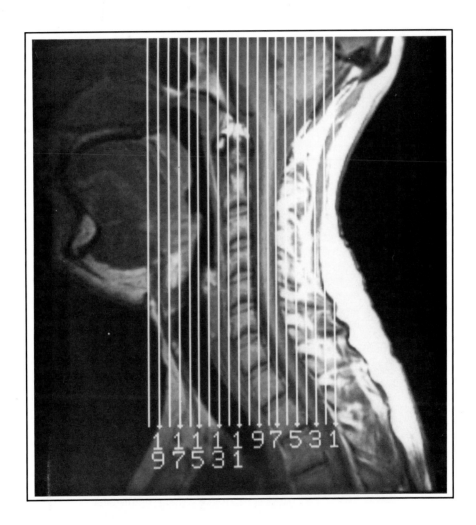

Key to the coronal planes of inspection for T1-weighted images.

# Figure 2-28

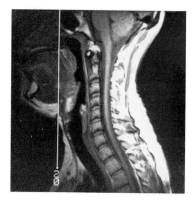

Although not part of the neck, there are several structures of interest in this coronal T1-weighted image. These include the orbit, where the optic nerve (cranial nerve II) and the medial and inferior rectus muscles are seen. In the nasal cavity, the superior, middle, and inferior nasal conchae are visible. Note that the nasal mucosa has become swollen and occludes the right nasal cavity. The hard palate, the alveolar parts of the maxilla, and mandible are seen with the tongue occupying the midline.

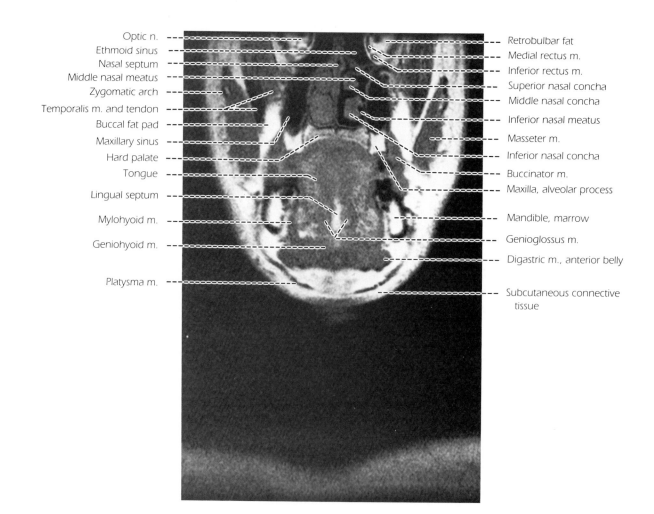

Optic n.
Ethmoid sinus
Nasal septum
Middle nasal meatus
Zygomatic arch
Temporalis m. and tendon
Buccal fat pad
Maxillary sinus
Hard palate
Tongue
Lingual septum
Mylohyoid m.
Geniohyoid m.
Platysma m.

Retrobulbar fat
Medial rectus m.
Inferior rectus m.
Superior nasal concha
Middle nasal concha
Inferior nasal meatus
Masseter m.
Inferior nasal concha
Buccinator m.
Maxilla, alveolar process
Mandible, marrow
Genioglossus m.
Digastric m., anterior belly
Subcutaneous connective tissue

The structural/functional condition of the nasal mucosa in this coronal T1-weighted image is as noted in the legend to Figure 2-28. In this section, the relationship between the masseter, mandible, and temporalis muscle can be seen. In addition, the parotid (Stenson's) duct can be found on the buccinator muscle. The duct pierces this muscle to gain access to the mouth. Note the appearance of the hyoid bone and ophthalmic artery in the orbit.

## Figure 2-29

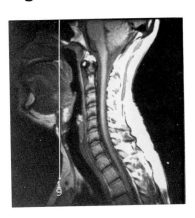

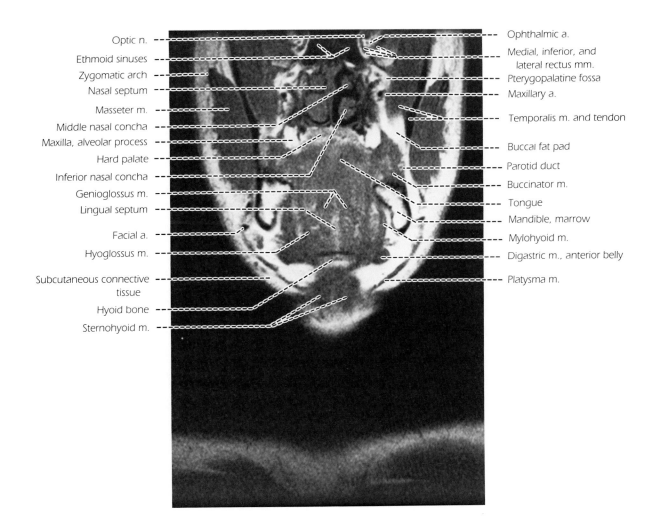

Optic n.
Ethmoid sinuses
Zygomatic arch
Nasal septum
Masseter m.
Middle nasal concha
Maxilla, alveolar process
Hard palate
Inferior nasal concha
Genioglossus m.
Lingual septum
Facial a.
Hyoglossus m.
Subcutaneous connective tissue
Hyoid bone
Sternohyoid m.

Ophthalmic a.
Medial, inferior, and lateral rectus mm.
Pterygopalatine fossa
Maxillary a.
Temporalis m. and tendon
Buccal fat pad
Parotid duct
Buccinator m.
Tongue
Mandible, marrow
Mylohyoid m.
Digastric m., anterior belly
Platysma m.

## Figure 2-30

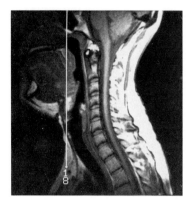

In this coronal T1-weighted image, all the muscles of mastication are represented: temporalis, masseter, and medial and lateral pterygoids. The hard palate, no longer visible in this section, has been replaced by the soft palate. The thyroid cartilage and sternohyoid and thyrohyoid muscles are seen. Note the submandibular gland beneath the mandible.

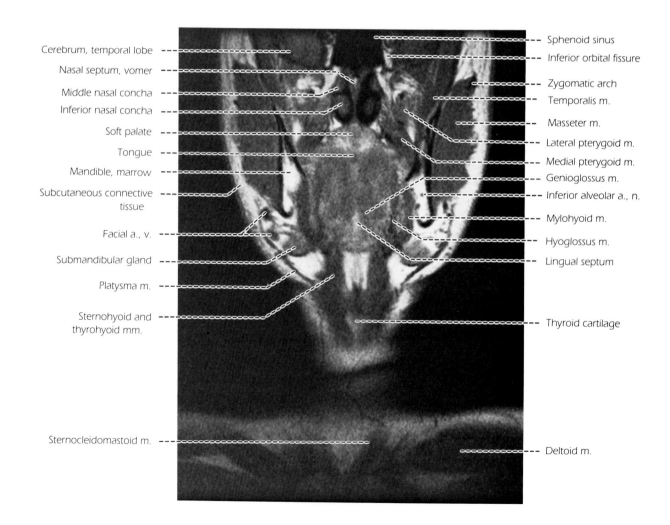

Cerebrum, temporal lobe

Nasal septum, vomer

Middle nasal concha

Inferior nasal concha

Soft palate

Tongue

Mandible, marrow

Subcutaneous connective tissue

Facial a., v.

Submandibular gland

Platysma m.

Sternohyoid and thyrohyoid mm.

Sternocleidomastoid m.

Sphenoid sinus

Inferior orbital fissure

Zygomatic arch

Temporalis m.

Masseter m.

Lateral pterygoid m.

Medial pterygoid m.

Genioglossus m.

Inferior alveolar a., n.

Mylohyoid m.

Hyoglossus m.

Lingual septum

Thyroid cartilage

Deltoid m.

Visible in this coronal T1-weighted image of the neck are the muscles of mastication: temporalis, lateral and medial pterygoids, and masseter. Note their relationship to the mandible. Note also the maxillary artery in the substance of the lateral pterygoid muscle. The sphenoid sinus is located above the nasopharynx and beneath the soft palate. The parotid gland is seen on the lateral margin of the masseter; the submandibular gland is beneath and medial to the mandible. The cut passes through the thyroid cartilage, and the larynx is exposed. The thyroid gland is identified. The facial artery and vein and the anterior jugular vein are also seen in this section. The inferior alveolar neurovascular bundle contains the inferior alveolar nerve, which is part of the mandibular division of the trigeminal nerve (cranial nerve V).

## Figure 2-31

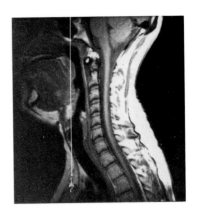

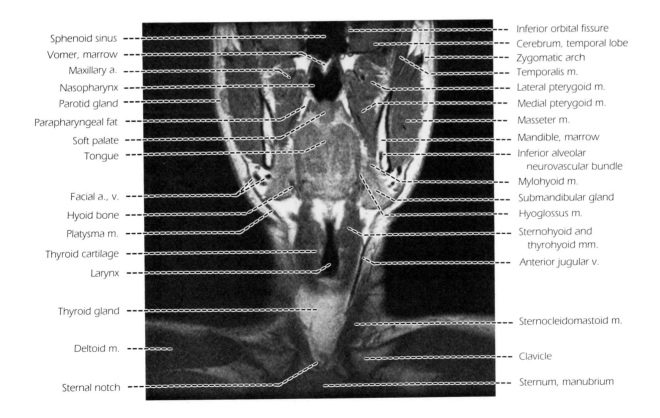

Sphenoid sinus
Vomer, marrow
Maxillary a.
Nasopharynx
Parotid gland
Parapharyngeal fat
Soft palate
Tongue
Facial a., v.
Hyoid bone
Platysma m.
Thyroid cartilage
Larynx
Thyroid gland
Deltoid m.
Sternal notch

Inferior orbital fissure
Cerebrum, temporal lobe
Zygomatic arch
Temporalis m.
Lateral pterygoid m.
Medial pterygoid m.
Masseter m.
Mandible, marrow
Inferior alveolar neurovascular bundle
Mylohyoid m.
Submandibular gland
Hyoglossus m.
Sternohyoid and thyrohyoid mm.
Anterior jugular v.
Sternocleidomastoid m.
Clavicle
Sternum, manubrium

# Figure 2-32

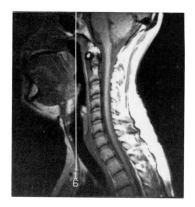

In this coronal T1-weighted image of the neck, the temporal lobe of the cerebrum can be seen lying on the floor of the middle cranial fossa. The muscles of mastication, which are described in the legend to Figure 2-31, are still present. The parotid and submandibular glands are also present. Note the palatine tonsils and the soft palate. The epiglottis is found in the pharynx, as well as the rima glottidis, the narrow space between the true vocal cords. Note the inferior thyroid veins.

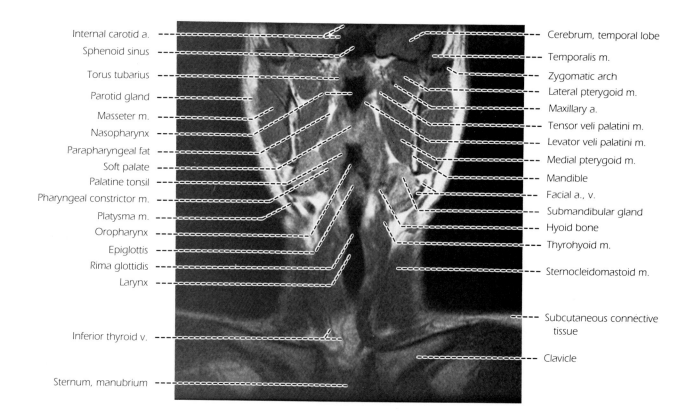

Internal carotid a. — Cerebrum, temporal lobe
Sphenoid sinus — Temporalis m.
Torus tubarius — Zygomatic arch
Parotid gland — Lateral pterygoid m.
Masseter m. — Maxillary a.
Nasopharynx — Tensor veli palatini m.
Parapharyngeal fat — Levator veli palatini m.
Soft palate — Medial pterygoid m.
Palatine tonsil — Mandible
Pharyngeal constrictor m. — Facial a., v.
Platysma m. — Submandibular gland
Oropharynx — Hyoid bone
Epiglottis — Thyrohyoid m.
Rima glottidis — Sternocleidomastoid m.
Larynx
— Subcutaneous connective tissue
Inferior thyroid v. — Clavicle
Sternum, manubrium

In this coronal T1-weighted image, the cavernous sinus containing the internal carotid artery is visible. The muscles of mastication found in this section include the lateral and medial pterygoids, masseter, and temporalis. Medial to the maxillary artery are the tensor and levator of the soft palate. Note the parotid gland and parotid (Stenson's) duct, located medially in the substance of the gland. The submandibular gland, still present, is located beneath the mandible. The true vocal ligament is seen at the rima glottidis beneath the cricoid cartilage.

## Figure 2-33

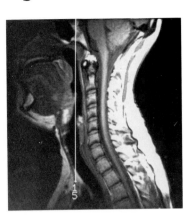

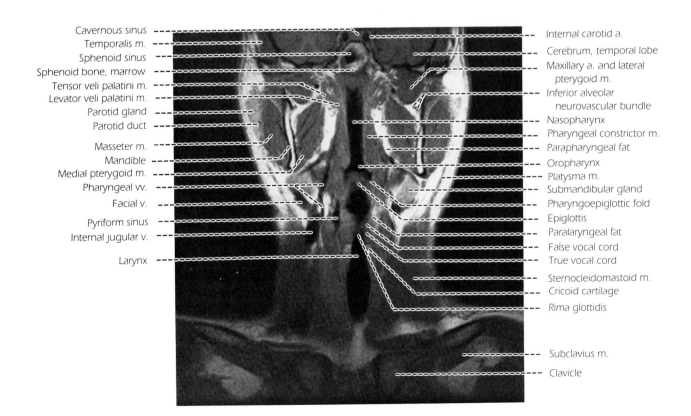

Cavernous sinus
Temporalis m.
Sphenoid sinus
Sphenoid bone, marrow
Tensor veli palatini m.
Levator veli palatini m.
Parotid gland
Parotid duct
Masseter m.
Mandible
Medial pterygoid m.
Pharyngeal vv.
Facial v.
Pyriform sinus
Internal jugular v.
Larynx

Internal carotid a.
Cerebrum, temporal lobe
Maxillary a. and lateral pterygoid m.
Inferior alveolar neurovascular bundle
Nasopharynx
Pharyngeal constrictor m.
Parapharyngeal fat
Oropharynx
Platysma m.
Submandibular gland
Pharyngoepiglottic fold
Epiglottis
Paralaryngeal fat
False vocal cord
True vocal cord
Sternocleidomastoid m.
Cricoid cartilage
Rima glottidis
Subclavius m.
Clavicle

# Figure 2-34

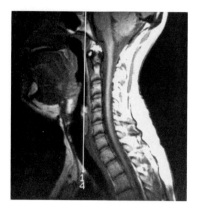

The blood vessels identified in this coronal T1-weighted image include the internal carotid, ascending pharyngeal, external carotid, common carotid, and maxillary arteries; the external and internal jugular, inferior thyroid, right brachiocephalic, facial, and maxillary veins; and the pterygoid plexus. The vocal fold is still present. Note the subclavius muscle, located beneath the clavicle.

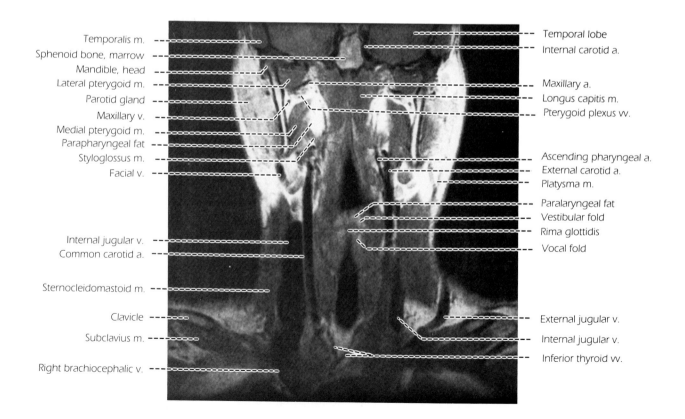

Temporalis m.
Sphenoid bone, marrow
Mandible, head
Lateral pterygoid m.
Parotid gland
Maxillary v.
Medial pterygoid m.
Parapharyngeal fat
Styloglossus m.
Facial v.

Internal jugular v.
Common carotid a.

Sternocleidomastoid m.

Clavicle
Subclavius m.

Right brachiocephalic v.

Temporal lobe
Internal carotid a.

Maxillary a.
Longus capitis m.
Pterygoid plexus vv.

Ascending pharyngeal a.
External carotid a.
Platysma m.

Paralaryngeal fat
Vestibular fold
Rima glottidis
Vocal fold

External jugular v.
Internal jugular v.
Inferior thyroid vv.

In this coronal T1-weighted image of the neck, the vertebral arteries are seen entering the sixth transverse foramen, the most common entry point (88 percent on left side, 92 percent on right side). Parts of the cochlea and semicircular canals are seen in the inner ear. The cervical vertebrae are identified. The atlantoaxial joint is clearly demonstrated. Note the anterior scalene muscle with the nerves of the brachial plexus coursing between the anterior scalene and the medial and posterior scalene muscles. The right and left subclavian arteries are shown with their vertebral, deep cervical, and transverse cervical branches. The common origin of the splenius capitis, longissimus capitis, and digastric muscles is shown, but the three muscles are not individually identified.

## Figure 2-37

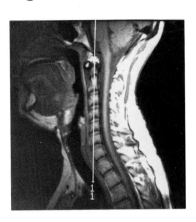

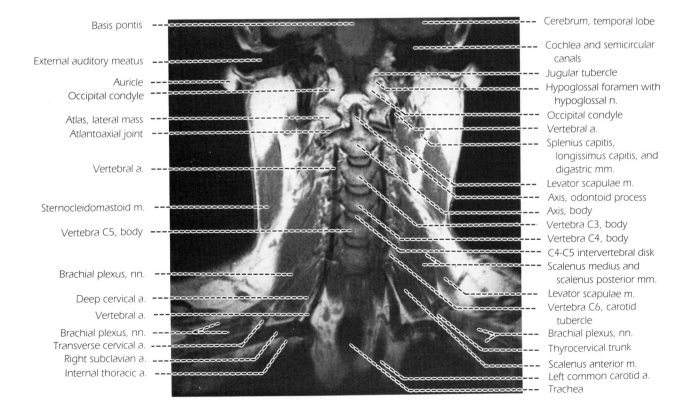

Basis pontis

External auditory meatus

Auricle
Occipital condyle

Atlas, lateral mass
Atlantoaxial joint

Vertebral a.

Sternocleidomastoid m.

Vertebra C5, body

Brachial plexus, nn.

Deep cervical a.
Vertebral a.
Brachial plexus, nn.
Transverse cervical a.
Right subclavian a.
Internal thoracic a.

Cerebrum, temporal lobe

Cochlea and semicircular canals
Jugular tubercle
Hypoglossal foramen with hypoglossal n.
Occipital condyle
Vertebral a.
Splenius capitis, longissimus capitis, and digastric mm.
Levator scapulae m.
Axis, odontoid process
Axis, body
Vertebra C3, body
Vertebra C4, body
C4-C5 intervertebral disk
Scalenus medius and scalenus posterior mm.
Levator scapulae m.
Vertebra C6, carotid tubercle
Brachial plexus, nn.
Thyrocervical trunk
Scalenus anterior m.
Left common carotid a.
Trachea

# Figure 2-38

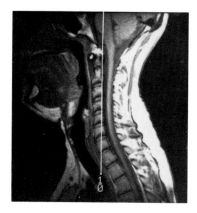

In this coronal T1-weighted image of the neck, numerous muscles can be identified including the obliquus capitis inferior and superior, levator scapulae, sternocleidomastoid, iliocostalis cervicis, longissimus cervicis, and scalenus medius and posterior. The digastric, longissimus capitis, and splenius capitis muscles have a very similar origin or insertion site on or near the mastoid process; hence the anatomic feature identified in the figure by that label could be any one of these three muscles. Note the seventh cervical nerve fibers of the brachial plexus leaving the intervertebral foramen.

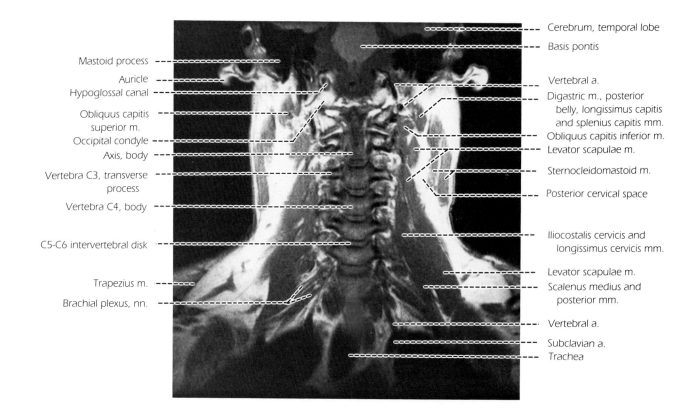

Cerebrum, temporal lobe

Basis pontis

Mastoid process

Auricle

Hypoglossal canal

Obliquus capitis superior m.

Occipital condyle

Axis, body

Vertebra C3, transverse process

Vertebra C4, body

C5-C6 intervertebral disk

Trapezius m.

Brachial plexus, nn.

Vertebral a.

Digastric m., posterior belly, longissimus capitis and splenius capitis mm.

Obliquus capitis inferior m.

Levator scapulae m.

Sternocleidomastoid m.

Posterior cervical space

Iliocostalis cervicis and longissimus cervicis mm.

Levator scapulae m.

Scalenus medius and posterior mm.

Vertebral a.

Subclavian a.

Trachea

In this coronal T1-weighted image of the neck, the spinal cord is seen lying in the vertebral canal surrounded by its membranes. The subarachnoid space containing cerebrospinal fluid is identified. An intervertebral foramen with nerve roots can be seen. At the level of vertebra T1, an articular pit with the head of the first rib is shown.

## Figure 2-39

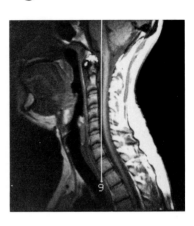

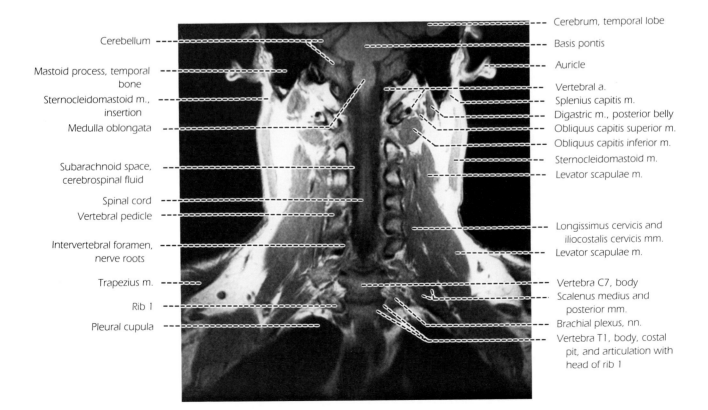

Cerebellum

Mastoid process, temporal bone

Sternocleidomastoid m., insertion

Medulla oblongata

Subarachnoid space, cerebrospinal fluid

Spinal cord

Vertebral pedicle

Intervertebral foramen, nerve roots

Trapezius m.

Rib 1

Pleural cupula

Cerebrum, temporal lobe

Basis pontis

Auricle

Vertebral a.

Splenius capitis m.

Digastric m., posterior belly

Obliquus capitis superior m.

Obliquus capitis inferior m.

Sternocleidomastoid m.

Levator scapulae m.

Longissimus cervicis and iliocostalis cervicis mm.

Levator scapulae m.

Vertebra C7, body

Scalenus medius and posterior mm.

Brachial plexus, nn.

Vertebra T1, body, costal pit, and articulation with head of rib 1

# Figure 2-40

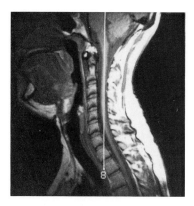

Visible in this coronal T1-weighted image of the neck are the muscles arising from or inserting into the mastoid process, including the sternocleidomastoid, digastric (posterior belly), splenius capitis, and longissimus capitis. Note the pedicles of the axis and the third cervical vertebra. The deep cervical and vertebral arteries are identified. The central canal of the spinal cord is exposed. The first thoracic vertebral body and the first rib are included in this section.

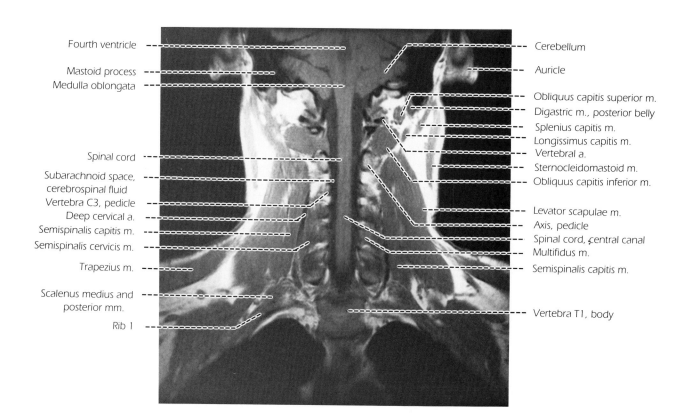

Several muscles described in previous sections can still be identified in this coronal T1-weighted image. These include the muscles arising from or inserting into the mastoid process, sternocleidomastoid, splenius capitis, longissimus capitis, and digastric (posterior belly); two suboccipital muscles, obliquus capitis inferior and superior; two semispinalis muscles, capitis and cervicis; and splenius cervicis. The levator scapulae arises from the posterior tubercles of the upper four cervical transverse processes and inserts onto the superior angle of the scapula. Note the hemifacets of vertebrae T2 and T3 for the head of rib 2, the superior articular process of T1, the inferior articular process of C7, and the costotransverse joint of vertebra T1 for rib 1.

## Figure 2-41

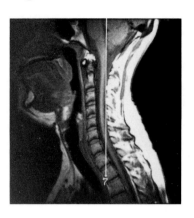

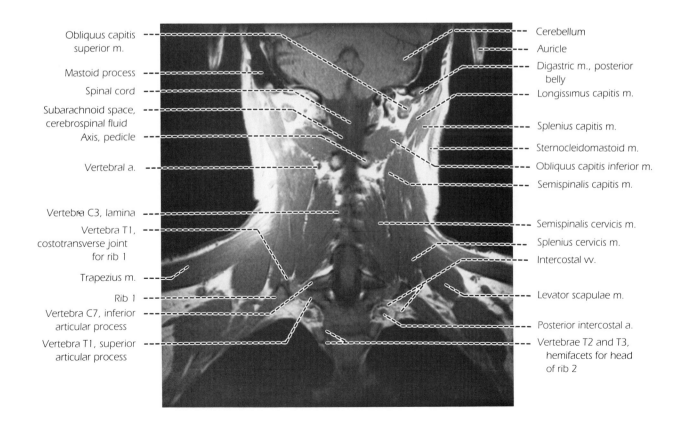

Obliquus capitis superior m.

Mastoid process

Spinal cord

Subarachnoid space, cerebrospinal fluid

Axis, pedicle

Vertebral a.

Vertebra C3, lamina

Vertebra T1, costotransverse joint for rib 1

Trapezius m.

Rib 1

Vertebra C7, inferior articular process

Vertebra T1, superior articular process

Cerebellum

Auricle

Digastric m., posterior belly

Longissimus capitis m.

Splenius capitis m.

Sternocleidomastoid m.

Obliquus capitis inferior m.

Semispinalis capitis m.

Semispinalis cervicis m.

Splenius cervicis m.

Intercostal vv.

Levator scapulae m.

Posterior intercostal a.

Vertebrae T2 and T3, hemifacets for head of rib 2

# Figure 2-42

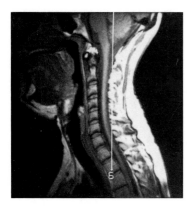

Visible in this coronal T1-weighted image are the bifid spinous processes, characteristic of the cervical region, on the axis and fifth and sixth vertebrae. The laminae can be seen on the seventh cervical vertebra.

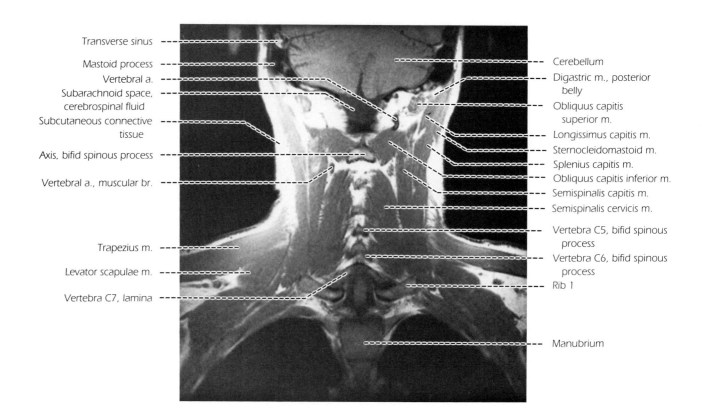

Transverse sinus

Mastoid process

Vertebral a.

Subarachnoid space, cerebrospinal fluid

Subcutaneous connective tissue

Axis, bifid spinous process

Vertebral a., muscular br.

Trapezius m.

Levator scapulae m.

Vertebra C7, lamina

Cerebellum

Digastric m., posterior belly

Obliquus capitis superior m.

Longissimus capitis m.

Sternocleidomastoid m.

Splenius capitis m.

Obliquus capitis inferior m.

Semispinalis capitis m.

Semispinalis cervicis m.

Vertebra C5, bifid spinous process

Vertebra C6, bifid spinous process

Rib 1

Manubrium

Visible in this coronal T1-weighted image are numerous muscles of the neck including the suboccipital rectus capitis posterior major and minor and the obliquus capitis inferior and superior. The mastoid process-related digastric, sternocleidomastoid, and splenius capitis and the interspinalis and the bifid spinous process muscles are also identified. The vertebral artery continues its almost ubiquitous presence in one location or another.

## Figure 2-43

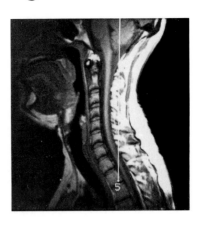

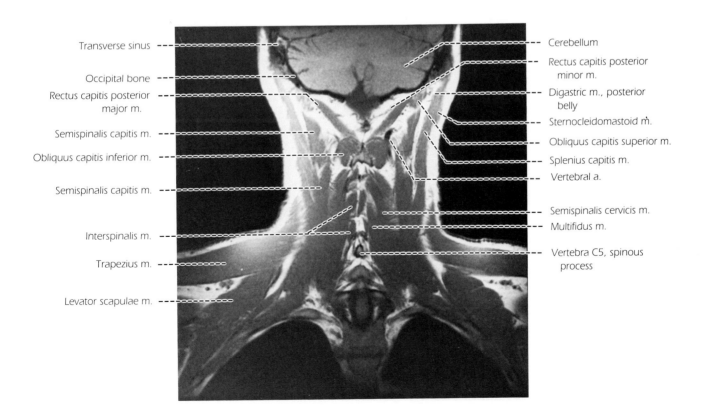

Transverse sinus

Occipital bone

Rectus capitis posterior major m.

Semispinalis capitis m.

Obliquus capitis inferior m.

Semispinalis capitis m.

Interspinalis m.

Trapezius m.

Levator scapulae m.

Cerebellum

Rectus capitis posterior minor m.

Digastric m., posterior belly

Sternocleidomastoid m.

Obliquus capitis superior m.

Splenius capitis m.

Vertebral a.

Semispinalis cervicis m.

Multifidus m.

Vertebra C5, spinous process

# Figure 2-44

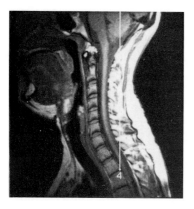

In this coronal T1-weighted image, the suprascapular and dorsal scapular arteries are visible beneath the trapezius and adjacent to the levator scapulae. These arteries supply the levator scapulae, rhomboids, supraspinatus, infraspinatus, and other muscles of the back. The occipital artery, which supplies the dorsum of the head, is also seen.

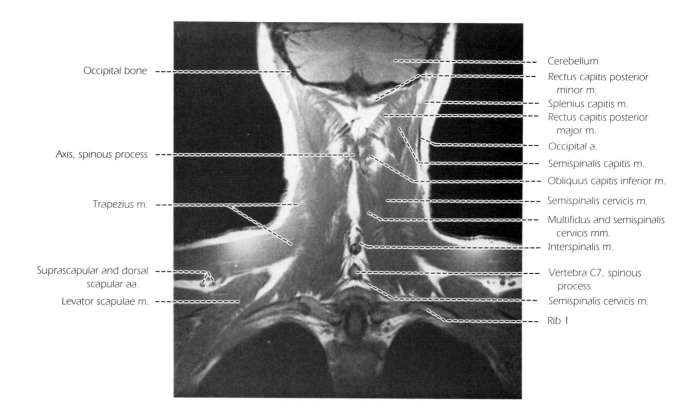

Occipital bone

Axis, spinous process

Trapezius m.

Suprascapular and dorsal scapular aa.

Levator scapulae m.

Cerebellum

Rectus capitis posterior minor m.

Splenius capitis m.

Rectus capitis posterior major m.

Occipital a.

Semispinalis capitis m.

Obliquus capitis inferior m.

Semispinalis cervicis m.

Multifidus and semispinalis cervicis mm.

Interspinalis m.

Vertebra C7, spinous process

Semispinalis cervicis m.

Rib 1

The major mass of muscle in this coronal T1-weighted image belongs to the trapezius, which originates from the superior nuchal line, external occipital protuberance, ligamentum nuchae, spinous process of the seventh cervical vertebra, the thoracic vertebrae and the corresponding supraspinous ligaments. It inserts onto the lateral third of the clavicle, acromion, and spine of the scapula. It is innervated by the spinal accessory nerve (cranial nerve XI) and the cervical plexus.

## Figure 2-45

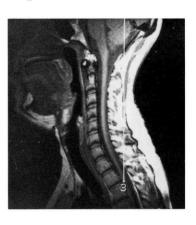

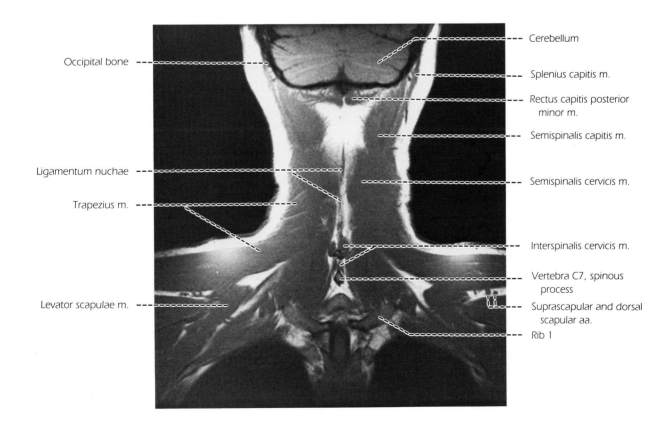

Cerebellum

Occipital bone

Splenius capitis m.

Rectus capitis posterior minor m.

Semispinalis capitis m.

Ligamentum nuchae

Semispinalis cervicis m.

Trapezius m.

Interspinalis cervicis m.

Vertebra C7, spinous process

Levator scapulae m.

Suprascapular and dorsal scapular aa.

Rib 1

# Figure 2-46

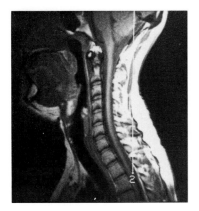

Coronal T1-weighted image of the neck showing the highly branched deep cervical artery, which lies behind the trapezius and semispinalis capitis.

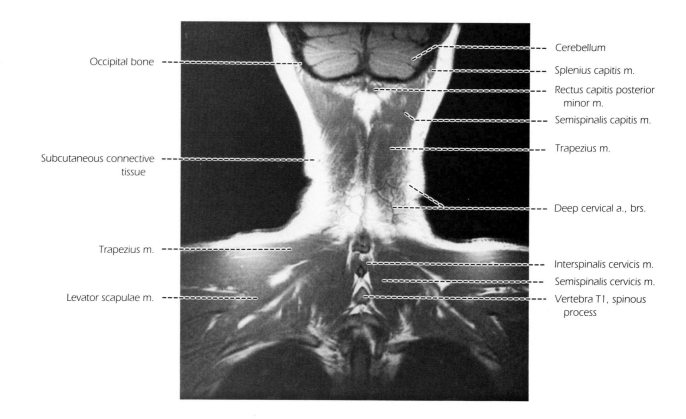

Occipital bone

Subcutaneous connective tissue

Trapezius m.

Levator scapulae m.

Cerebellum

Splenius capitis m.

Rectus capitis posterior minor m.

Semispinalis capitis m.

Trapezius m.

Deep cervical a., brs.

Interspinalis cervicis m.

Semispinalis cervicis m.

Vertebra T1, spinous process

In this coronal T1-weighted image of the neck are seen remnants of cervical and head muscles. Note the cerebellum and the occipital lobe of the cerebrum. The trapezius is spread out on the shoulders.

## Figure 2-47

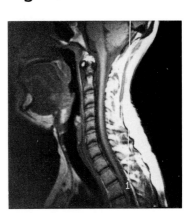

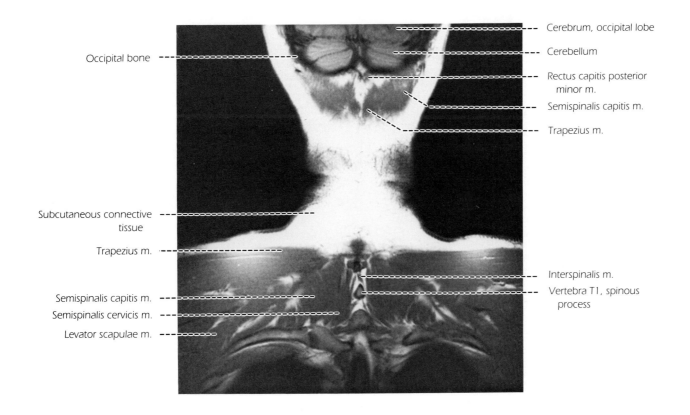

Occipital bone

Subcutaneous connective tissue

Trapezius m.

Semispinalis capitis m.
Semispinalis cervicis m.
Levator scapulae m.

Cerebrum, occipital lobe

Cerebellum

Rectus capitis posterior minor m.

Semispinalis capitis m.

Trapezius m.

Interspinalis m.
Vertebra T1, spinous process

# Figure 2-48

Coronal T2-weighted image of the neck showing the relationship between the masseter and medial pterygoid muscles and the mandible. The maxillary artery lies medial to the lateral pterygoid muscle. Note the submandibular gland below and medial to the mandible and the parotid above and lateral to the mandible.

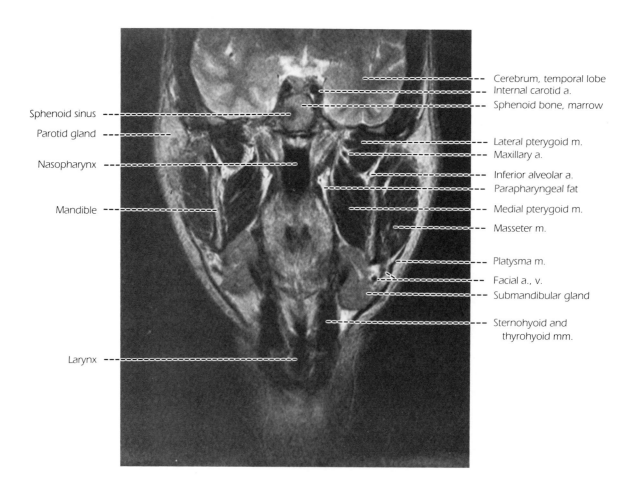

# Figure 2-49

In this coronal T2-weighted image of the neck the inferior alveolar artery is identified. The inferior alveolar artery, vein, and nerve enter the mandibular foramen to supply the lower jaw and teeth. The other arterial vessel identified in this section is the internal carotid. The section cuts the nasopharynx, oropharynx, and larynx. The epiglottis and pharyngoepitlottic fold are shown. A small slice of tensor veli palatini muscle can be seen.

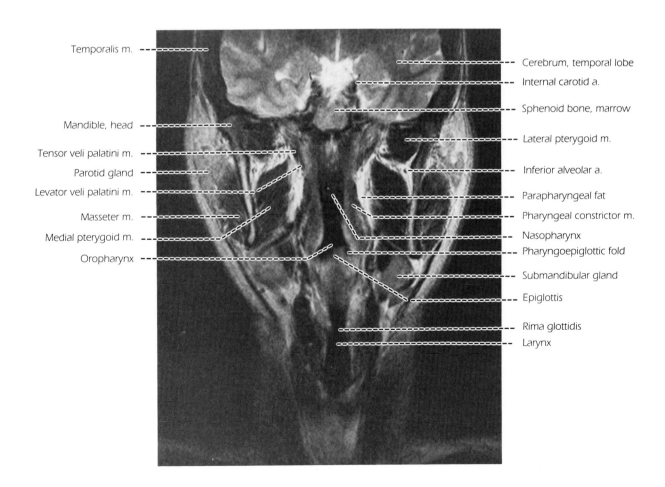

Temporalis m.

Mandible, head

Tensor veli palatini m.

Parotid gland

Levator veli palatini m.

Masseter m.

Medial pterygoid m.

Oropharynx

Cerebrum, temporal lobe

Internal carotid a.

Sphenoid bone, marrow

Lateral pterygoid m.

Inferior alveolar a.

Parapharyngeal fat

Pharyngeal constrictor m.

Nasopharynx

Pharyngoepiglottic fold

Submandibular gland

Epiglottis

Rima glottidis

Larynx

# Figure 2-50

Visible in this coronal T2-weighted image of the neck are the cochlea and semicircular canals. The full extent of the parotid glands can also be appreciated in this section.

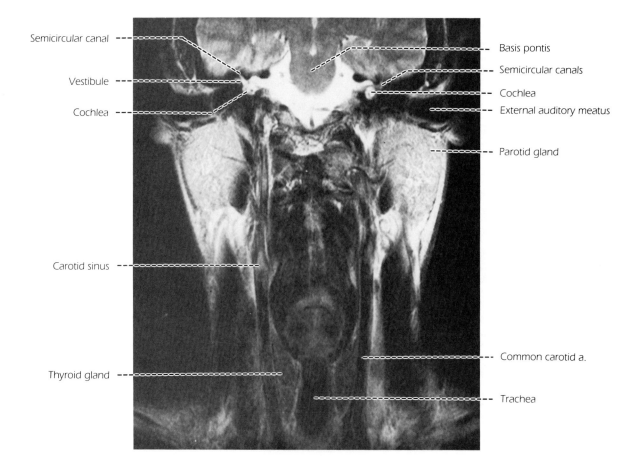

Semicircular canal

Vestibule

Cochlea

Basis pontis

Semicircular canals

Cochlea

External auditory meatus

Parotid gland

Carotid sinus

Common carotid a.

Thyroid gland

Trachea

In this coronal T2-weighted image a zygapophyseal joint between the atlas and axis is identified. Note the vestibule, semicircular canals, and the facial and vestibulocochlear nerves (cranial nerves VII and VIII).

## Figure 2-51

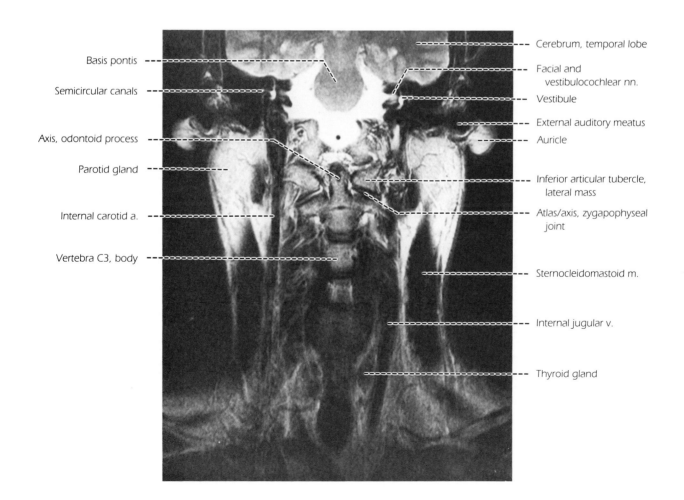

Basis pontis

Semicircular canals

Axis, odontoid process

Parotid gland

Internal carotid a.

Vertebra C3, body

Cerebrum, temporal lobe

Facial and vestibulocochlear nn.

Vestibule

External auditory meatus

Auricle

Inferior articular tubercle, lateral mass

Atlas/axis, zygapophyseal joint

Sternocleidomastoid m.

Internal jugular v.

Thyroid gland

# Figure 2-52

In this coronal T2-weighted image of the neck the transverse foramina in cervical vertebrae 2, 3, and 4 are clearly seen. The vertebral arteries fill these foramina. Typically, the vertebral artery enters the sixth transverse foramen. Note the insertion of the sterno-cleidomastoid muscle on the mastoid process.

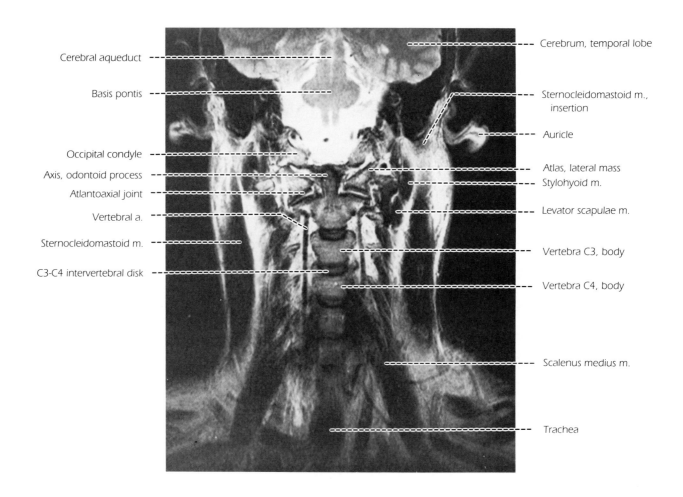

Cerebral aqueduct

Basis pontis

Occipital condyle

Axis, odontoid process

Atlantoaxial joint

Vertebral a.

Sternocleidomastoid m.

C3-C4 intervertebral disk

Cerebrum, temporal lobe

Sternocleidomastoid m., insertion

Auricle

Atlas, lateral mass

Stylohyoid m.

Levator scapulae m.

Vertebra C3, body

Vertebra C4, body

Scalenus medius m.

Trachea

Coronal T2-weighted image of the neck demonstrating bundles of nerve fibers that will form the brachial plexus of nerves. The brachial plexus is usually formed from the fifth through eighth cervical and first thoracic spinal nerves. The spinal nerves along with the subclavian artery usually leave the neck between scalenus anterior and scalenus medius, although they may pierce scalenus anterior.

Figure 2-53

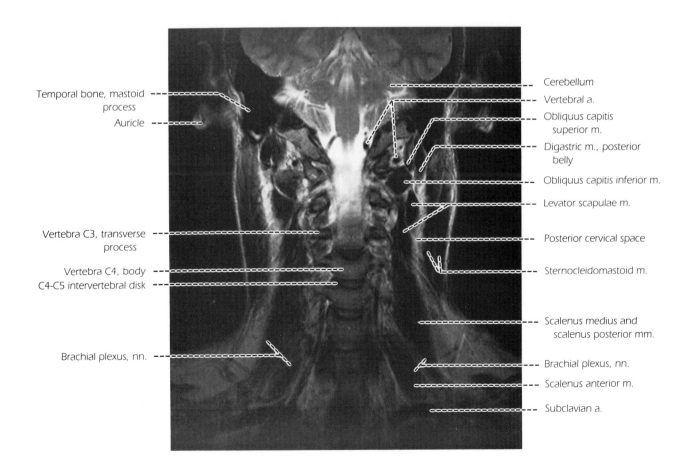

Temporal bone, mastoid process

Auricle

Vertebra C3, transverse process

Vertebra C4, body

C4-C5 intervertebral disk

Brachial plexus, nn.

Cerebellum

Vertebral a.

Obliquus capitis superior m.

Digastric m., posterior belly

Obliquus capitis inferior m.

Levator scapulae m.

Posterior cervical space

Sternocleidomastoid m.

Scalenus medius and scalenus posterior mm.

Brachial plexus, nn.

Scalenus anterior m.

Subclavian a.

# Figure 2-54

In this coronal T2-weighted image of the neck the vertebral foramen, filled with cerebrospinal fluid, is seen surrounding and supporting the spinal cord. Note the nerves that form the brachial plexus, the dura entering the intervertebral (neural) foramen, and nerve fibers in the intervertebral foramen.

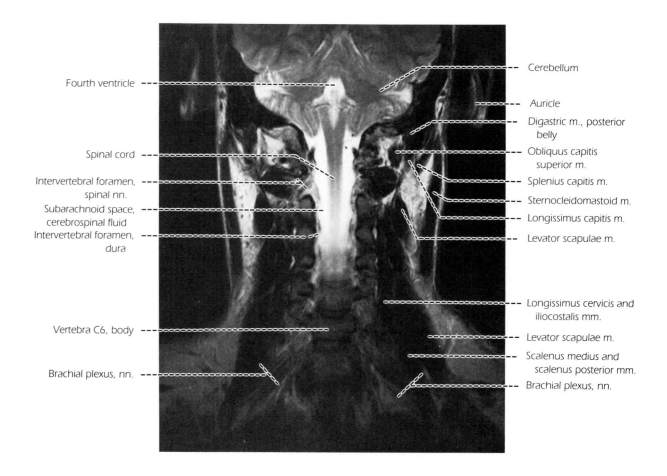

Fourth ventricle

Spinal cord

Intervertebral foramen, spinal nn.

Subarachnoid space, cerebrospinal fluid

Intervertebral foramen, dura

Vertebra C6, body

Brachial plexus, nn.

Cerebellum

Auricle

Digastric m., posterior belly

Obliquus capitis superior m.

Splenius capitis m.

Sternocleidomastoid m.

Longissimus capitis m.

Levator scapulae m.

Longissimus cervicis and iliocostalis mm.

Levator scapulae m.

Scalenus medius and scalenus posterior mm.

Brachial plexus, nn.

# SAGITTAL VIEWS

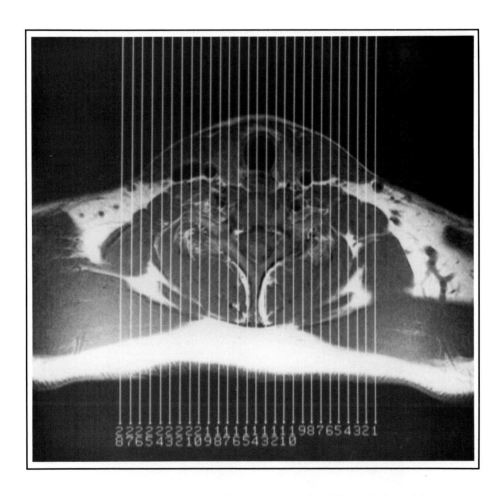

Key to the sagittal planes of inspection for T1-weighted images.

# Figure 2-55

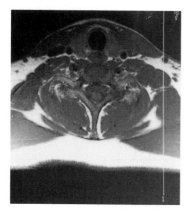

In this sagittal T1-weighted image, muscles of the neck and head region include the trapezius, levator scapulae, and scalenes (anterior, middle, and posterior). The trunks of the brachial plexus are located between the anterior and middle scalenes. Muscles related to the thorax and upper limb include the rhomboideus minor and major, intercostal, serratus posterior superior, subclavius, and pectoralis major. Note the intercostal vein, artery, and nerve at the level of rib 3.

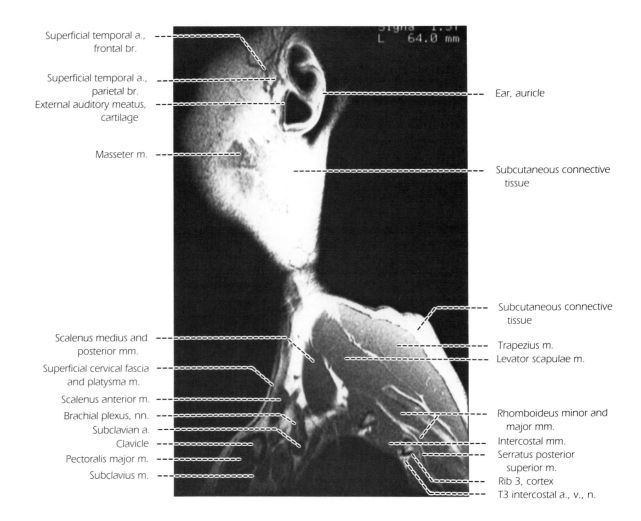

Important blood vessels in the sagittal T1-weighted image of the neck identified here include the superficial temporal (frontal and parietal branches), subclavian, and intercostal arteries, and the external jugular, subclavian, and intercostal veins. Elements of the brachial plexus of nerves are seen along with their relationship to the anterior and middle scalene muscles. The sternocleidomastoid, trapezius, levator scapulae, rhomboideus minor and major, and serratus posterior superior muscles are also identified.

## Figure 2-56

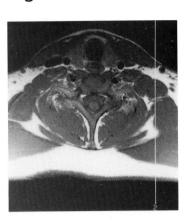

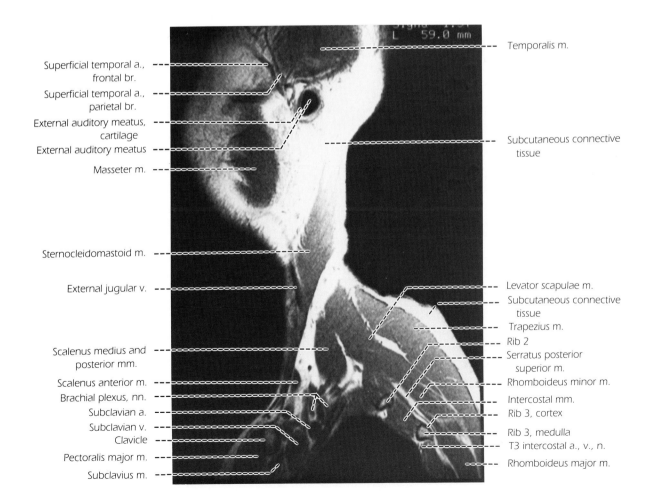

# Figure 2-57

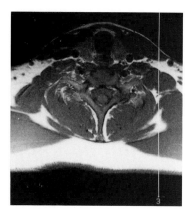

Sagittal T1-weighted image of the neck showing the trunks that form the brachial plexus as well as their relationship to muscles and blood vessels in the neck. The parotid gland appears for the first time. Muscles of the head that are present in this section include the temporalis and masseter. Muscles of the shoulder and upper thorax include the levator scapulae, the two rhomboids, serratus posterior superior, and trapezius. The first three ribs are present. Pectoralis major, a muscle of the arm, is identified.

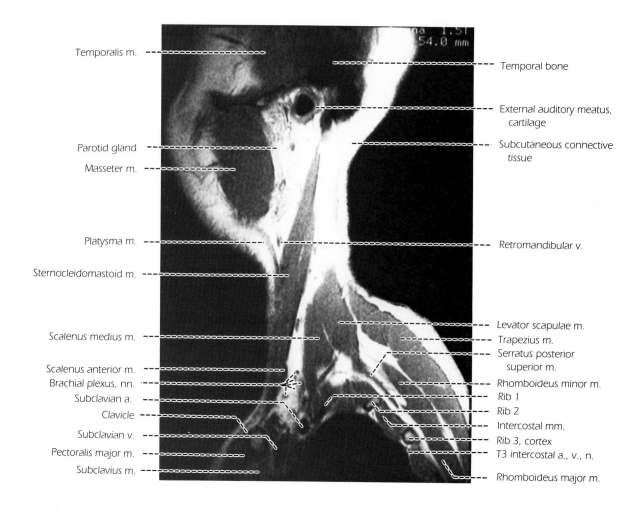

Temporalis m.

Parotid gland

Masseter m.

Platysma m.

Sternocleidomastoid m.

Scalenus medius m.

Scalenus anterior m.

Brachial plexus, nn.

Subclavian a.

Clavicle

Subclavian v.

Pectoralis major m.

Subclavius m.

Temporal bone

External auditory meatus, cartilage

Subcutaneous connective tissue

Retromandibular v.

Levator scapulae m.

Trapezius m.

Serratus posterior superior m.

Rhomboideus minor m.

Rib 1

Rib 2

Intercostal mm.

Rib 3, cortex

T3 intercostal a., v., n.

Rhomboideus major m.

In this sagittal T1-weighted image, muscles associated with the neck include the platysma, scalenus medius and anterior, levator scapulae, trapezius, iliocostalis cervicis, and longissimus cervicis. The subclavian artery and the nerves of the brachial plexus are shown. The section includes the apex of the lung; clavicle; intercostal, rhomboideus minor and major, subclavius, and pectoralis major muscles; ribs 1, 2, and 3; and an intercostal neurovascular bundle. The face is represented by two facial muscles, the platysma and zygomaticus major. The masseter muscle and the parotid gland are also present. Note the external auditory meatus.

## Figure 2-58

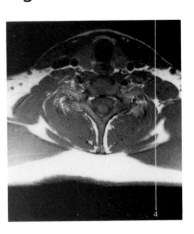

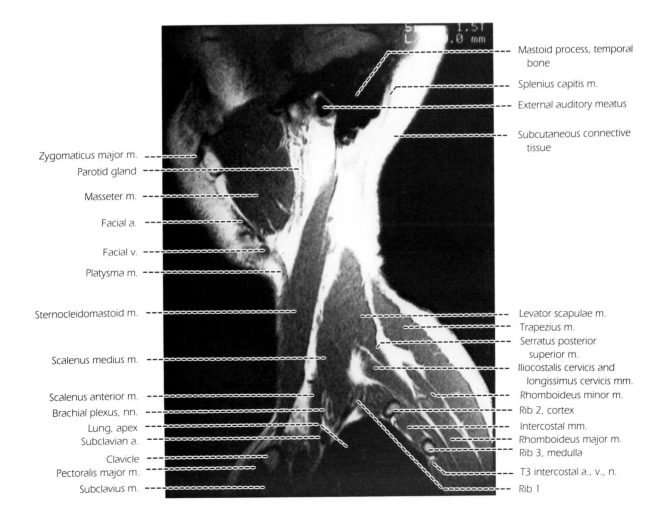

Mastoid process, temporal bone

Splenius capitis m.

External auditory meatus

Subcutaneous connective tissue

Zygomaticus major m.

Parotid gland

Masseter m.

Facial a.

Facial v.

Platysma m.

Sternocleidomastoid m.

Scalenus medius m.

Scalenus anterior m.

Brachial plexus, nn.

Lung, apex

Subclavian a.

Clavicle

Pectoralis major m.

Subclavius m.

Levator scapulae m.

Trapezius m.

Serratus posterior superior m.

Iliocostalis cervicis and longissimus cervicis mm.

Rhomboideus minor m.

Rib 2, cortex

Intercostal mm.

Rhomboideus major m.

Rib 3, medulla

T3 intercostal a., v., n.

Rib 1

## Figure 2-59

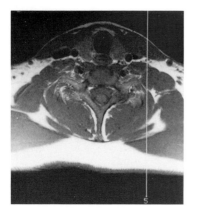

In this sagittal T1-weighted image of the neck, the important muscles include the splenius capitis, iliocostalis cervicis, longissimus cervicis, splenius cervicis, the three scalenes (anterior, middle, and posterior), sternocleidomastoid, and platysma. Note the nerves destined to form the brachial plexus including cervical nerves V through VIII and thoracic nerve 1. Note the cervical and spinal accessory (cranial nerve XI) nerves in the posterior triangle. The triangle is formed by the posterior border of sternocleidomastoid anteriorly, the anterior border of trapezius posteriorly, and the cranial part of the clavicle inferiorly. Note the first three ribs. The temporal lobe of the brain is exposed along with the transverse sinus.

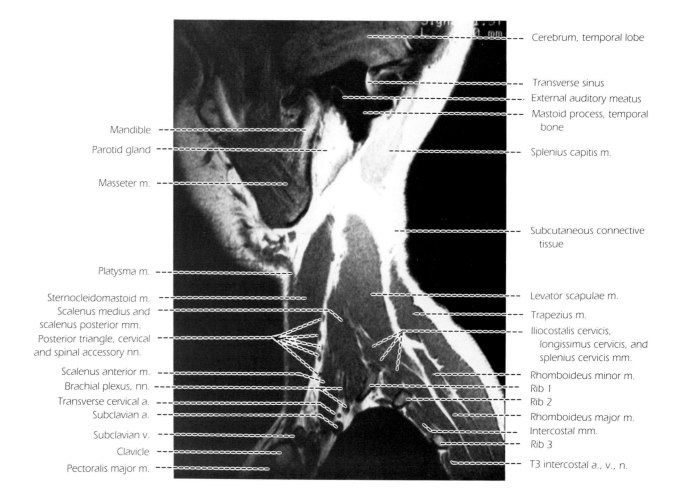

Muscles of the neck visible in this sagittal T1-weighted image include the platysma, scalenes (anterior, middle, and posterior), iliocostalis cervicis, longissimus cervicis, splenius cervicis, and levator scapulae. The temporomandibular joint and submandibular gland make their first appearance in this section. Several important blood vessels are present including the facial, subclavian, and occipital arteries and the facial and subclavian veins. Ribs 1,2, and 3 are present, and the three intercostal muscles are identified in their external, internal, and innermost layers.

## Figure 2-60

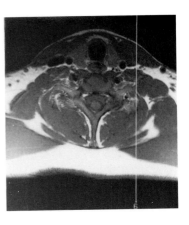

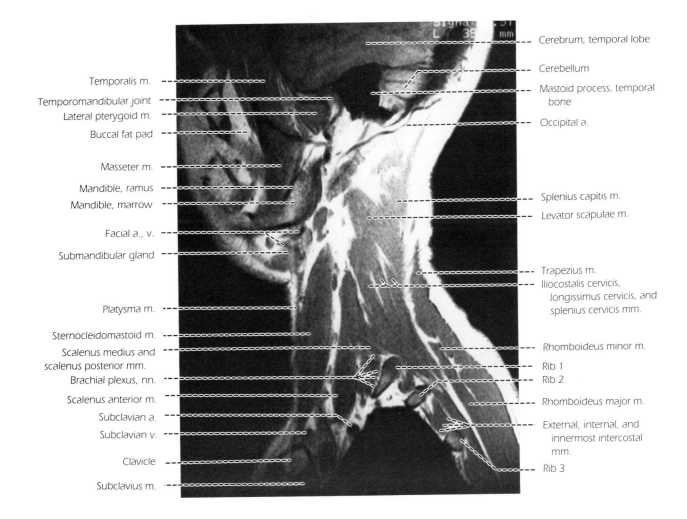

Temporalis m.

Temporomandibular joint

Lateral pterygoid m.

Buccal fat pad

Masseter m.

Mandible, ramus

Mandible, marrow

Facial a., v.

Submandibular gland

Platysma m.

Sternocleidomastoid m.

Scalenus medius and scalenus posterior mm.

Brachial plexus, nn.

Scalenus anterior m.

Subclavian a.

Subclavian v.

Clavicle

Subclavius m.

Cerebrum, temporal lobe

Cerebellum

Mastoid process, temporal bone

Occipital a.

Splenius capitis m.

Levator scapulae m.

Trapezius m.

Iliocostalis cervicis, longissimus cervicis, and splenius cervicis mm.

Rhomboideus minor m.

Rib 1

Rib 2

Rhomboideus major m.

External, internal, and innermost intercostal mm.

Rib 3

## Figure 2-61

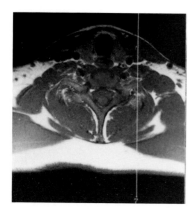

In this sagittal T1-weighted image of the neck, muscles include the splenius cervicis, iliocostalis cervicis, longissimus cervicis, scalenes (anterior, middle, and posterior), and platysma. Muscles of the head include the digastric (posterior belly), suboccipital, obliquus capitis superior and inferior, and sternocleidomastoid. Muscles of mastication include the medial and lateral pterygoids and the temporalis. Note the submandibular gland and the direct course of the internal jugular vein. Elements of the brachial plexus are still lodged between the anterior and middle scalene muscles. The apex of the left lung is in the pleural cavity.

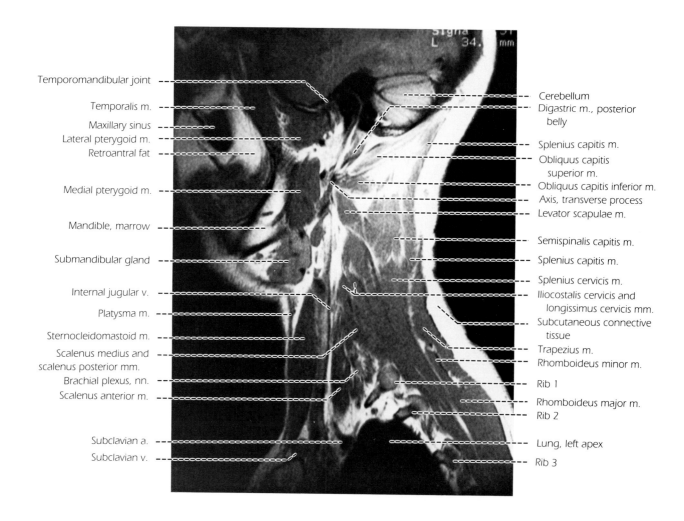

Temporomandibular joint
Temporalis m.
Maxillary sinus
Lateral pterygoid m.
Retroantral fat
Medial pterygoid m.
Mandible, marrow
Submandibular gland
Internal jugular v.
Platysma m.
Sternocleidomastoid m.
Scalenus medius and scalenus posterior mm.
Brachial plexus, nn.
Scalenus anterior m.
Subclavian a.
Subclavian v.

Cerebellum
Digastric m., posterior belly
Splenius capitis m.
Obliquus capitis superior m.
Obliquus capitis inferior m.
Axis, transverse process
Levator scapulae m.
Semispinalis capitis m.
Splenius capitis m.
Splenius cervicis m.
Iliocostalis cervicis and longissimus cervicis mm.
Subcutaneous connective tissue
Trapezius m.
Rhomboideus minor m.
Rib 1
Rhomboideus major m.
Rib 2
Lung, left apex
Rib 3

In this sagittal T1-weighted image, the structure making its first appearance is the cochlea. The other structures have been seen in previous sections because of their length or breadth. The muscles of the neck include the splenius cervicis, longissimus cervicis, and iliocostalis cervicis. Muscles concerned with the support of the head include the superior and inferior oblique, semispinalis capitis, splenius capitis, sternocleidomastoid, and trapezius. The transverse process of the axis is seen. The other bony structure is the mandible. Muscles that insert into the mandible include the masseter, lateral and medial pterygoids, and temporalis.

Figure 2-62

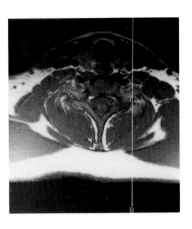

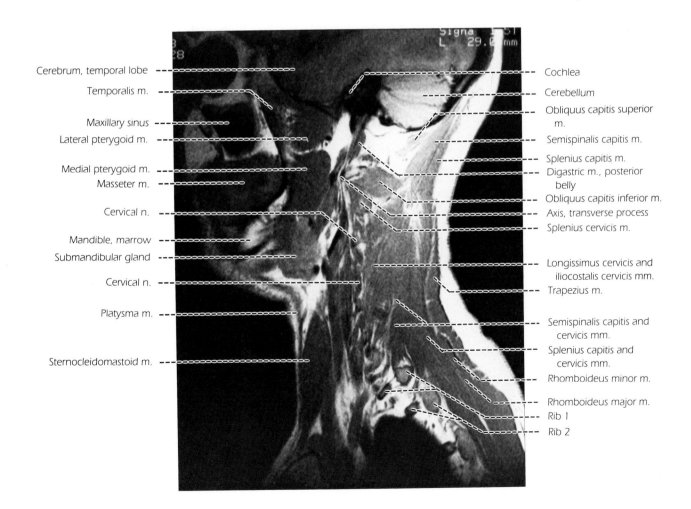

Cerebrum, temporal lobe

Temporalis m.

Maxillary sinus

Lateral pterygoid m.

Medial pterygoid m.

Masseter m.

Cervical n.

Mandible, marrow

Submandibular gland

Cervical n.

Platysma m.

Sternocleidomastoid m.

Cochlea

Cerebellum

Obliquus capitis superior m.

Semispinalis capitis m.

Splenius capitis m.

Digastric m., posterior belly

Obliquus capitis inferior m.

Axis, transverse process

Splenius cervicis m.

Longissimus cervicis and iliocostalis cervicis mm.

Trapezius m.

Semispinalis capitis and cervicis mm.

Splenius capitis and cervicis mm.

Rhomboideus minor m.

Rhomboideus major m.

Rib 1

Rib 2

# Figure 2-63

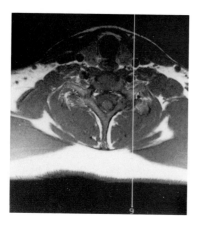

Structures appearing for the first time in this sagittal T1-weighted image of the neck include the facial and vestibulocochlear nerves (cervical nerves VII and VIII), vertebral artery, zygapophyseal joints of the vertebral column with their inferior and superior articular processes, first and second molar teeth, inferior orbital foramen, and eyeball (globe).

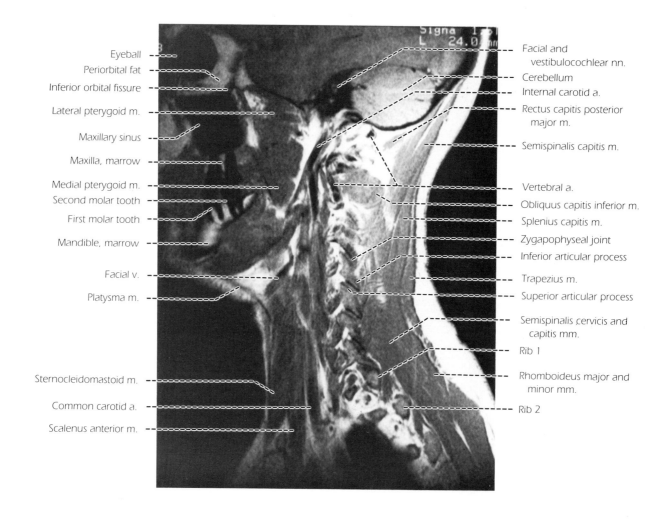

In this sagittal T1-weighted image of the neck, structures and/or relationships seen for the first time include the internal carotid artery in its S-shape configuration; first and second premolar teeth; pterygopalatine fossa; pterygopalatine ganglion (one of two parasympathetic ganglia of the facial nerve [cranial nerve VII] in the head); maxillary artery; optic nerve (cranial nerve XI); and foramen rotundum, through which the maxillary division of the trigeminal nerve (cranial nerve V) leaves the cranium.

## Figure 2-64

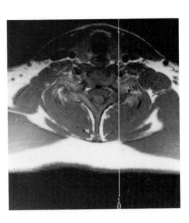

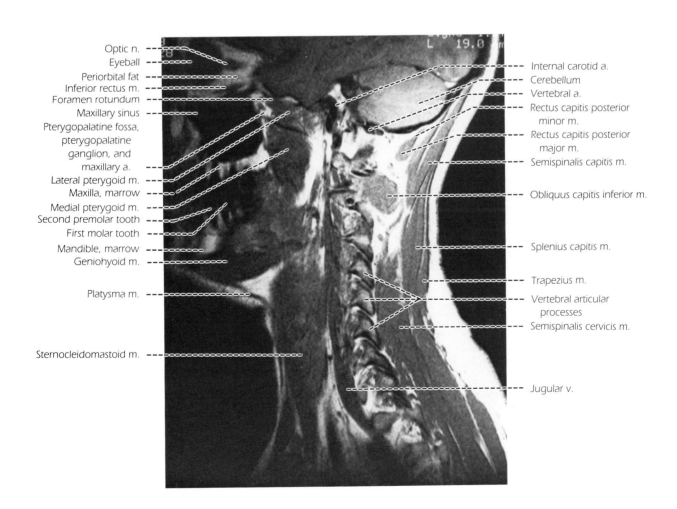

Optic n.
Eyeball
Periorbital fat
Inferior rectus m.
Foramen rotundum
Maxillary sinus
Pterygopalatine fossa, pterygopalatine ganglion, and maxillary a.
Lateral pterygoid m.
Maxilla, marrow
Medial pterygoid m.
Second premolar tooth
First molar tooth
Mandible, marrow
Geniohyoid m.
Platysma m.
Sternocleidomastoid m.

Internal carotid a.
Cerebellum
Vertebral a.
Rectus capitis posterior minor m.
Rectus capitis posterior major m.
Semispinalis capitis m.
Obliquus capitis inferior m.
Splenius capitis m.
Trapezius m.
Vertebral articular processes
Semispinalis cervicis m.
Jugular v.

# Figure 2-65

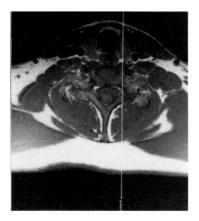

In this sagittal T1-weighted image of the neck, structures appearing for the first time include the odontoid process of the axis; intervertebral canal, containing nerve roots; pyriform sinus; tongue; first premolar tooth; and the lateral rectus muscle, one of six intrinsic eye muscles exclusively innervated by the abducens nerve (cranial nerve VI).

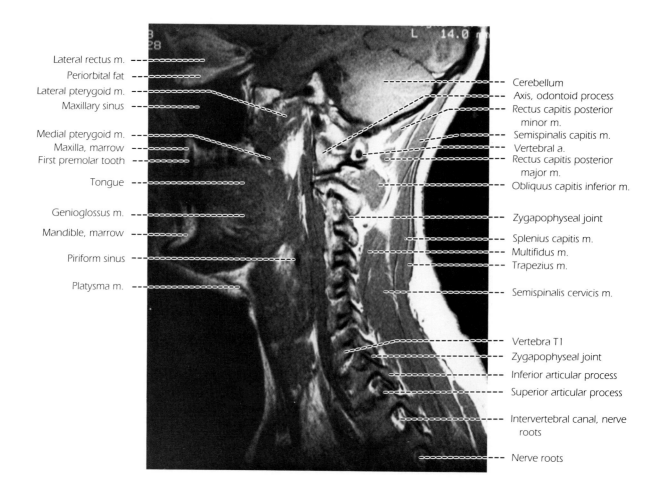

Lateral rectus m.
Periorbital fat
Lateral pterygoid m.
Maxillary sinus

Medial pterygoid m.
Maxilla, marrow
First premolar tooth

Tongue

Genioglossus m.

Mandible, marrow

Piriform sinus

Platysma m.

Cerebellum
Axis, odontoid process
Rectus capitis posterior minor m.
Semispinalis capitis m.
Vertebral a.
Rectus capitis posterior major m.
Obliquus capitis inferior m.

Zygapophyseal joint

Splenius capitis m.
Multifidus m.
Trapezius m.

Semispinalis cervicis m.

Vertebra T1
Zygapophyseal joint
Inferior articular process
Superior articular process
Intervertebral canal, nerve roots
Nerve roots

In this sagittal T1-weighted image of the neck, the structures or topographic relationships seen for the first time include the transverse sinus, posterior arch of the atlas, intervertebral disks, vertebral laminae, ligamentum flavum, esophagus, larynx, sternohyoid and sternothyroid muscles, pre-epiglottic fat, geniohyoid muscle, hyoid bone, and epiglottis.

## Figure 2-66

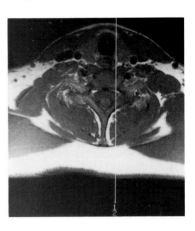

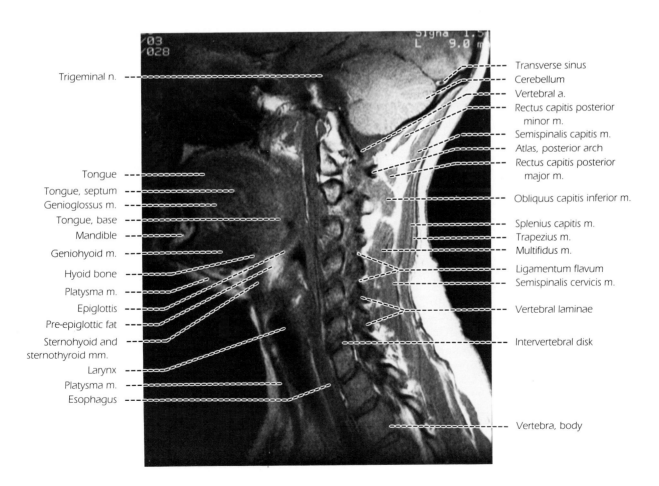

# Figure 2-67

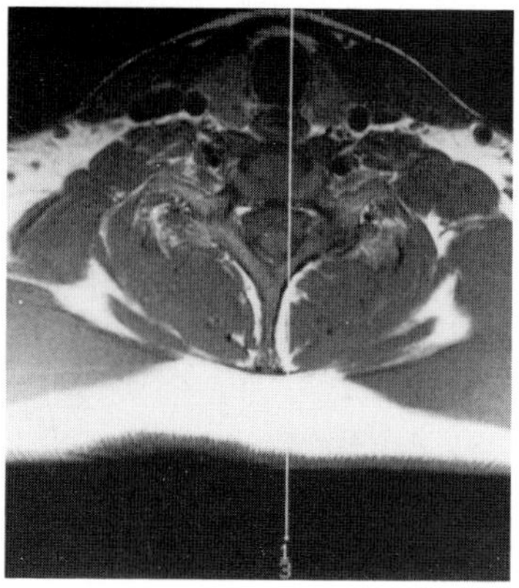

In this sagittal T1-weighted image of the neck, structures and topographic relationships seen for the first time include the bone marrow of the basiocciput, anterior arch of the atlas, odontoid process of the axis, ligamentum nuchae, spinal cord, supraspinal ligament, anterior and posterior longitudinal ligaments, mandible, vallecula, prevertebral fat, inferior and middle conchae, and sphenoid sinus.

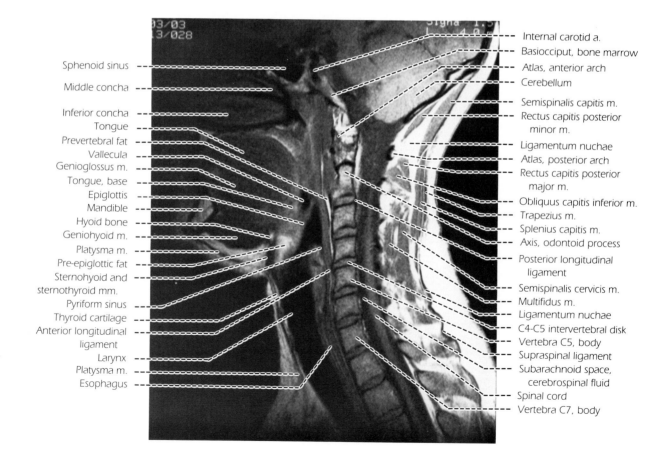

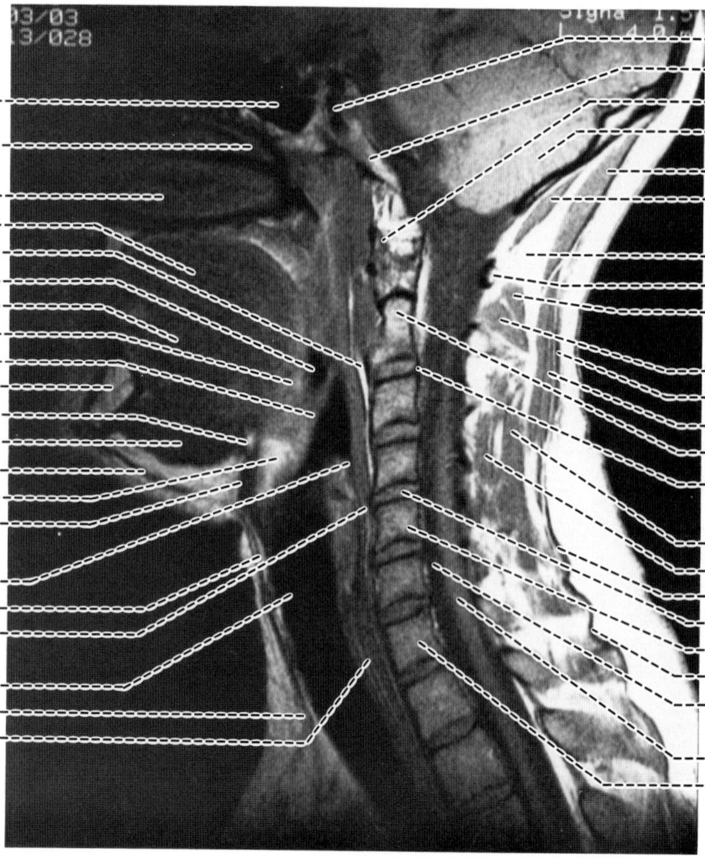
Sphenoid sinus
Middle concha
Inferior concha
Tongue
Prevertebral fat
Vallecula
Genioglossus m.
Tongue, base
Epiglottis
Mandible
Hyoid bone
Geniohyoid m.
Platysma m.
Pre-epiglottic fat
Sternohyoid and sternothyroid mm.
Pyriform sinus
Thyroid cartilage
Anterior longitudinal ligament
Larynx
Platysma m.
Esophagus
Internal carotid a.
Basiocciput, bone marrow
Atlas, anterior arch
Cerebellum
Semispinalis capitis m.
Rectus capitis posterior minor m.
Ligamentum nuchae
Atlas, posterior arch
Rectus capitis posterior major m.
Obliquus capitis inferior m.
Trapezius m.
Splenius capitis m.
Axis, odontoid process
Posterior longitudinal ligament
Semispinalis cervicis m.
Multifidus m.
Ligamentum nuchae
C4-C5 intervertebral disk
Vertebra C5, body
Supraspinal ligament
Subarachnoid space, cerebrospinal fluid
Spinal cord
Vertebra C7, body

In this sagittal T1-weighted image, structures and topographic relationships seen for the first time include the basis pontis; cerebellar tonsil; body of the axis; interspinalis muscle; thyroid cartilage; cricoid cartilage; epiglottis and its free edge, body, and petiolus; vallecula; uvula; and hard palate.

## Figure 2-68

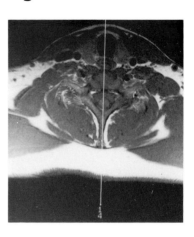

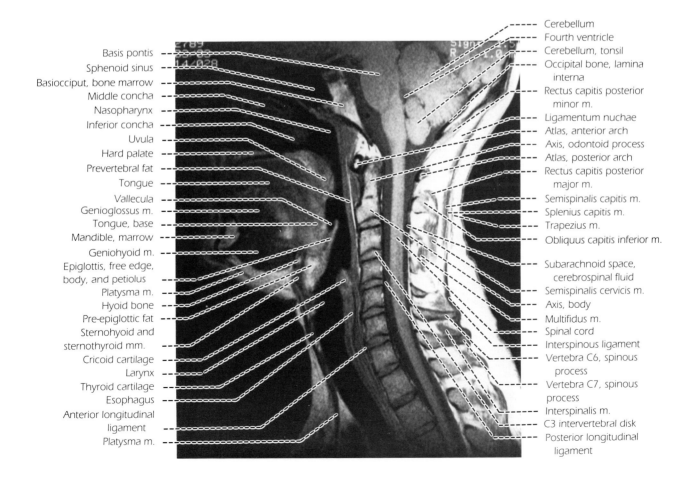

Basis pontis
Sphenoid sinus
Basiocciput, bone marrow
Middle concha
Nasopharynx
Inferior concha
Uvula
Hard palate
Prevertebral fat
Tongue
Vallecula
Genioglossus m.
Tongue, base
Mandible, marrow
Geniohyoid m.
Epiglottis, free edge, body, and petiolus
Platysma m.
Hyoid bone
Pre-epiglottic fat
Sternohyoid and sternothyroid mm.
Cricoid cartilage
Larynx
Thyroid cartilage
Esophagus
Anterior longitudinal ligament
Platysma m.

Cerebellum
Fourth ventricle
Cerebellum, tonsil
Occipital bone, lamina interna
Rectus capitis posterior minor m.
Ligamentum nuchae
Atlas, anterior arch
Axis, odontoid process
Atlas, posterior arch
Rectus capitis posterior major m.
Semispinalis capitis m.
Splenius capitis m.
Trapezius m.
Obliquus capitis inferior m.
Subarachnoid space, cerebrospinal fluid
Semispinalis cervicis m.
Axis, body
Multifidus m.
Spinal cord
Interspinous ligament
Vertebra C6, spinous process
Vertebra C7, spinous process
Interspinalis m.
C3 intervertebral disk
Posterior longitudinal ligament

# Figure 2-69

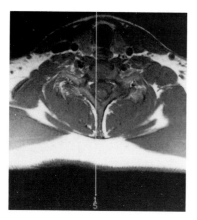

In this sagittal T1-weighted image of the neck, structures or topographic relationships seen for the first time include the fourth ventricle, occipital bone (lamina interna), body of the axis, nasopharynx, vomer, and hypophysis (pituitary gland).

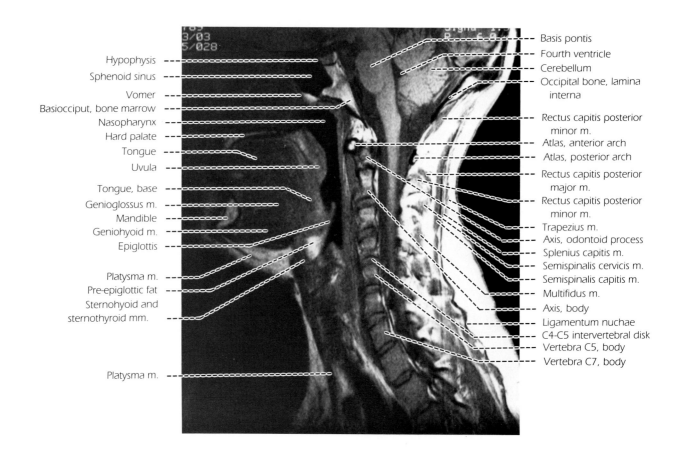

The section depicted in this sagittal T1-weighted image of the neck corresponds structurally to Figure 2-66.

## Figure 2-70

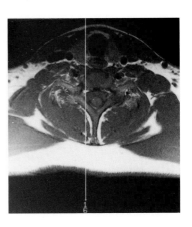

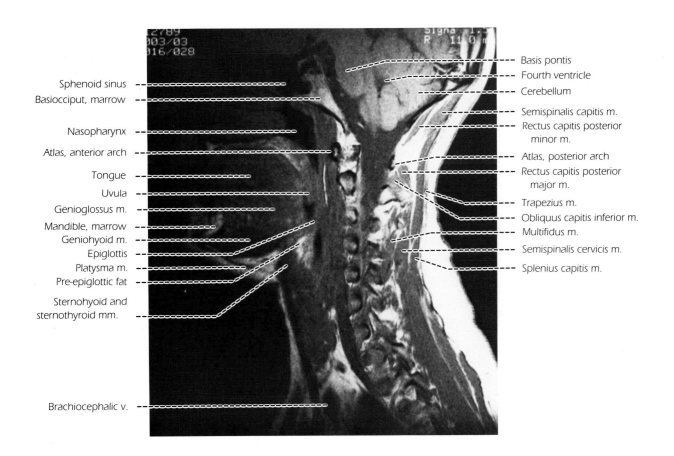

Sphenoid sinus
Basiocciput, marrow

Nasopharynx

Atlas, anterior arch

Tongue
Uvula
Genioglossus m.
Mandible, marrow
Geniohyoid m.
Epiglottis
Platysma m.
Pre-epiglottic fat

Sternohyoid and
sternothyroid mm.

Brachiocephalic v.

Basis pontis
Fourth ventricle
Cerebellum

Semispinalis capitis m.
Rectus capitis posterior
minor m.

Atlas, posterior arch
Rectus capitis posterior
major m.

Trapezius m.
Obliquus capitis inferior m.
Multifidus m.
Semispinalis cervicis m.
Splenius capitis m.

# Figure 2-71

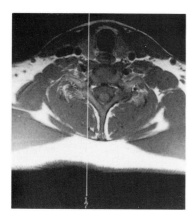

The muscles visible in this sagittal T1-weighted image of the neck include the semispinalis capitis, splenius capitis, trapezius, multifidus, semispinalis cervicis, and platysma. The suboccipital muscles include the rectus capitis posterior major and obliquus capitis inferior. Note the zygapophyseal joint. The internal carotid artery is visible in the carotid canal.

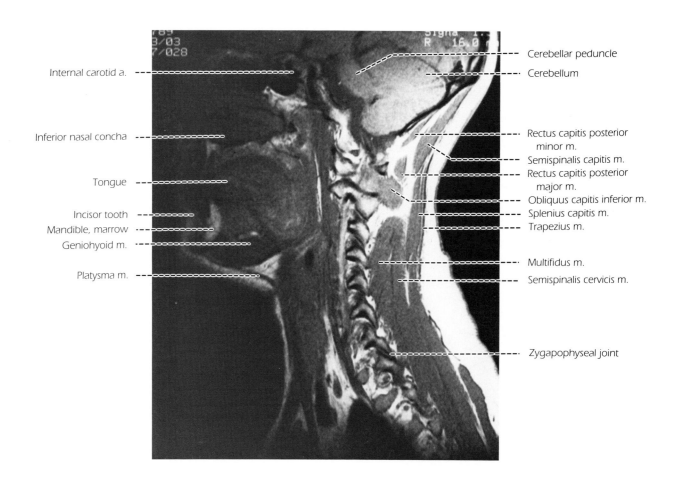

Internal carotid a.

Inferior nasal concha

Tongue

Incisor tooth
Mandible, marrow
Geniohyoid m.

Platysma m.

Cerebellar peduncle
Cerebellum

Rectus capitis posterior minor m.
Semispinalis capitis m.
Rectus capitis posterior major m.
Obliquus capitis inferior m.
Splenius capitis m.
Trapezius m.

Multifidus m.
Semispinalis cervicis m.

Zygapophyseal joint

In this sagittal T1-weighted image of the neck, the trigeminal nerve (cranial nerve V) is identified. Note the vertebral artery in the transverse foramen of the axis. The superior and inferior articular processes of a zygapophyseal joint are shown.

## Figure 2-72

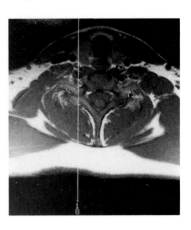

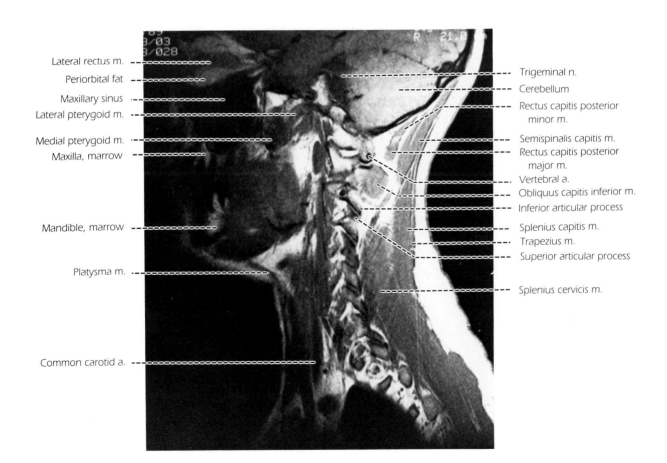

Lateral rectus m.
Periorbital fat
Maxillary sinus
Lateral pterygoid m.

Medial pterygoid m.
Maxilla, marrow

Mandible, marrow

Platysma m.

Common carotid a.

Trigeminal n.
Cerebellum
Rectus capitis posterior minor m.

Semispinalis capitis m.
Rectus capitis posterior major m.
Vertebral a.
Obliquus capitis inferior m.
Inferior articular process
Splenius capitis m.
Trapezius m.
Superior articular process

Splenius cervicis m.

# Figure 2-73

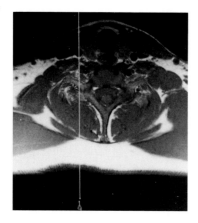

Sagittal T1-weighted image of the neck showing the orbit, which contains the eyeball, superior and inferior rectus muscles, optic nerve (cranial nerve I), and periorbital fat. In the mouth region, note the maxillary sinus, the teeth in the mandible, and the medial and lateral pterygoids, which are chewing and grinding muscles. The facial vein is identified. The tightly layered dorsal neck and head muscles include the semispinalis capitis, splenius capitis, semispinalis cervicis, and trapezius. The suboccipital muscles include the rectus capitis posterior major and minor and inferior oblique. Note the numerous roots of cervical nerves.

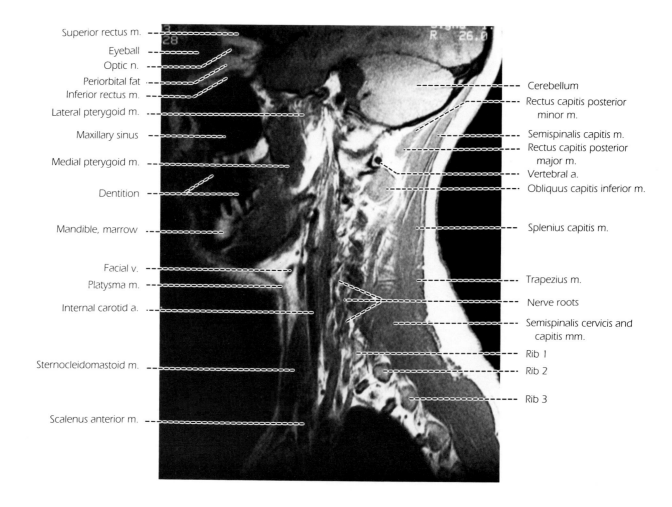

Visible in this sagittal T1-weighted image of the neck are the cochlea and semicircular canals, which are supplied by the vestibulocochlear nerve (cranial nerve VIII) and its companion nerve, the facial (cranial nerve VII). Lateral to the vertebrae the strong muscles of the back of the neck dominate this region. Muscles found in this section include, in the suboccipital group, the rectus capitis major and obliquus capitis inferior; and in the head and neck group, the semispinalis capitis and cervicis, splenius capitis and cervicis, longissimus capitis and cervicis, and trapezius. Sternocleidomastoid and platysma appear anteriorly. Note the appearance of the first two ribs, the apex of the lung in the pleural cupola (cervical pleura), and the submandibular gland.

## Figure 2-74

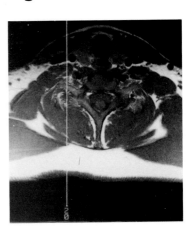

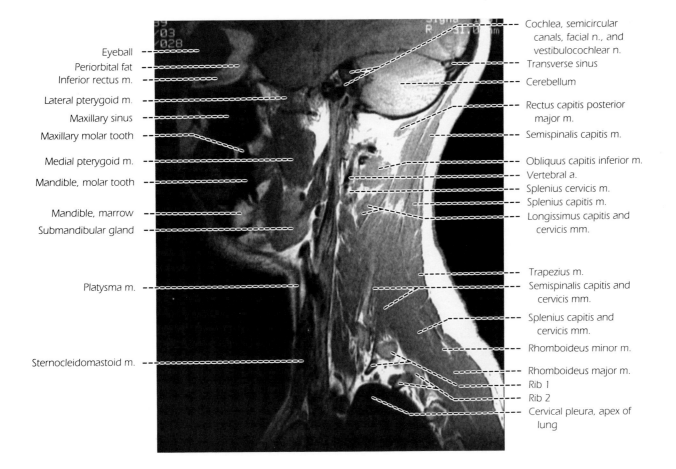

Eyeball

Periorbital fat

Inferior rectus m.

Lateral pterygoid m.

Maxillary sinus

Maxillary molar tooth

Medial pterygoid m.

Mandible, molar tooth

Mandible, marrow

Submandibular gland

Platysma m.

Sternocleidomastoid m.

Cochlea, semicircular canals, facial n., and vestibulocochlear n.

Transverse sinus

Cerebellum

Rectus capitis posterior major m.

Semispinalis capitis m.

Obliquus capitis inferior m.

Vertebral a.

Splenius cervicis m.

Splenius capitis m.

Longissimus capitis and cervicis mm.

Trapezius m.

Semispinalis capitis and cervicis mm.

Splenius capitis and cervicis mm.

Rhomboideus minor m.

Rhomboideus major m.

Rib 1

Rib 2

Cervical pleura, apex of lung

# Figure 2-75

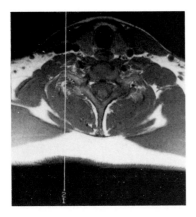

In this sagittal T1-weighted image of the neck, identifiable suboccipital muscles include the rectus capitis posterior major and obliquus capitis inferior and superior. In this section, the scalenes (anterior, middle, and posterior) are identified. Rhomboideus major and minor and levator scapulae are the three medial scapular muscles. Note the position of the subclavian and internal carotid arteries.

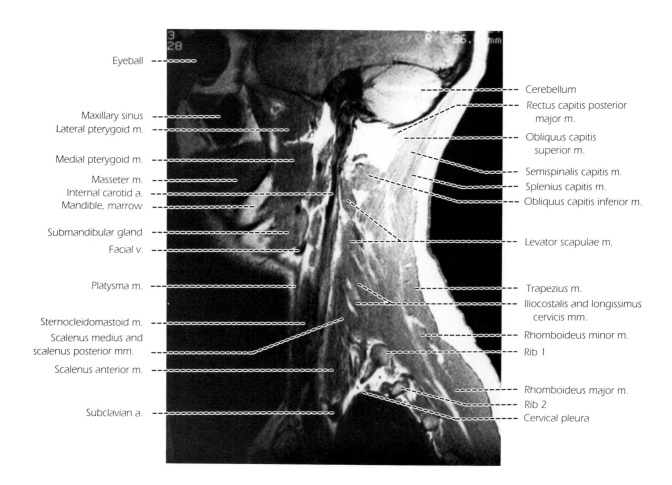

In this sagittal T1-weighted image, the tortuous facial artery can be seen beneath the mandible, both the subclavian artery and vein are present, and the three scalenes (anterior, middle, and posterior) can also be seen. The submandibular gland is diminishing in size.

## Figure 2-76

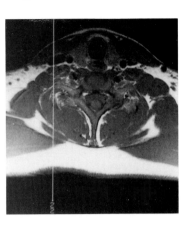

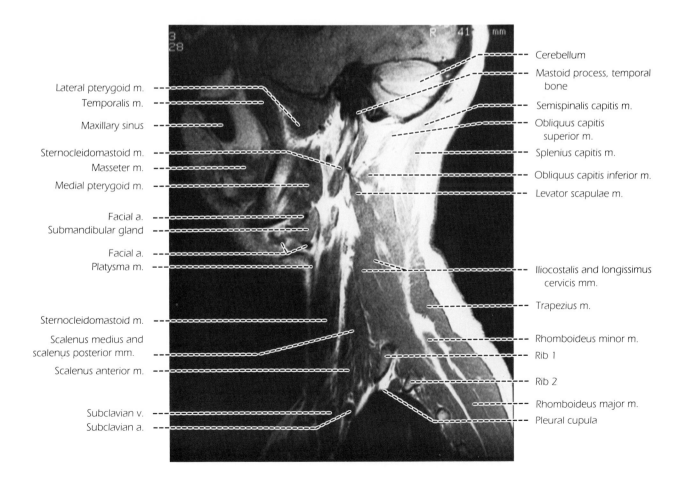

Lateral pterygoid m.
Temporalis m.
Maxillary sinus
Sternocleidomastoid m.
Masseter m.
Medial pterygoid m.
Facial a.
Submandibular gland
Facial a.
Platysma m.
Sternocleidomastoid m.
Scalenus medius and scalenus posterior mm.
Scalenus anterior m.
Subclavian v.
Subclavian a.

Cerebellum
Mastoid process, temporal bone
Semispinalis capitis m.
Obliquus capitis superior m.
Splenius capitis m.
Obliquus capitis inferior m.
Levator scapulae m.
Iliocostalis and longissimus cervicis mm.
Trapezius m.
Rhomboideus minor m.
Rib 1
Rib 2
Rhomboideus major m.
Pleural cupula

# Figure 2-77

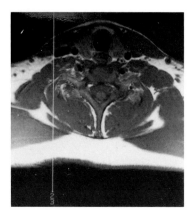

In this sagittal T1-weighted image of the neck, the facial artery has crossed the mandible and is in its typical cranial/medial course. Note the position of the subclavian artery between the anterior and middle scalene muscles. It will soon be accompanied by nerve trunks, which will form the brachial plexus.

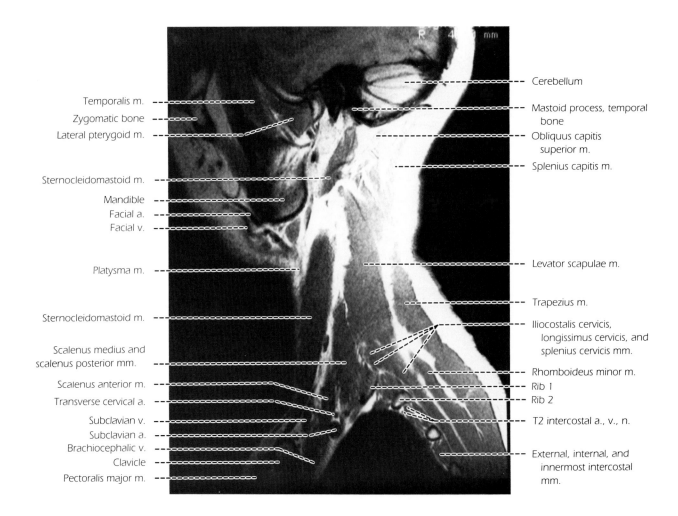

Sagittal T1-weighted image of the neck showing the nerve roots, cut in cross section, that accompany the subclavian artery; these and others will form the brachial plexus. The position of the nerve roots and subclavian artery between the anterior and middle scalene muscles is the usual configuration. They will pass over the first rib and under the clavicle.

## Figure 2-78

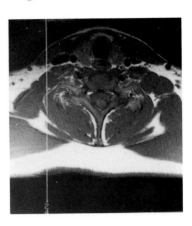

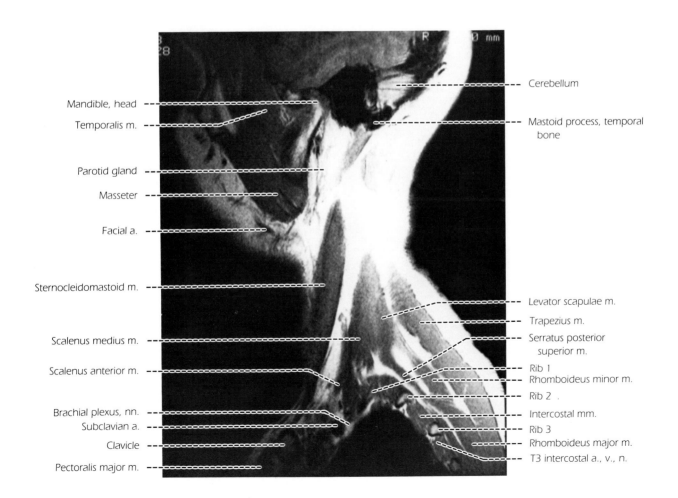

Cerebellum

Mandible, head

Temporalis m.

Mastoid process, temporal bone

Parotid gland

Masseter

Facial a.

Sternocleidomastoid m.

Levator scapulae m.

Trapezius m.

Scalenus medius m.

Serratus posterior superior m.

Scalenus anterior m.

Rib 1

Rhomboideus minor m.

Rib 2 .

Intercostal mm.

Brachial plexus, nn.

Subclavian a.

Rib 3

Clavicle

Rhomboideus major m.

T3 intercostal a., v., n.

Pectoralis major m.

# Figure 2-79

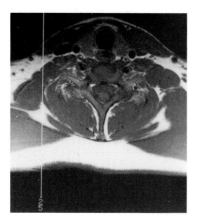

Sagittal T1-weighted image of the neck showing the progress of the cervical and thoracic nerves that form the brachial plexus. Here the nerves lie in front of the medial and posterior scalene muscles and are topographically related to the subclavian artery. Once again, the parotid gland appears on the right side of the face.

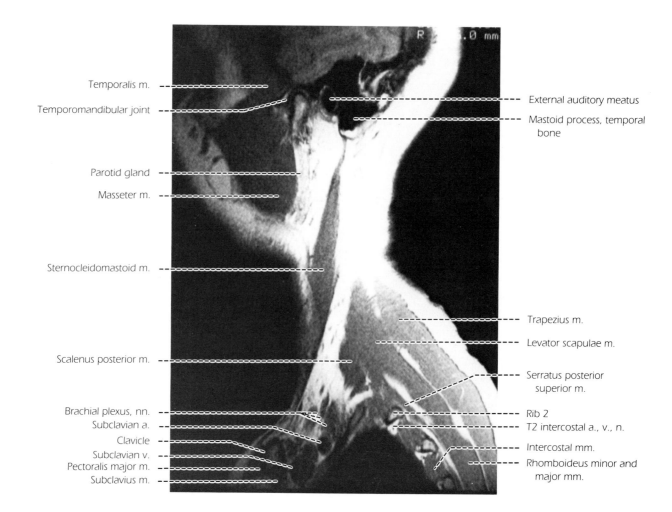

Temporalis m.
Temporomandibular joint
Parotid gland
Masseter m.
Sternocleidomastoid m.
Scalenus posterior m.
Brachial plexus, nn.
Subclavian a.
Clavicle
Subclavian v.
Pectoralis major m.
Subclavius m.

External auditory meatus
Mastoid process, temporal bone
Trapezius m.
Levator scapulae m.
Serratus posterior superior m.
Rib 2
T2 intercostal a., v., n.
Intercostal mm.
Rhomboideus minor and major mm.

In this sagittal T1-weighted image, trunks of the brachial plexus are found anterior to the scalenus posterior and dorsal and cranial to the subclavian artery in the neck region. The sternocleidomastoid is seen inserting into the mastoid process of the temporal bone.

## Figure 2-80

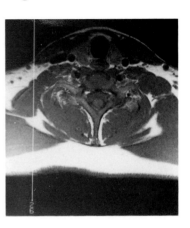

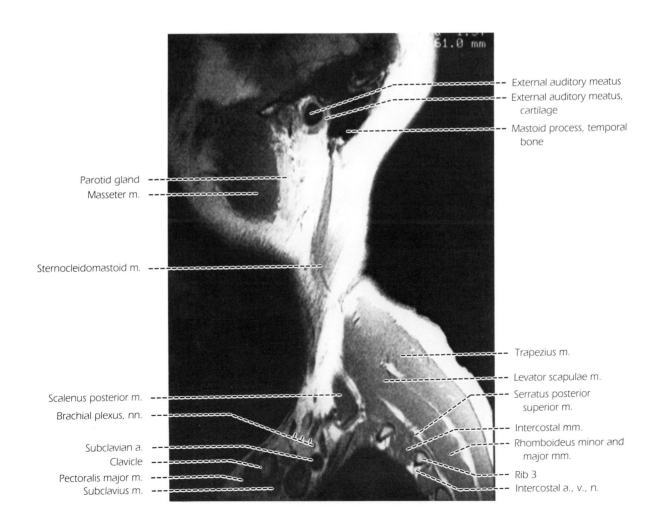

External auditory meatus
External auditory meatus, cartilage
Mastoid process, temporal bone

Parotid gland
Masseter m.

Sternocleidomastoid m.

Trapezius m.
Levator scapulae m.
Scalenus posterior m.
Serratus posterior superior m.
Brachial plexus, nn.
Intercostal mm.
Rhomboideus minor and major mm.
Subclavian a.
Clavicle
Rib 3
Pectoralis major m.
Subclavius m.
Intercostal a., v., n.

# Figure 2-81

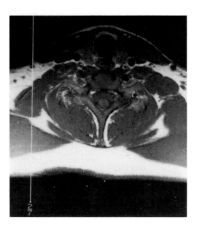

Sagittal T1-weighted image of the neck showing the topographic relationship between the nerves that form the brachial plexus and the subclavian artery. The clavicle is also shown. These structures cross the cranial surface of the first rib.

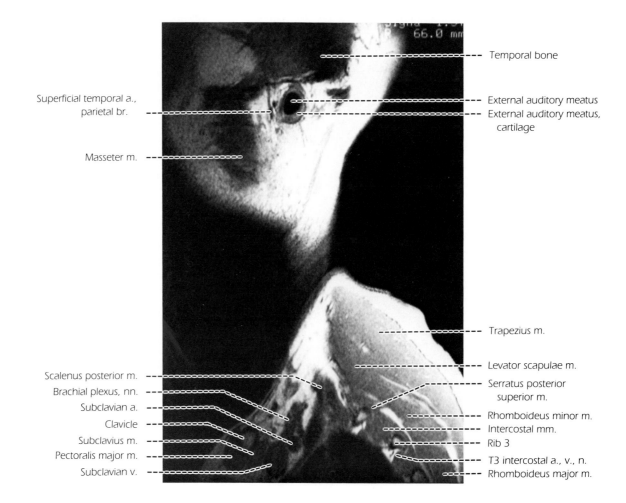

Of major interest in this sagittal T1-weighted image are the nerves that form the brachial plexus and their topographic relationship with the posterior scalene muscle and the subclavian artery. The superficial temporal artery and its frontal and parietal branches are seen at the level of the external auditory meatus. Note the pleural cupula.

## Figure 2-82

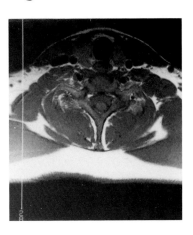

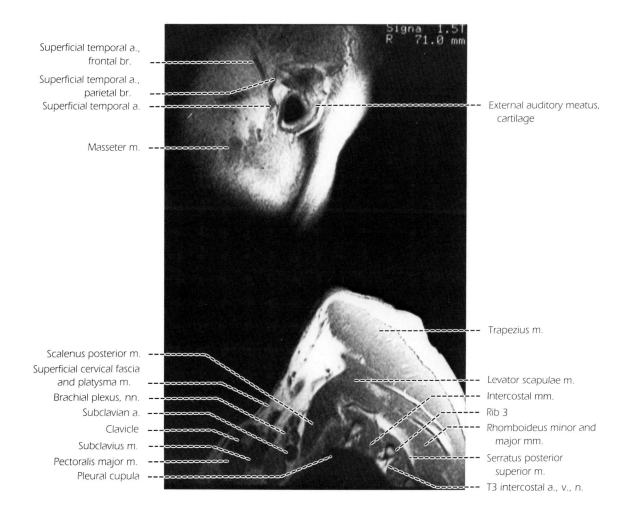

Superficial temporal a., frontal br.

Superficial temporal a., parietal br.

Superficial temporal a.

Masseter m.

External auditory meatus, cartilage

Trapezius m.

Scalenus posterior m.

Superficial cervical fascia and platysma m.

Brachial plexus, nn.

Subclavian a.

Clavicle

Subclavius m.

Pectoralis major m.

Pleural cupula

Levator scapulae m.

Intercostal mm.

Rib 3

Rhomboideus minor and major mm.

Serratus posterior superior m.

T3 intercostal a., v., n.

## Figure 2-83

In this axial T2-weighted image of the neck, the muscles include the platysma, sternohyoid, and sternothyroid in the visceral compartment; the three scalenes and longus colli in the prevertebral region; and the iliocostalis cervicis, longissimus cervicis, splenius cervicis, and multifidus in the vertebral region. The body, arch, and spinous process of the fifth cervical vertebra are seen. The thyroid gland extends above the level of the trachea to the infraglottic region of the larynx and is found at the level of the cricoid cartilage in this section.

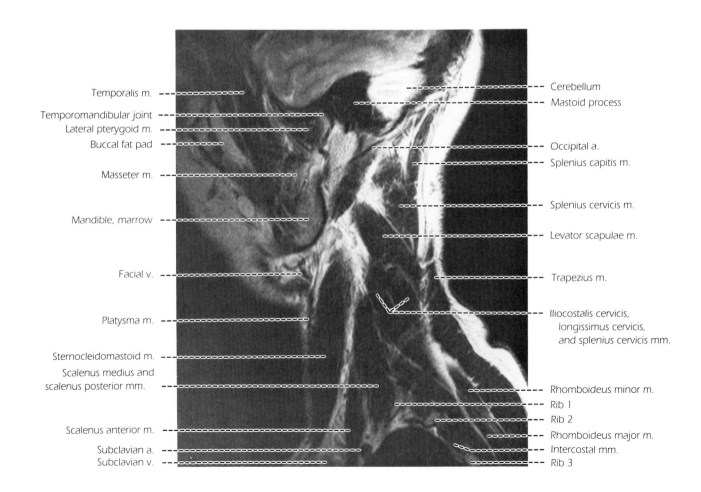

Temporalis m.

Temporomandibular joint
Lateral pterygoid m.
Buccal fat pad

Masseter m.

Mandible, marrow

Facial v.

Platysma m.

Sternocleidomastoid m.
Scalenus medius and
scalenus posterior mm.

Scalenus anterior m.
Subclavian a.
Subclavian v.

Cerebellum
Mastoid process

Occipital a.
Splenius capitis m.

Splenius cervicis m.

Levator scapulae m.

Trapezius m.

Iliocostalis cervicis,
longissimus cervicis,
and splenius cervicis mm.

Rhomboideus minor m.
Rib 1
Rib 2
Rhomboideus major m.
Intercostal mm.
Rib 3

In this sagittal T2-weighted image of the neck, the muscles include the rectus capitis posterior major, semispinalis capitis, obliquus capitis inferior, spinalis capitis, trapezius, spinalis cervicis and capitis, and sternocleidomastoid. The inferior orbital fissure, periorbital fat, lens, and eyeball (globe) are present. The facial and vestibulocochlear nerves (cranial nerves VII and VIII) are closely associated with the cochlea and vestibular apparatus in the inner ear.

**Figure 2-84**

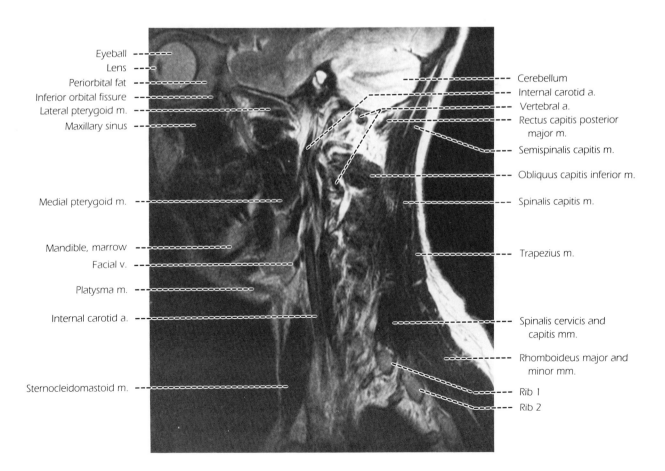

## Figure 2-85

In this sagittal T2-weighted image of the neck, the zygapophyseal joints of the vertebral column can be seen. In addition, the superior and inferior articular processes and two intervertebral foramina containing nerve roots are identified. Note the structural detail seen in the cerebellum.

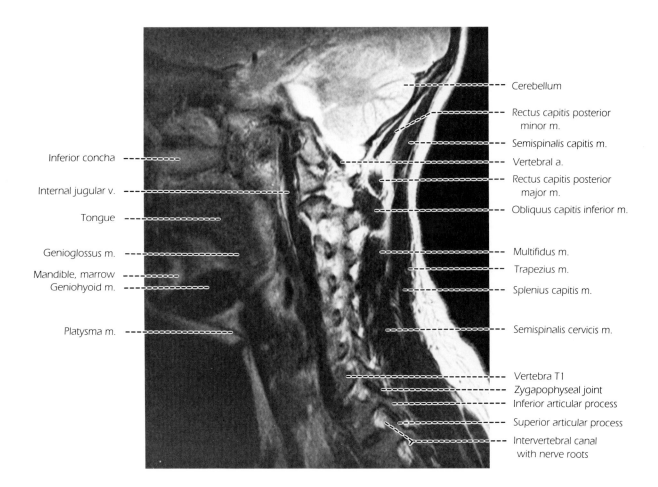

Inferior concha

Internal jugular v.

Tongue

Genioglossus m.

Mandible, marrow
Geniohyoid m.

Platysma m.

Cerebellum

Rectus capitis posterior
minor m.

Semispinalis capitis m.

Vertebral a.

Rectus capitis posterior
major m.

Obliquus capitis inferior m.

Multifidus m.

Trapezius m.

Splenius capitis m.

Semispinalis cervicis m.

Vertebra T1
Zygapophyseal joint
Inferior articular process
Superior articular process
Intervertebral canal
with nerve roots

In this sagittal T2-weighted image of the neck, the pharynx and larynx are well visualized. The nasal concha, hard palate, tongue, uvula, base of the tongue, vallecula, epiglottis, hyoid bone, and cricoid and thyroid cartilages are visible. The subarachnoid space filled with cerebrospinal fluid and the spinal cord are located in the vertebral foramen. The intervertebral disks, spinous processes, anterior and posterior longitudinal ligaments, ligamentum nuchae, and interspinalis muscles are also seen.

# Figure 2-86

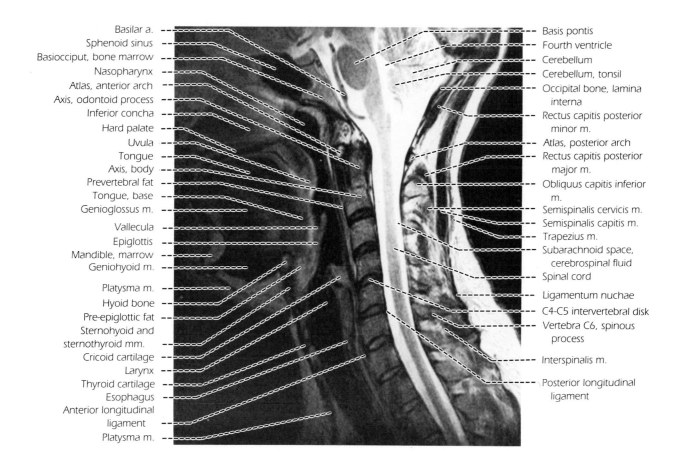

Basilar a.
Sphenoid sinus
Basiocciput, bone marrow
Nasopharynx
Atlas, anterior arch
Axis, odontoid process
Inferior concha
Hard palate
Uvula
Tongue
Axis, body
Prevertebral fat
Tongue, base
Genioglossus m.

Vallecula
Epiglottis
Mandible, marrow
Geniohyoid m.

Platysma m.
Hyoid bone
Pre-epiglottic fat
Sternohyoid and
sternothyroid mm.
Cricoid cartilage
Larynx
Thyroid cartilage
Esophagus
Anterior longitudinal
ligament
Platysma m.

Basis pontis
Fourth ventricle
Cerebellum
Cerebellum, tonsil
Occipital bone, lamina
interna
Rectus capitis posterior
minor m.
Atlas, posterior arch
Rectus capitis posterior
major m.
Obliquus capitis inferior
m.
Semispinalis cervicis m.
Semispinalis capitis m.
Trapezius m.
Subarachnoid space,
cerebrospinal fluid
Spinal cord

Ligamentum nuchae
C4-C5 intervertebral disk
Vertebra C6, spinous
process

Interspinalis m.

Posterior longitudinal
ligament

# Figure 2-87

In this sagittal T2-weighted image of the neck, the following structures in the vertebral column are identified: the anterior and posterior arches of the atlas, odontoid process of the axis; intervertebral disk (C4-C5), anterior and posterior longitudinal ligaments, ligamentum nuchae, body of vertebrae C5 and C7, and interspinous ligament. Contained within the vertebral foramen, the spinal cord and the subarachnoid space containing cerebrospinal fluid are visible. On the visceral anterior side, the epiglottis, hyoid bone, thyroid cartilage, larynx, and esophagus are seen. In the nasal cavity, note the middle and inferior conchae, and in the larynx, note the epiglottis at the base of the tongue.

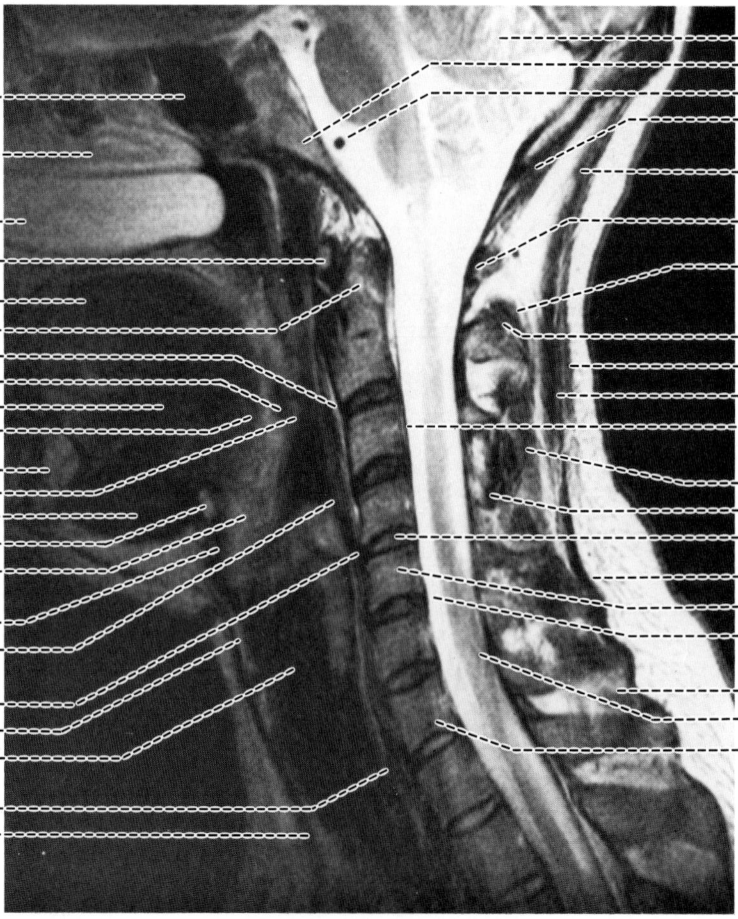

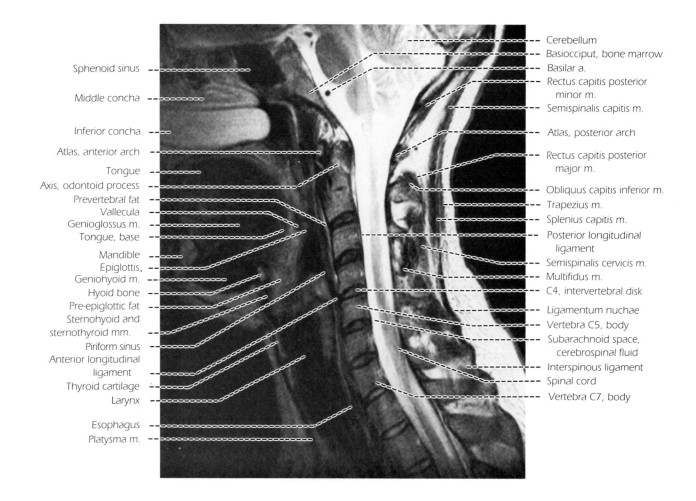

Sphenoid sinus
Middle concha
Inferior concha
Atlas, anterior arch
Tongue
Axis, odontoid process
Prevertebral fat
Vallecula
Genioglossus m.
Tongue, base
Mandible
Epiglottis
Geniohyoid m.
Hyoid bone
Pre-epiglottic fat
Sternohyoid and sternothyroid mm.
Piriform sinus
Anterior longitudinal ligament
Thyroid cartilage
Larynx
Esophagus
Platysma m.
Cerebellum
Basiocciput, bone marrow
Basilar a.
Rectus capitis posterior minor m.
Semispinalis capitis m.
Atlas, posterior arch
Rectus capitis posterior major m.
Obliquus capitis inferior m.
Trapezius m.
Splenius capitis m.
Posterior longitudinal ligament
Semispinalis cervicis m.
Multifidus m.
C4, intervertebral disk
Ligamentum nuchae
Vertebra C5, body
Subarachnoid space, cerebrospinal fluid
Interspinous ligament
Spinal cord
Vertebra C7, body

# 3

# CRANIAL NERVES

## Figure 3-1

Midsagittal T1-weighted image showing the olfactory bulb and optic nerve. The olfactory bulb is located under the frontal lobe. The optic nerve (cranial nerve II) is ventral to the hypothalamus. The pituitary gland is ventral to the optic nerve and dorsal to the sphenoid sinus. The basilar artery is ventral to the pons. Other structures seen in this section include the thalamus and corpus callosum.

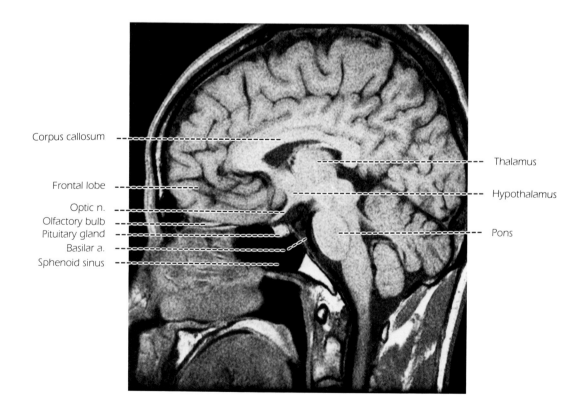

Parasagittal T1-weighted image showing the optic nerve (cranial nerve II) ventral to the diencephalon. Other structures seen in this section include the corpus callosum, cerebellum, and basis pontis.

Figure 3-2

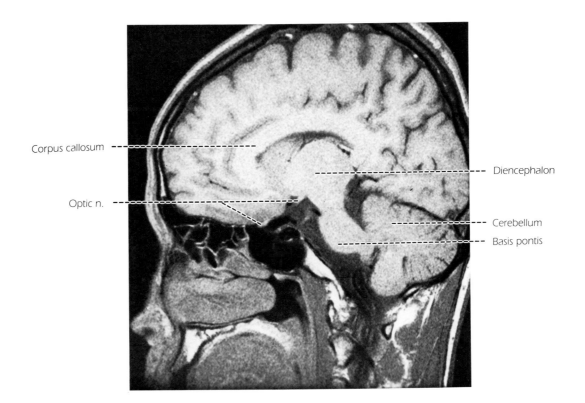

Corpus callosum

Optic n.

Diencephalon

Cerebellum

Basis pontis

## Figure 3-3

Midsagittal T1-weighted image showing the optic nerve (cranial nerve II) beneath the hypothalamus. The mamillary body is in the caudal part of the hypothalamus. Dorsal to the hypothalamus is the thalamus. The pituitary gland is ventral to the optic nerve.

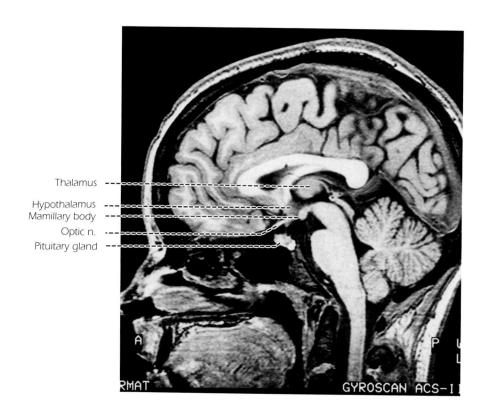

Thalamus

Hypothalamus
Mamillary body

Optic n.

Pituitary gland

Figure 3-4

Parasagittal T1-weighted image showing the optic nerve (cranial nerve II), optic chiasma, and pituitary gland. The optic chiasma is ventral to the hypothalamus. The pituitary stalk links the hypothalamus with the pituitary gland. The anterior and posterior lobes are seen within the pituitary gland. The posterior lobe is characterized by high signal intensity.

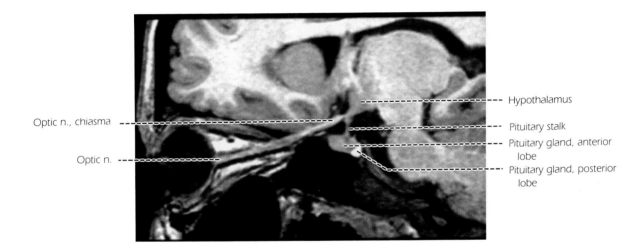

Optic n., chiasma

Optic n.

Hypothalamus

Pituitary stalk

Pituitary gland, anterior lobe

Pituitary gland, posterior lobe

## Figure 3-5

Coronal T1-weighted image showing the optic nerve (cranial nerve II) ventral to the third ventricle. The internal carotid artery is medial to the temporal lobe. Other structures seen in this section include the head of the caudate nucleus, putamen, and anterior limb of the internal capsule.

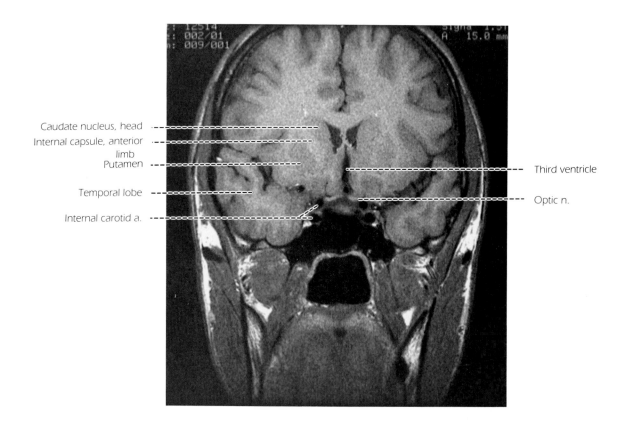

Coronal T1-weighted image showing the optic nerve (cranial nerve II) and the pituitary gland. Other structures seen in this section include the head of the caudate nucleus, putamen, lateral ventricle, and temporal lobe.

Figure 3-6

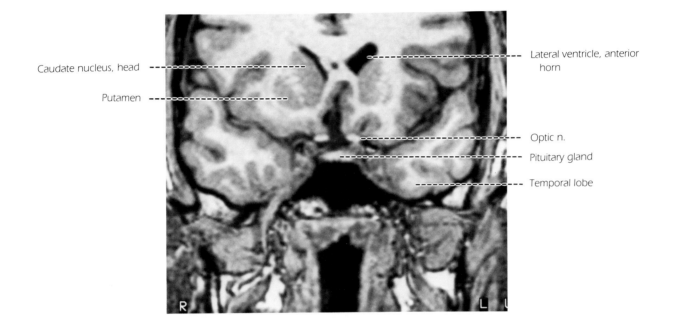

Caudate nucleus, head

Putamen

Lateral ventricle, anterior horn

Optic n.

Pituitary gland

Temporal lobe

# Figure 3-7

Axial T1-weighted image showing the optic nerve (cranial nerve II) inside and outside the optic canal, optic chiasma, optic tract, and optic radiation. The latter is located lateral to the trigone of the lateral ventricle. The mamillary bodies are seen ventral to the midbrain.

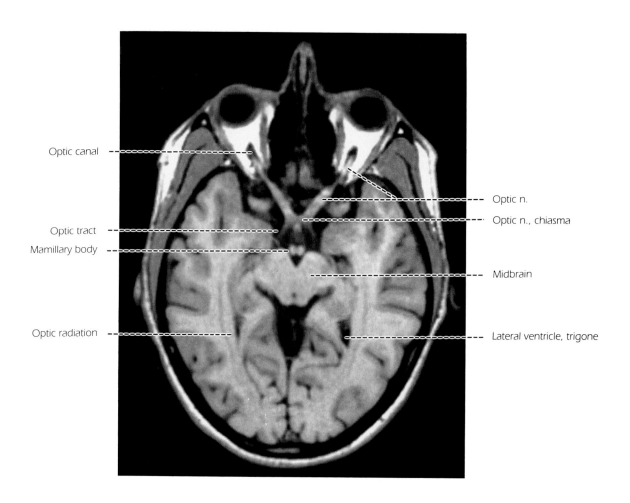

Axial T1-weighted image showing the optic nerve (cranial nerve II), optic chiasma, and optic tract. Other structures seen in this section include the temporal lobe, pineal gland, and trigone of the lateral ventricle.

## Figure 3-8

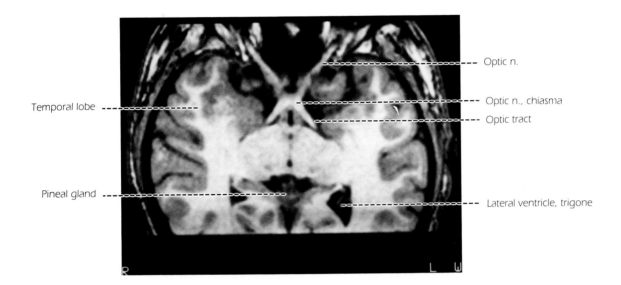

## Figure 3-9

Parasagittal T1-weighted image showing the oculomotor nerve (cranial nerve III) ventral to the midbrain. Rostral to the midbrain is the mamillary body. Other structures seen in this section include the corpus callosum and thalamus.

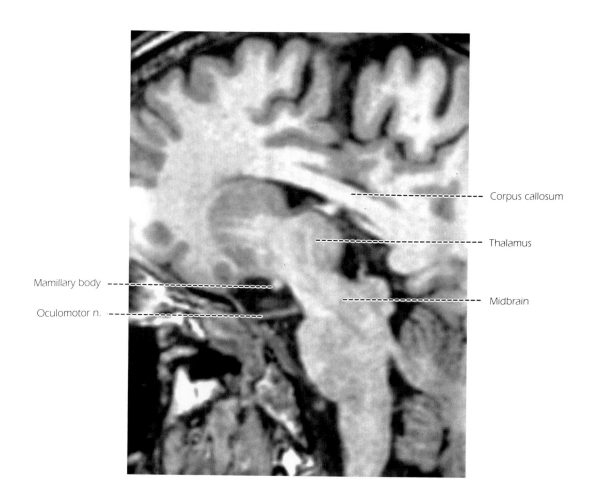

Corpus callosum

Thalamus

Mamillary body

Oculomotor n.

Midbrain

Axial T1-weighted image showing the trochlear nerve (cranial nerve IV) coursing around the pons. Other structures seen in this section include the optic nerve (cranial nerve II) and internal carotid artery.

Figure 3-10

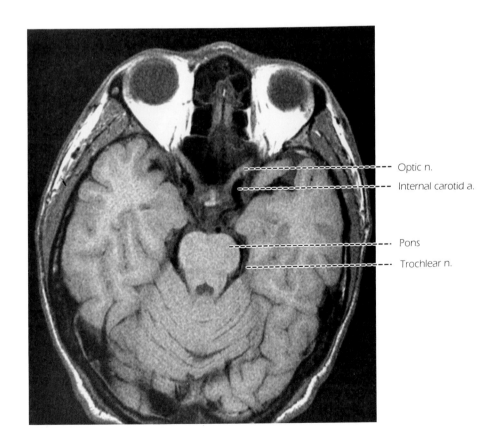

Optic n.

Internal carotid a.

Pons

Trochlear n.

## Figure 3-11

Axial T1-weighted image showing the trochlear nerve (cranial nerve IV) coursing lateral to the pons. Other structures seen in this section include the optic nerve (cranial nerve II), temporal lobe, fourth ventricle, and cerebellum.

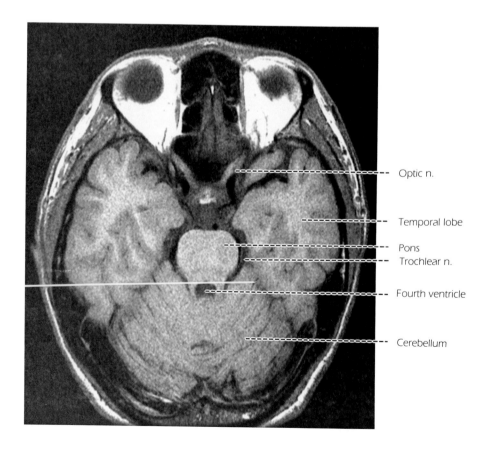

Optic n.

Temporal lobe

Pons
Trochlear n.

Fourth ventricle

Cerebellum

Axial T2-weighted image showing the trigeminal nerve (cranial nerve V) leaving the pons. The basilar artery is ventral to the pons. Dorsal to the pons and separating it from the cerebellum is the fourth ventricle. The internal carotid artery and Meckel's cavity are medial to the temporal lobe. The bright signal intensity of the eyeball and the low signal intensity of the lens are apparent.

Figure 3-12

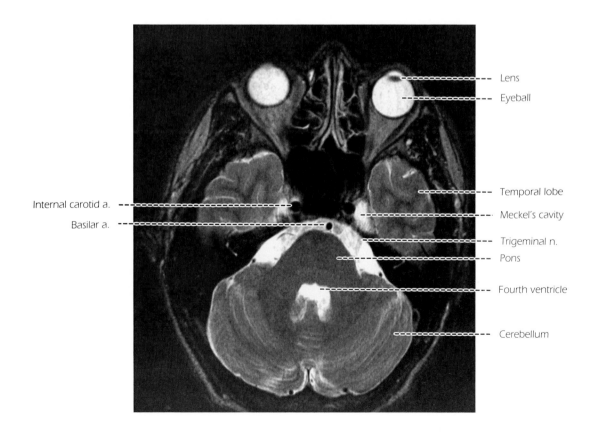

Lens
Eyeball

Internal carotid a.
Basilar a.

Temporal lobe
Meckel's cavity
Trigeminal n.
Pons
Fourth ventricle
Cerebellum

## Figure 3-13

Axial T2-weighted image showing the trigeminal nerve (cranial nerve V) leaving the pons. Ventral to the pons is the basilar artery. Dorsal to the pons is the fourth ventricle. The cerebellum is superior to the fourth ventricle. The internal carotid artery and Meckel's cavity are medial to the temporal lobe.

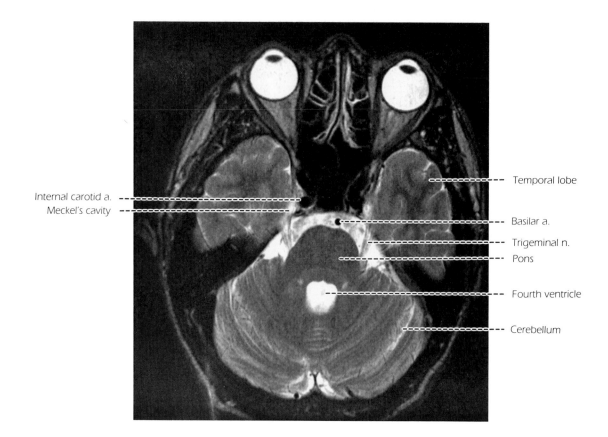

Axial T1-weighted image showing the trigeminal nerve (cranial nerve V) exiting from the pons. The fourth ventricle separates the cerebellum and the pons. Medial to the temporal lobe is the internal carotid artery.

Figure 3-14

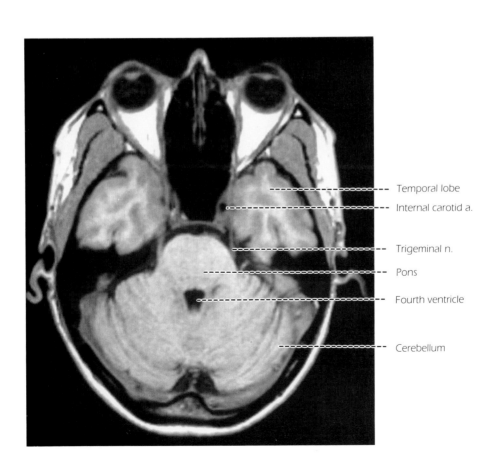

Temporal lobe

Internal carotid a.

Trigeminal n.

Pons

Fourth ventricle

Cerebellum

## Figure 3-15

Axial T1-weighted image showing the trigeminal nerve (cranial nerve V) exiting from the pons. The internal carotid artery is seen medial to the temporal lobe.

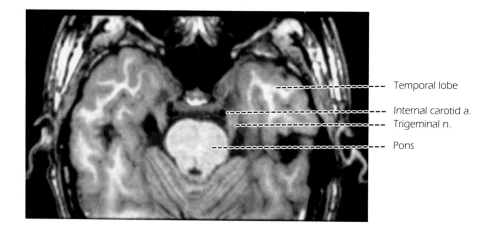

Temporal lobe

Internal carotid a.

Trigeminal n.

Pons

Sagittal T1-weighted image showing the abducens nerve (cranial nerve VI) leaving the brain stem at the pontomedullary junction.

Figure 3-16

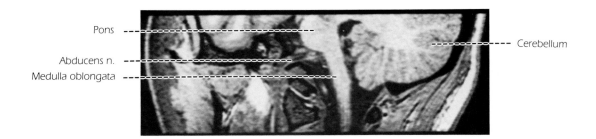

## Figure 3-17

Axial T1-weighted image showing the facial and vestibulocochlear nerves (cranial nerves VII and VIII). Other structures related to these two nerves include the geniculate ganglion, cochlea, vestibule, and greater superficial petrosal nerve.

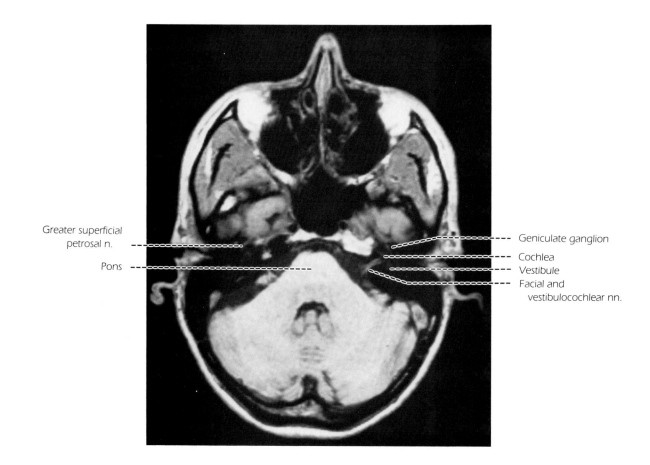

Greater superficial petrosal n.

Pons

Geniculate ganglion

Cochlea

Vestibule

Facial and vestibulocochlear nn.

Parasagittal T1-weighted image showing the vertical part of the facial nerve (cranial nerve VII) rostral to the cerebellum. The temporal lobe is seen.

Figure 3-18

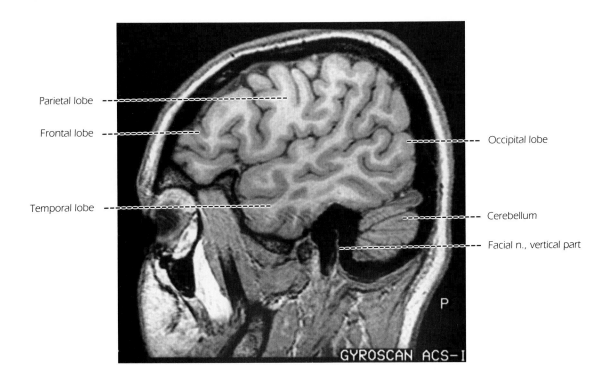

Parietal lobe

Frontal lobe

Occipital lobe

Temporal lobe

Cerebellum

Facial n., vertical part

P

GYROSCAN ACS-I

# Figure 3-19

Parasagittal T1-weighted image showing the facial and vestibulocochlear nerves (cranial nerves VII and VIII) emanating from the pons. Other structures seen in this section include the occipital lobe, cerebellum, fourth ventricle, and medulla oblongata.

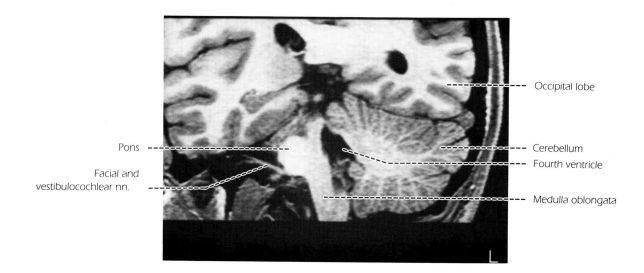

Parasagittal T1-weighted image showing the glosso-pharyngeal, vagus, and spinal accessory nerves (cranial nerves IX, X, and XI) exiting from the medulla oblongata. Rostral to the medulla oblongata is the pons, and caudal to it is the spinal cord. The fourth ventricle and cerebellum are also seen.

## Figure 3-20

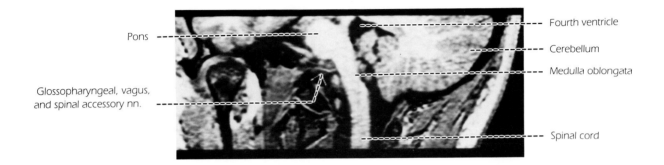

Pons

Glossopharyngeal, vagus, and spinal accessory nn.

Fourth ventricle

Cerebellum

Medulla oblongata

Spinal cord

## Figure 3-21

Axial T1-weighted image of the brain stem showing the glossopharyngeal, vagus, and spinal accessory nerves (cranial nerves IX, X, and XI) exiting from the lateral part of the medulla oblongata.

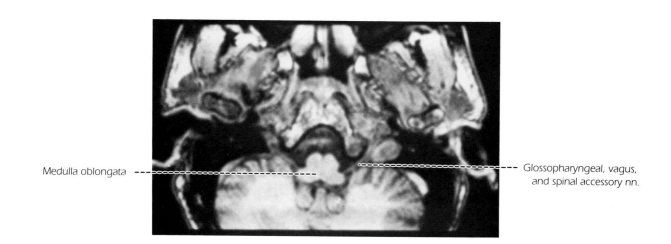

Medulla oblongata ----- ----- Glossopharyngeal, vagus, and spinal accessory nn.

Axial T1-weighted image of the brain stem showing the glossopharyngeal, vagus, and spinal accessory nerves (cranial nerves IV, X, and XI) exiting from the lateral surface of the medulla oblongata.

# Figure 3-22

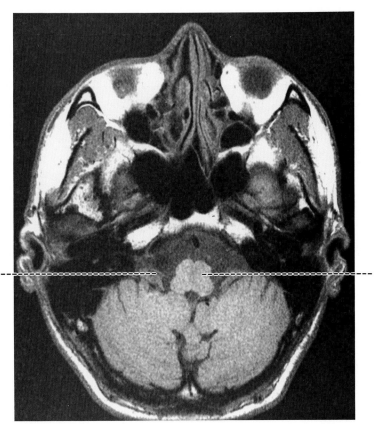

Glossopharyngeal, vagus, and spinal accessory nn.          Medulla oblongata

# Figure 3-23

Axial T1-weighted image showing the hypoglossal nerve (cranial nerve XII) in the hypoglossal canal. A neuroma of the left hypoglossal nerve is seen. Other structures identified are the medulla oblongata, cerebellum, and internal occipital protuberance.

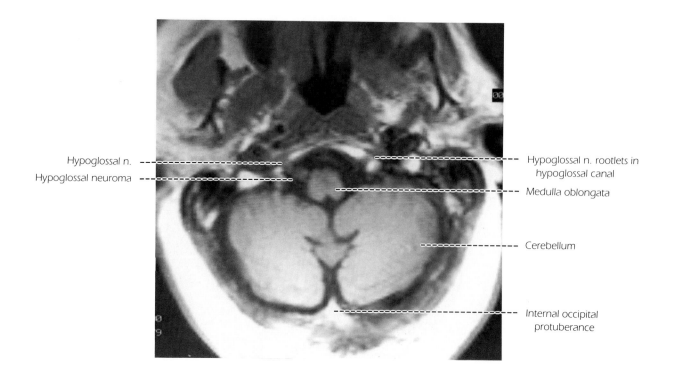

# 4

# GADOLINIUM-ENHANCED IMAGES

## Figure 4-1

Two gadolinium-enhanced images of the brain. The upper image is a midsagittal section, and the lower is an anterior coronal section. In the midsagittal section, vascular channels such as the great cerebral vein (Galen's vein), straight sinus, and arachnoid granulations are seen. Other important structures include the corpus callosum, thalamus, hypothalamus, optic nerve (cranial nerve II), cerebellum, pons, medulla oblongata, and frontal lobe. The fourth ventricle is located between the cerebellum and the pons. Non-neural structures present in this section include the pharyngeal recess, epiglottis, root of the tongue with the genioglossus muscle, lingual septum, uvula, sphenoid sinus, nasal septum, and sella turcica. In the frontal coronal section are seen muscles of extraocular movement including the superior rectus, superior oblique, lateral rectus, medial rectus, inferior oblique, and inferior rectus. The middle and inferior conchae of the nose are seen.

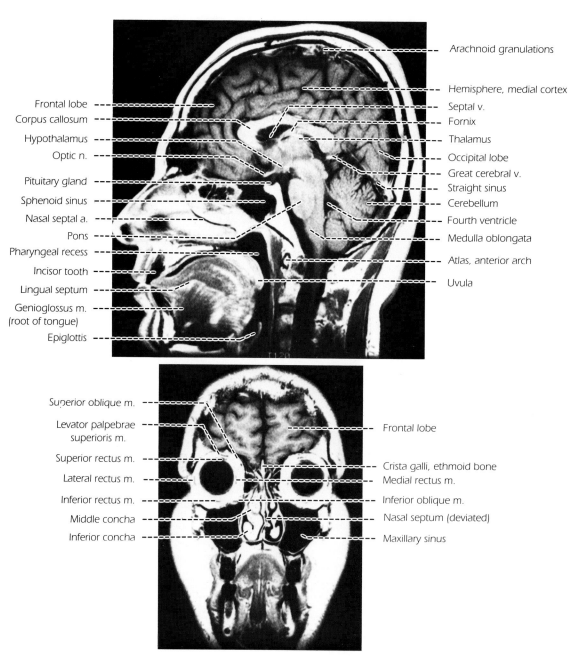

Upper image labels:
Frontal lobe
Corpus callosum
Hypothalamus
Optic n.
Pituitary gland
Sphenoid sinus
Nasal septal a.
Pons
Pharyngeal recess
Incisor tooth
Lingual septum
Genioglossus m. (root of tongue)
Epiglottis

Arachnoid granulations
Hemisphere, medial cortex
Septal v.
Fornix
Thalamus
Occipital lobe
Great cerebral v.
Straight sinus
Cerebellum
Fourth ventricle
Medulla oblongata
Atlas, anterior arch
Uvula

Lower image labels:
Superior oblique m.
Levator palpebrae superioris m.
Superior rectus m.
Lateral rectus m.
Inferior rectus m.
Middle concha
Inferior concha

Frontal lobe
Crista galli, ethmoid bone
Medial rectus m.
Inferior oblique m.
Nasal septum (deviated)
Maxillary sinus

Two axial gadolinium-enhanced images. The upper section shows the cerebellar hemisphere, cerebellar vermis, and medulla oblongata. Non-neural structures seen in this section include the nasolacrimal duct, maxillary sinus, head of the mandible (condylar process), petrous part of the temporal bone, zygomatic arch, coronoid process of the mandible, and temporalis muscle. The internal carotid artery is also seen. In the lower section, the cerebellar hemisphere and the cerebellar tonsil are seen adjacent to the medulla oblongata. Non-neural structures include the nasal septum, temporalis muscle, coronoid process of the mandible, torus tubarius, head of the mandible, maxillary sinus, nasopharynx, pharyngeal recess (Rosenmüller's fossa), jugular bulb, and internal carotid artery. Muscles include the masseter, temporalis, lateral pterygoid, and longus capitis.

Figure 4-2

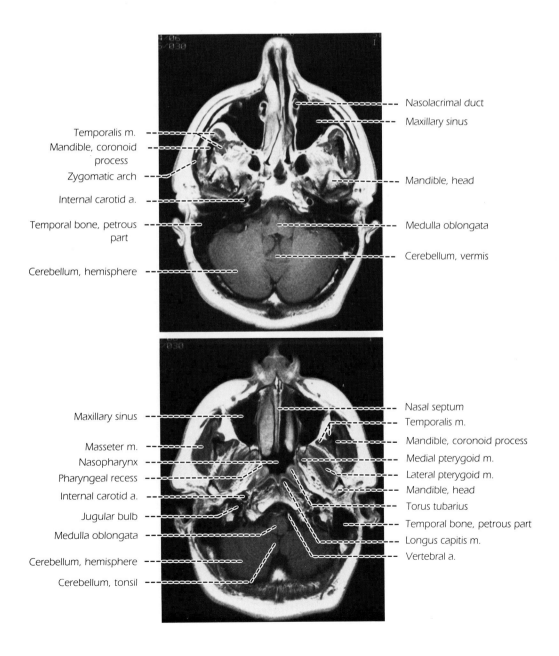

# Figure 4-3

Two axial gadolinium-enhanced images. The upper section is through the midbrain. The lower section is through the temporal lobe, cerebellum, and pons. Neural structures seen in the upper section include the orbital and rectus gyri of the frontal lobes; optic nerve (cranial nerve II), chiasma, and tract; cerebral peduncle; cerebral aqueduct of the midbrain; infundibular recess; and pituitary (hypophyseal) stalk. Non-neural structures include the crista galli, lens, and posterior chamber of the eyeball (globe). The mamillary body is caudal to the pituitary stalk. In the lower section, the basis pontis is seen within the pons. The superior cerebellar peduncle connects the cerebellum and pons. The fourth ventricle is located between the cerebellum and pons. The temporal poles are seen on both sides. Non-neural structures include the nasolacrimal duct and ethmoid sinus.

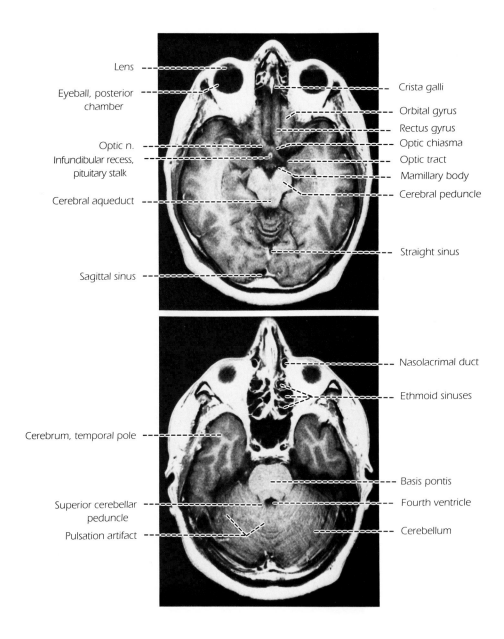

Two coronal gadolinium-enhanced images. The upper section is at the level of the splenium of the corpus callosum. The lower section is at the level of the body of the corpus callosum anteriorly. In the upper section, vascular channels include the superior sagittal sinus, basal vein (Rosenthal's vein), and vertebral artery. Neural structures include the posterior horn of the lateral ventricle, splenium of the corpus callosum, cingulate sulcus, superior and inferior colliculi, and fourth ventricle. In the lower section, the corpus callosum is seen capping the body of the lateral ventricle. The septum pellucidum separates the two cavities of the lateral ventricle. The insular cortex is seen inside the lateral fissure. The optic tract is dorsal to the pituitary (hypophyseal) stalk. The internal carotid artery and cavernous sinus are well visualized. Non-neural structures include the ramus of the mandible, lateral pterygoid muscle, and Meckel's cavity.

Figure 4-4

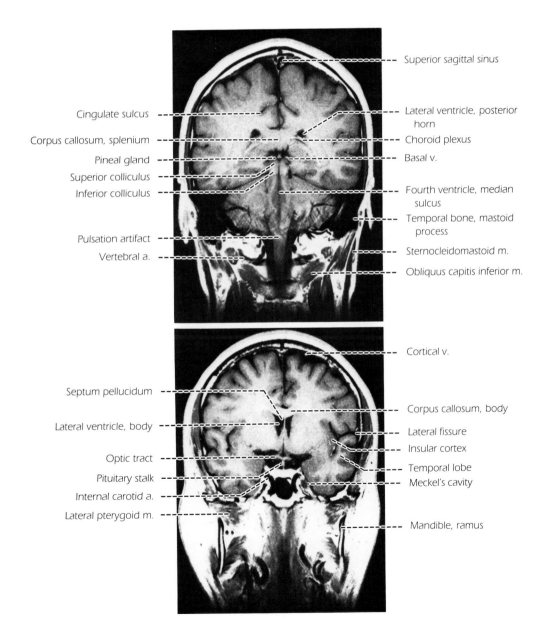

# Figure 4-5

Two gadolinium-enhanced coronal images through the rostral part of the brain. In the upper section, the corpus callosum is seen capping the anterior horn of the lateral ventricle. The two anterior horns are separated by the septum pellucidum. The lateral fissure is seen separating the frontal and temporal lobes of the cerebrum. Non-neural structures include the pharyngeal recess, torus tubarius, uvula, soft palate, palatine tonsil, oropharynx, mandible, nasopharynx, and zygomatic arch. Muscles seen in this section include the lateral pterygoid, masseter, and medial pterygoid. In the lower section, the corpus callosum is again seen capping the lateral ventricles. The septum pellucidum separates the two lateral ventricles. The caudate nucleus forms the lateral wall of the lateral ventricle. The anterior limb of the internal capsule separates the two parts of the lentiform nucleus, the caudate from the putamen. Beneath the optic chiasma is the pituitary gland. The internal carotid artery and the cavernous sinus are well enhanced.

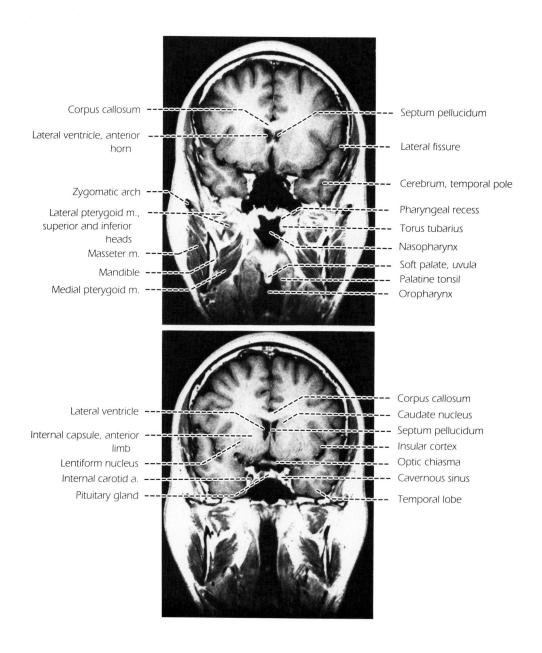

Corpus callosum
Lateral ventricle, anterior horn
Zygomatic arch
Lateral pterygoid m., superior and inferior heads
Masseter m.
Mandible
Medial pterygoid m.

Septum pellucidum
Lateral fissure
Cerebrum, temporal pole
Pharyngeal recess
Torus tubarius
Nasopharynx
Soft palate, uvula
Palatine tonsil
Oropharynx

Lateral ventricle
Internal capsule, anterior limb
Lentiform nucleus
Internal carotid a.
Pituitary gland

Corpus callosum
Caudate nucleus
Septum pellucidum
Insular cortex
Optic chiasma
Cavernous sinus
Temporal lobe

Two gadolinium-enhanced axial images. The upper one is at the level of the genu and splenium of the corpus callosum. The lower one is at the level of the pineal gland. In the upper section, the corpus callosum is seen capping the lateral ventricles. The two cavities of the lateral ventricle are separated by the septum pellucidum. Beneath the septum pellucidum are the columns of the fornix. The caudate nucleus is in the lateral wall of the lateral ventricle. The caudate nucleus is separated from the putamen by the anterior limb of the internal capsule. The thalamus is seen on each side of the midline. The choroid plexus and the internal cerebral vein are well enhanced. In the lower section, the pineal gland is seen in the caudal part of the brain. Beneath the pineal gland is the habenular commissure. The insular cortex is seen deep within the lateral fissure. Lateral to the insular cortex is the transverse gyrus of Heschl. The third ventricle is seen in the midline. The hippocampus is within the temporal horn of the lateral ventricle. The optic radiation is found lateral to the posterior horn of the lateral ventricle.

Figure 4-6

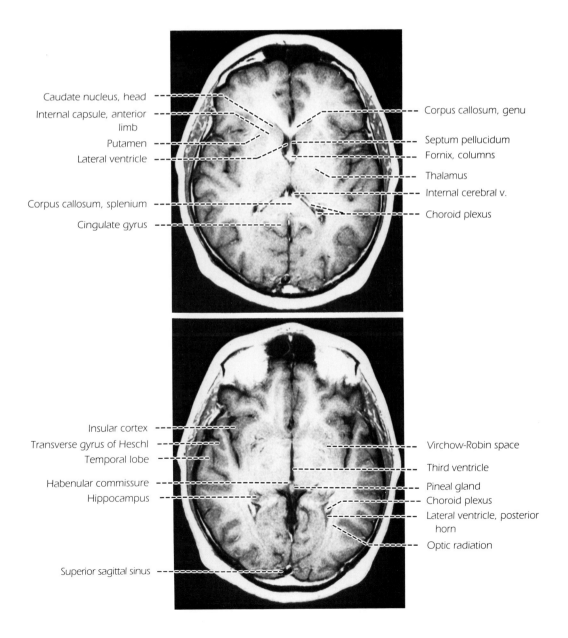

Caudate nucleus, head

Internal capsule, anterior limb

Putamen

Lateral ventricle

Corpus callosum, splenium

Cingulate gyrus

Corpus callosum, genu

Septum pellucidum

Fornix, columns

Thalamus

Internal cerebral v.

Choroid plexus

Insular cortex

Transverse gyrus of Heschl

Temporal lobe

Habenular commissure

Hippocampus

Superior sagittal sinus

Virchow-Robin space

Third ventricle

Pineal gland

Choroid plexus

Lateral ventricle, posterior horn

Optic radiation

# 5

# MR
# ANGIOGRAPHY

# HEAD

## Figure 5-1

MRA showing components of the anterior and posterior circulations. The anterior cerebral, middle cerebral, and posterior communicating arteries arise from the internal carotid artery. The two anterior cerebral arteries are joined by the anterior communicating artery. The posterior communicating artery connects the internal carotid with the posterior cerebral artery. The ascending frontal, posterior parietal, and angular arteries, branches of the middle cerebral artery, are seen. Branches of the posterior cerebral artery seen in this image include the anterior inferior temporal, posterior inferior temporal, and the parieto-occipital arteries. The superior cerebellar artery, a branch of the basilar artery, is seen.

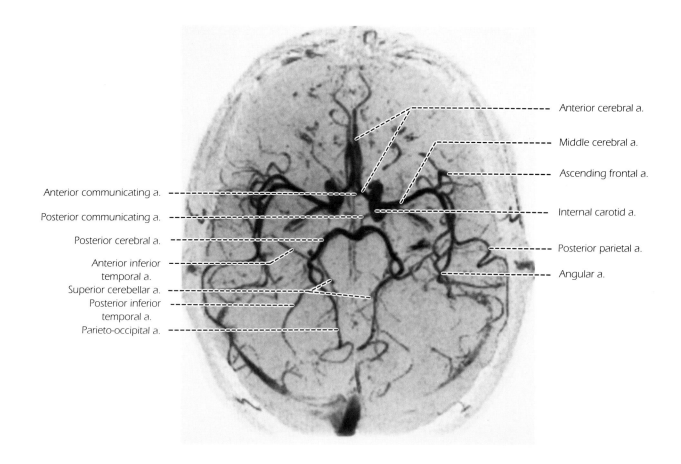

Anterior cerebral a.

Middle cerebral a.

Ascending frontal a.

Anterior communicating a.

Posterior communicating a.

Internal carotid a.

Posterior cerebral a.

Posterior parietal a.

Anterior inferior temporal a.

Angular a.

Superior cerebellar a.

Posterior inferior temporal a.

Parieto-occipital a.

Figure 5-2

Lateral view of MRA showing branches of the anterior, middle, and posterior cerebral arteries. The anterior cerebral artery continues around the corpus callosum as the pericallosal artery. Branches of the anterior cerebral artery seen in this image include the precentral, paracentral, anterior internal frontal, middle internal frontal, and posterior internal frontal arteries. Branches of the middle cerebral artery seen in this image include the anterior parietal, posterior parietal, posterior temporal, central, and orbital frontal arteries. Branches of the posterior cerebral artery include the calcarine, parieto-occipital, posterior inferior temporal, and anterior inferior temporal arteries.

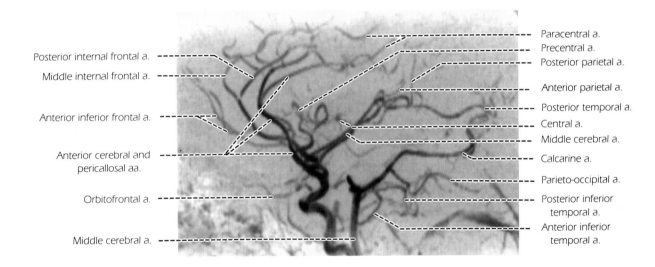

Posterior internal frontal a.

Middle internal frontal a.

Anterior inferior frontal a.

Anterior cerebral and pericallosal aa.

Orbitofrontal a.

Middle cerebral a.

Paracentral a.
Precentral a.
Posterior parietal a.

Anterior parietal a.

Posterior temporal a.

Central a.

Middle cerebral a.

Calcarine a.

Parieto-occipital a.

Posterior inferior temporal a.

Anterior inferior temporal a.

# Figure 5-3

MRA showing the internal carotid, middle cerebral, and anterior cerebral arteries. The middle meningeal artery, a branch of the external carotid artery, is also seen. The petrous, cavernous, and intracranial parts of the internal carotid artery are visualized. The anterior cerebral artery continues as the pericallosal artery. The ascending frontal and posterior parietal arteries, branches of the middle cerebral artery, are seen.

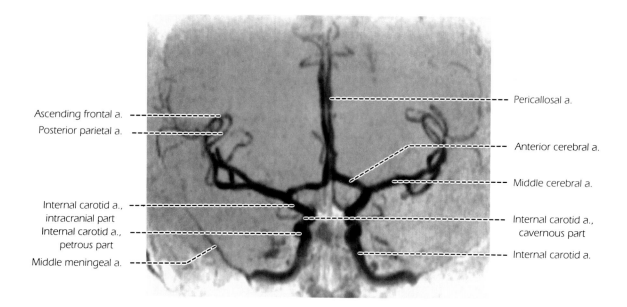

MRA showing components of the posterior circulation. The basilar artery with its two terminal branches, the superior cerebellar and posterior cerebral arteries, are seen. Several branches of the posterior cerebral artery are visualized including the anterior inferior temporal, posterior inferior temporal, calcarine, parieto-occipital, and middle temporal arteries. The middle temporal artery is best seen in axial frontal views such as this one.

Figure 5-4

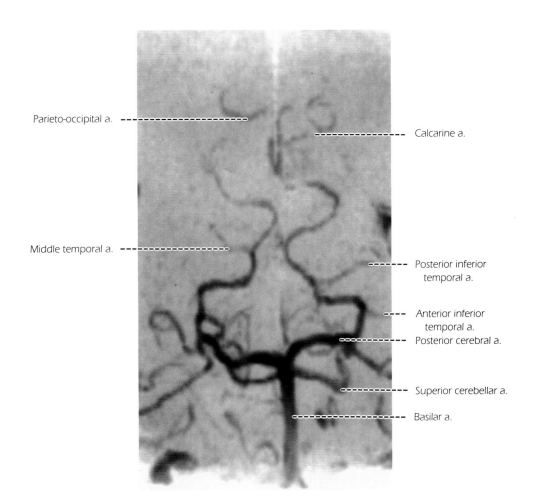

Parieto-occipital a.

Calcarine a.

Middle temporal a.

Posterior inferior temporal a.

Anterior inferior temporal a.

Posterior cerebral a.

Superior cerebellar a.

Basilar a.

# Figure 5-5

MR venogram showing the superficial and deep venous drainage of the brain. The superior sagittal sinus courses along the superior margin of the falx cerebri and drains into the confluence of sinuses (torcular herophili). The septal and thalamostriate veins are seen draining into the internal cerebral vein. The internal cerebral vein and basal vein in turn drain into the great cerebral vein (Galen's vein). The great cerebral vein drains into the straight sinus at the junction of the falx cerebri and tentorium cerebelli. The straight sinus empties into the confluence of sinuses. The two transverse sinuses arise from the confluence of sinuses. The transverse sinus is continuous with the sigmoid sinus at the occipital petrosal junction. The sigmoid sinus drains into the internal jugular vein. A small venous channel, the occipital sinus, is seen draining into the confluence of sinuses. The superior and inferior petrosal sinuses drain into the sigmoid sinus. Other venous channels seen in this section include the anterior insular vein, draining the surface of the insular cortex, olfactory vein, frontorbital vein, and marginal sinus.

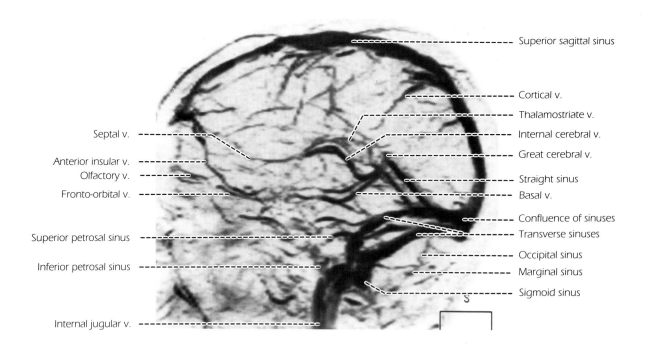

MR venogram showing the drainage of the superior sagittal sinus into the confluence of sinuses. The transverse sinus arises from the confluence of sinuses and is continuous with the sigmoid sinus. The latter drains into the internal jugular vein. Some cortical veins are also seen.

Figure 5-6

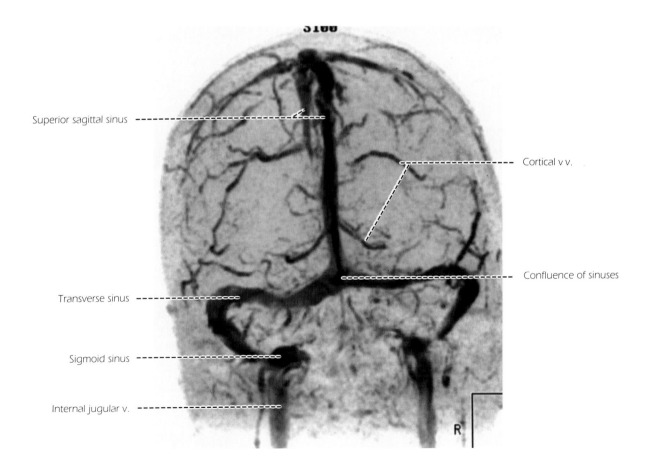

Superior sagittal sinus

Transverse sinus

Sigmoid sinus

Internal jugular v.

Cortical v v.

Confluence of sinuses

# Figure 5-7

MR venogram showing the drainage of the superior sagittal and straight sinuses into the confluence of sinuses. The transverse sinus arises from the confluence of sinuses and is continuous with the sigmoid sinus. The latter drains into the internal jugular vein.

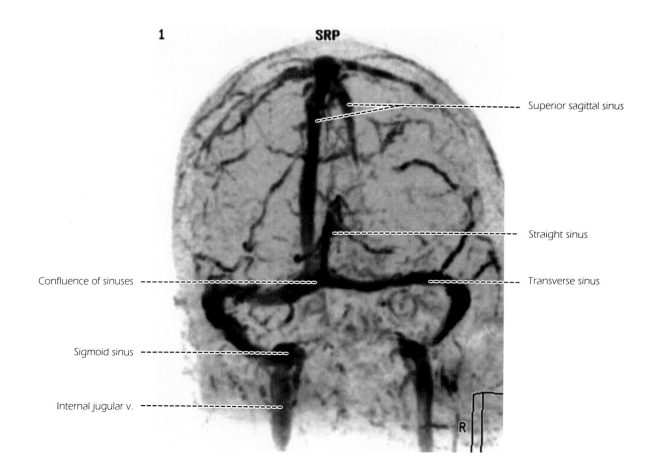

1                     SRP

Superior sagittal sinus

Straight sinus

Confluence of sinuses

Transverse sinus

Sigmoid sinus

Internal jugular v.

R

MR venogram showing the internal cerebral vein and the great cerebral vein draining into the straight sinus. The straight sinus in turn drains into the confluence of sinuses. The transverse sinus arises from the confluence of sinuses and is continuous with the sigmoid sinus. The superior sagittal sinus is seen draining into the confluence of sinuses. The superior and inferior petrosal sinuses are seen draining into the sigmoid sinus. The petrosal vein, a short but large vein located at the anterior and lateral edge of the cerebellar hemisphere, is seen draining into the superior petrosal sinus. The inferior hemispheric vein, which drains the cerebellum, empties into the petrosal vein. The tentorial sinus is also seen.

## Figure 5-8

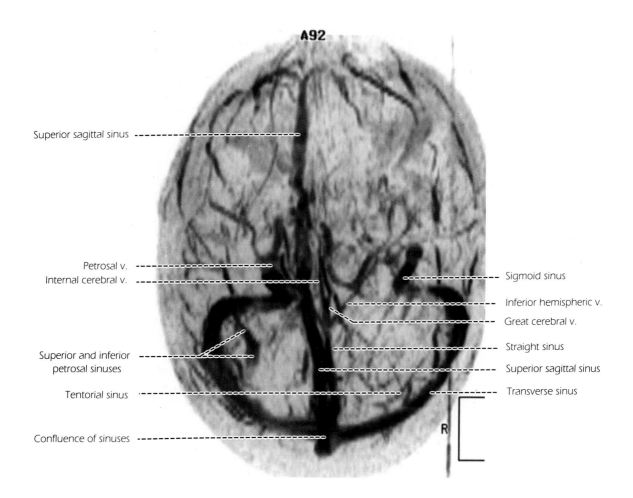

## Figure 5-9

MR venogram showing several vessels that drain the posterior fossa. These include the petrosal, brachial, great horizontal fissure, lateral anastomotic mesencephalic, inferior hemispheric, precentral cerebellar, and inferior anastomotic veins. The frontal polar and superficial middle cerebral veins, which drain the cerebral hemispheres, are also seen. The precentral vein is an unpaired midline vessel that drains into the great cerebral vein. The lateral anastomotic mesencephalic vein is so named because it anastomoses the superior with the anterior group of cerebellar veins. Several sinuses are seen in this image including the sigmoid sinus, transverse sinus, tentorial sinus, confluence of sinuses, and superior and lateral petrosal sinuses. The internal cerebral vein is also seen.

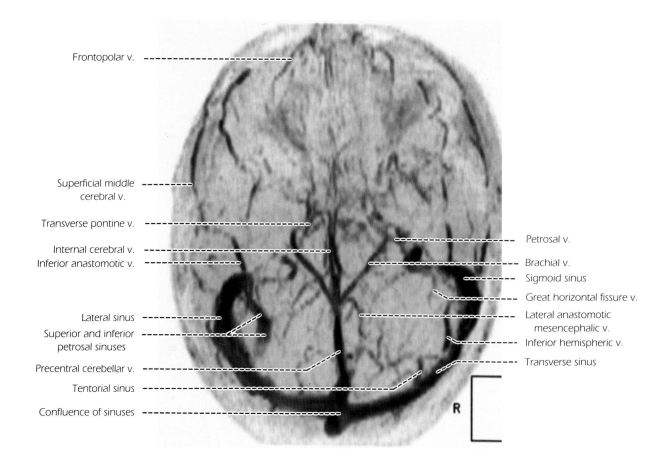

Frontopolar v.

Superficial middle cerebral v.

Transverse pontine v.

Internal cerebral v.

Inferior anastomotic v.

Lateral sinus

Superior and inferior petrosal sinuses

Precentral cerebellar v.

Tentorial sinus

Confluence of sinuses

Petrosal v.

Brachial v.

Sigmoid sinus

Great horizontal fissure v.

Lateral anastomotic mesencephalic v.

Inferior hemispheric v.

Transverse sinus

R

# NECK

# Figure 5-10

MRA showing the common carotid arteries and their bifurcation into external and internal carotid arteries. The vertebral artery is also seen. The superficial temporal, maxillary, facial, and lingual arteries, branches of the external carotid artery, are seen.

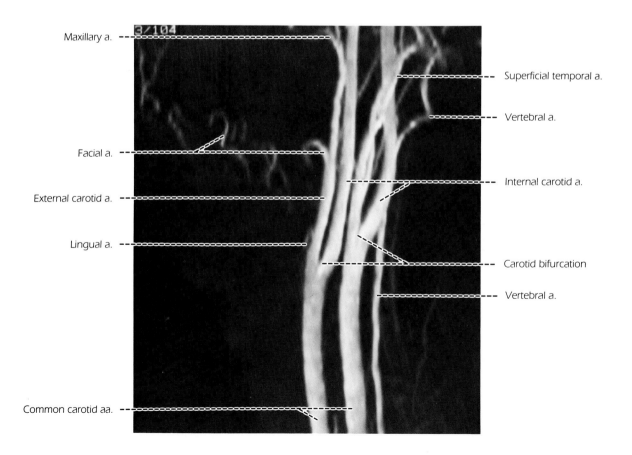

Maxillary a.

Superficial temporal a.

Vertebral a.

Facial a.

Internal carotid a.

External carotid a.

Lingual a.

Carotid bifurcation

Vertebral a.

Common carotid aa.

MRA showing the common carotid arteries and their bifurcation into external and internal carotid arteries. Several branches of the external carotid artery are seen including the superficial temporal, inferior pharyngeal, transverse facial, facial, and lingual arteries. The vertebral artery is also seen.

Figure 5-11

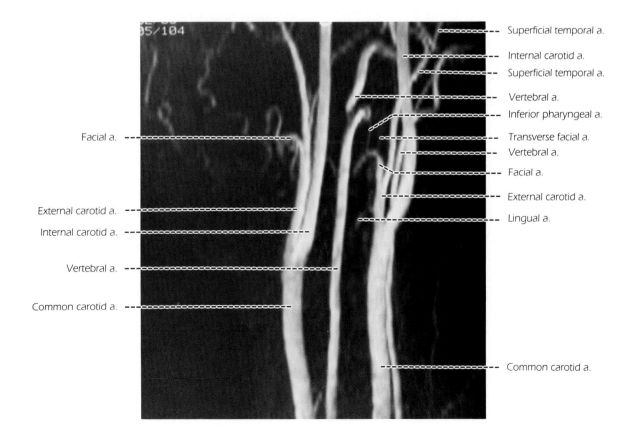

Superficial temporal a.

Internal carotid a.

Superficial temporal a.

Vertebral a.

Inferior pharyngeal a.

Transverse facial a.

Vertebral a.

Facial a.

External carotid a.

Lingual a.

Common carotid a.

Facial a.

External carotid a.

Internal carotid a.

Vertebral a.

Common carotid a.

## Figure 5-12

MRA showing the common carotid arteries and their bifurcation into external and internal carotid arteries. Several branches of the external carotid artery are visualized including the ascending pharyngeal, facial, lingual, and superior thyroid arteries. The internal vertebral plexus of veins is seen. The vertebral arteries are also seen.

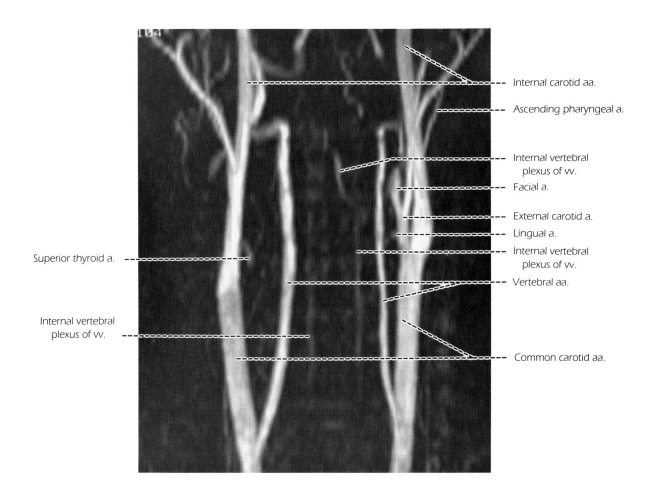

Internal carotid aa.

Ascending pharyngeal a.

Internal vertebral plexus of vv.

Facial a.

External carotid a.

Lingual a.

Internal vertebral plexus of vv.

Vertebral aa.

Common carotid aa.

Superior thyroid a.

Internal vertebral plexus of vv.

MRA showing the common carotid arteries and their bifurcation into external and internal carotid arteries. The vertebral arteries and the anterior spinal artery, a branch of the vertebral artery, are seen. Several branches of the external carotid artery are visualized including the facial, lingual, and superior thyroid arteries.

# Figure 5-13

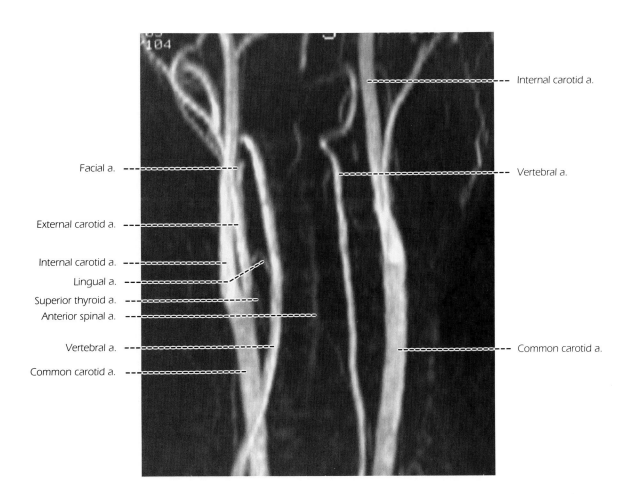

Facial a.

External carotid a.

Internal carotid a.
Lingual a.

Superior thyroid a.
Anterior spinal a.

Vertebral a.

Common carotid a.

Internal carotid a.

Vertebral a.

Common carotid a.

## Figure 5-14

MRA showing the common carotid arteries and their bifurcation into internal and external carotid arteries. The vertebral arteries are also seen. The facial artery, a branch of the external carotid artery, is visualized.

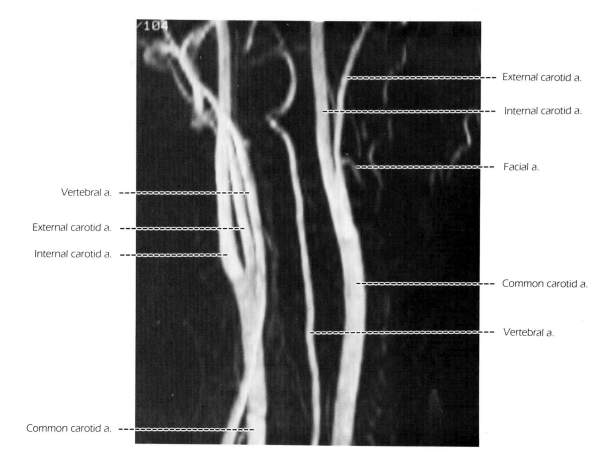

Vertebral a.

External carotid a.

Internal carotid a.

Common carotid a.

External carotid a.

Internal carotid a.

Facial a.

Common carotid a.

Vertebral a.

MRA showing the common carotid arteries and their bifurcation into external and internal carotid arteries. The vertebral arteries are also seen. Several branches of the external carotid artery are identified including the lingual, superior thyroid, and facial arteries.

# Figure 5-15

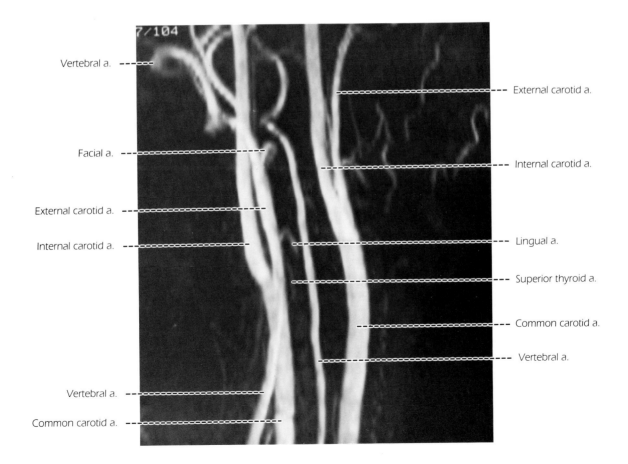

## Figure 5-16

MR venogram showing the internal and external jugular veins in the neck. Several other venous channels are seen including the deep cervical vein, vertebral venous plexus, and cervical plexus of veins.

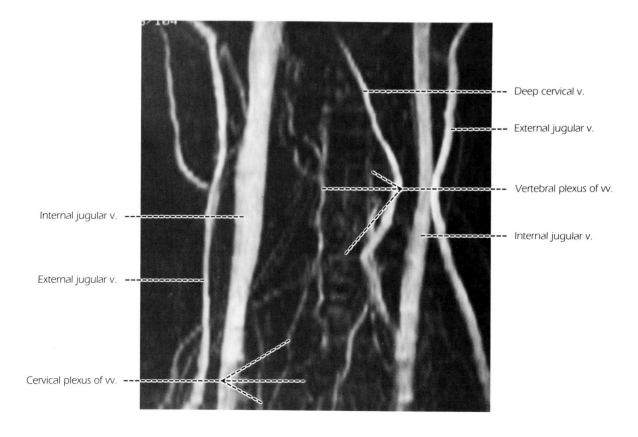

Deep cervical v.

External jugular v.

Vertebral plexus of vv.

Internal jugular v.

Internal jugular v.

External jugular v.

Cervical plexus of vv.

MR venogram showing several veins in the neck.
These include the internal and external jugular veins,
anterior jugular vein, and vertebral plexus of veins.

# Figure 5-17

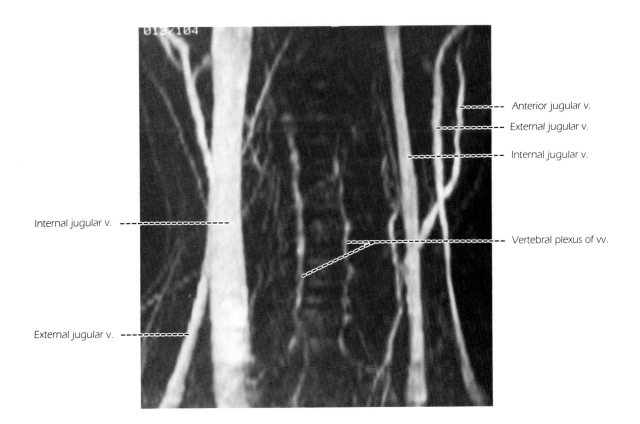

Internal jugular v. --------

External jugular v. --------

Anterior jugular v.

External jugular v.

Internal jugular v.

Vertebral plexus of vv.

## Figure 5-18

MR venogram showing venous channels in the neck. These include the internal and external jugular veins and vertebral plexus of veins.

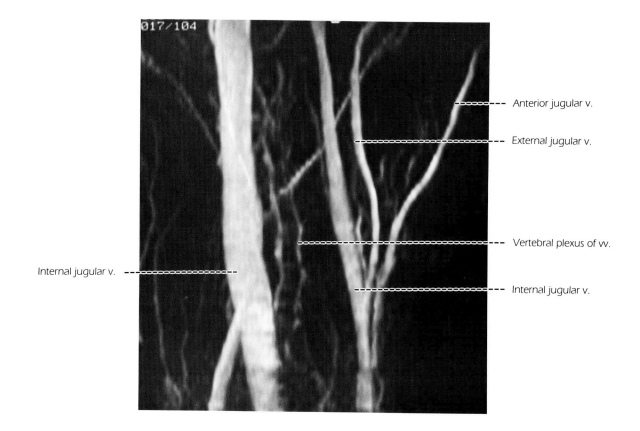

017/104

Anterior jugular v.

External jugular v.

Vertebral plexus of v.

Internal jugular v.

Internal jugular v.

MR venogram of the neck veins showing the external and internal jugular veins, transverse cervical vein, and cervical plexus of veins.

Figure 5-19

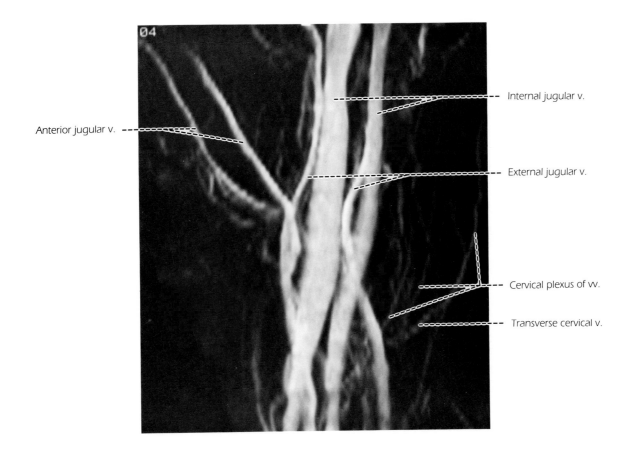

## Figure 5-20

MR venogram showing a number of venous channels in the neck. These include the external and internal jugular veins, anterior jugular veins, cervical plexus of veins, and transverse cervical vein.

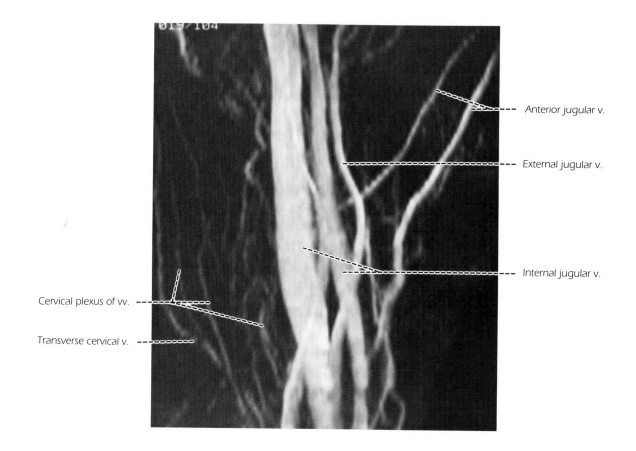

Anterior jugular v.

External jugular v.

Internal jugular v.

Cervical plexus of vv.

Transverse cervical v.

MR venogram showing a number of cervical venous channels. These include the external and internal jugular veins, veins draining the thyroid gland, anterior jugular vein, transverse cervical vein, and posterior cervical plexus of veins.

Figure 5-21

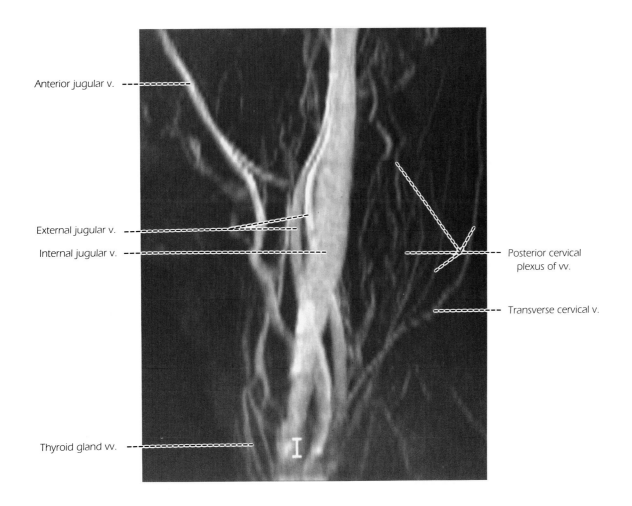

Anterior jugular v.

External jugular v.

Internal jugular v.

Posterior cervical plexus of vv.

Transverse cervical v.

Thyroid gland vv.

# INDEX